Challenges & Updates in Pediatric Pathology

Editor

JESSICA L. DAVIS

SURGICAL PATHOLOGY CLINICS

www.surgpath.theclinics.com

Consulting Editor
JASON L. HORNICK

December 2020 • Volume 13 • Number 4

ELSEVIER

1600 John F. Kennedy Boulevard • Suite 1800 • Philadelphia, Pennsylvania, 19103-2899

http://www.theclinics.com

SURGICAL PATHOLOGY CLINICS Volume 13, Number 4
December 2020 ISSN 1875-9181, ISBN-13: 978-0-323-77578-6

Editor: Katerina Heidhausen
Developmental Editor: Donald Mumford

Surgical Pathology Clinics (ISSN 1875-9181) is published quarterly by Elsevier Inc., 360 Park Avenue South, New York, NY 10010. Months of issue are March, June, September, and December. Business and Editorial Office: Elsevier Inc., 1600 John F. Kennedy Blvd., Ste. 1800, Philadelphia, PA 19103-2899. Accounting and Circulation Offices: Elsevier Inc., 3251 Riverport Lane, Maryland Heights, MO 63043. Periodicals postage paid at New York, NY and at additional mailing offices. Subscription prices are $219.00 per year (US individuals), $294.00 per year (US institutions), $100.00 per year (US students/residents), $272.00 per year (Canadian individuals), $335.00 per year (Canadian Institutions), $263.00 per year (foreign individuals), $335.00 per year (foreign institutions), and $120.00 per year (international students/residents), $100.00 per year (Canadian students/residents). Foreign air speed delivery is included in all *Clinics'* subscription prices. All prices are subject to change without notice. **POSTMASTER:** Send address changes to *Surgical Pathology Clinics*, Elsevier, 3251 Riverport Lane, Maryland Heights, MO 63043. **Customer Service: 1-800-654-2452 (US). From outside the United States, call 1-314-447-8871. Fax: 1-314-447-8029. E-mail:** JournalsCustomerServiceusa@elsevier.com **(for print support)** and JournalsOnlineSupport-usa@elsevier.com **(for online support).**

Reprints. For copies of 100 or more, of articles in this publication, please contact the Commercial Reprints Department, Elsevier Inc., 360 Park Avenue South, New York, NY 10010-1710. Tel. 212-633-3874; Fax: 212-633-3820; E-mail: reprints@elsevier.com.

Surgical Pathology Clinics of North America is covered in *MEDLINE/PubMed (Index Medicus)*.

Contributors

CONSULTING EDITOR

JASON L. HORNICK, MD, PhD
Director of Surgical Pathology and
Immunohistochemistry, Brigham and Women's
Hospital, Professor of Pathology, Harvard
Medical School, Boston, Massachusetts, USA

EDITOR

JESSICA L. DAVIS, MD
Associate Professor, Director of Surgical
Pathology, Department of Pathology, Oregon
Health & Science University, Portland, Oregon,
USA

AUTHORS

ALYAA AL-IBRAHEEMI, MD
Department of Pathology, Staff Pathologist,
Boston Children's Hospital, Boston,
Massachusetts, USA

MICHAEL A. ARNOLD, MD, PhD
Medical Director of Anatomic Pathology,
Children's Hospital Colorado, Associate
Professor of Pathology, University of Colorado,
Anschutz Medical Campus, Aurora, Aurora,
Colorado, USA

SONJA CHEN, MBBS
Assistant Professor of Pathology, Warren
Alpert Medical School of Brown University,
Pediatric and Surgical Pathologist, Lifespan
Academic Medical Center, Rhode Island
Hospital, Providence, Rhode Island, USA

SOO-JIN CHO, MD, PhD
Associate Professor, Department of Pathology,
University of California San Francisco, San
Francisco, California, USA

BONNIE L. COLE, MD
Clinical Associate Professor University of
Washington School of Medicine, Department
of Laboratory Medicine and Pathology, Seattle,
Washington, USA

NAHIR CORTES-SANTIAGO, MD, PhD
Assistant Professor, Department of Pathology
and Immunology, Baylor College of Medicine,
Department of Pathology, Texas Children's
Hospital, Houston, Texas, USA

JESSICA L. DAVIS, MD
Associate Professor, Director of Surgical
Pathology, Department of Pathology, Oregon
Health & Science University, Portland,
Oregon, USA

GAIL H. DEUTSCH, MD
Professor, Department of Pathology,
University of Washington School of Medicine,
Department of Laboratories, Seattle
Children's Hospital, Seattle, Washington,
USA

MEGAN K. DISHOP, MD
Department of Pathology and Laboratory
Medicine, Phoenix Children's Hospital,
Phoenix, Arizona, USA

MELANIE H. HAKAR, DO
Neuropathology Fellow, Department of Pathology, Oregon Health & Science University, Portland, Oregon, USA

SAMUEL HWANG, MD
Pediatric Pathology Fellow, Seattle Children's Hospital, University of Washington, Seattle, Washington, USA

JASON A. JARZEMBOWSKI, MD, PhD
Vice Chair and Professor, Department of Pathology, Medical College of Wisconsin, Medical Director, Pathology and Laboratory Medicine, Children's Wisconsin, Milwaukee, Wisconsin, USA

RAJ P. KAPUR, MD, PhD
Professor, Department of Pathology, Seattle Children's Hospital, University of Washington, Seattle, Washington, USA

JILL LIPSETT, BMBS, PhD, FRCPA, FISQua
Department of Anatomical Pathology, S.A. Pathology, Women's and Children's Hospital, North Adelaide, South Australia, Australia

ANITA NAGY, MD, FRCPath
Clinical Fellow, Division of Pathology, Hospital for Sick Children, Toronto, Ontario, Canada

LAUREN N. PARSONS, MD
Assistant Professor, Medical College of Wisconsin, Staff Pathologist, Children's Hospital of Wisconsin, Milwaukee, Wisconsin, USA

CHRISTOPHER R. PIERSON, MD, PhD
Associate Professor of Pathology and Anatomy, Departments of Pathology, and Biomedical Education & Anatomy, The Ohio State University, Neuropathologist, Nationwide Children's Hospital, Department of Pathology and Laboratory Medicine, Columbus, Ohio, USA

ERIN R. RUDZINSKI, MD
Clinical Associate Professor, Director of Anatomic Pathology, Department of Laboratories, Seattle Children's Hospital, Seattle, Washington, USA

PIERRE RUSSO, MD
Professor, Department of Pathology and Laboratory Medicine, Director, Division of Anatomic Pathology, The University of Pennsylvania School of Medicine, The Children's Hospital of Philadelphia, Philadelphia, Pennsylvania, USA

GINO R. SOMERS, MBBS, PhD, FRCPA
Division Head, Pathology, Hospital for Sick Children, Professor, Department of Laboratory Medicine and Pathobiology, University of Toronto, Toronto, Ontario, Canada

AMY L. TREECE, MD
Department of Pathology, Pediatric and Molecular Pathologist, Children's Hospital Colorado, Assistant Professor, University of Colorado School of Medicine, Aurora, Colorado, USA

MATTHEW D. WOOD, MD, PhD
Assistant Professor, Department of Pathology, Oregon Health & Science University and Knight Cancer Institute, Portland, Oregon, USA

Contents

Preface   xi

Jessica L. Davis

Advances and Pitfalls in the Diagnosis of Hirschsprung Disease   567

Samuel Hwang and Raj P. Kapur

Surgical pathology for Hirschsprung disease (HSCR) occasionally is difficult, especially for those who encounter the disorder infrequently. This article reviews pathologic features of HSCR, considers various specimens the pathologist is required to evaluate, and discusses useful ancillary tests. Potential diagnostic pitfalls are highlighted, and helpful hints are provided to successfully navigate challenging situations. Finally, the article looks forward to new ancillary tests on the horizon and future topics for HSCR research.

Updates in Pediatric Congenital Enteropathies: Differential Diagnosis, Testing, and Genetics   581

Pierre Russo

Congenital enteropathies comprise a heterogeneous group of disorders typically resulting in severe diarrhea and intestinal failure. Recent advances in and more widespread application of genetic testing have allowed more accurate diagnosis of these entities as well as identification of new disorders, provided a deeper understanding of intestinal pathophysiology through genotype-phenotype correlations, and permitted the exploration of more specific therapies to diseases that have heretofore been resistant to conventional treatments. The therapeutic armamentarium for these disorders now includes intestinal and hematopoietic stem cell transplantation, specific targeted therapy, such as the use of interleukin-1 receptor antagonists and, in some cases, gene therapy.

Pediatric Liver Tumors: Updates in Classification   601

Soo-Jin Cho

Malignant primary liver tumors are rare in children, accounting for 1% to 2% of pediatric solid tumors. Yet a wide histologic spectrum is seen, particularly in hepatoblastoma, the most common malignant liver tumor in children. Furthermore, there can be significant morphologic overlap with hepatocellular carcinoma, the second most common pediatric liver malignancy, and tumors with hybrid features of hepatoblastoma and hepatocellular carcinoma are also reported (currently placed in the provisional category of malignant hepatocellular neoplasm, not otherwise specified). This review provides detailed morphologic descriptions and updates in the evolving clinical context of these tumors, and presents recent molecular advances that may further help in accurate classification of these tumors, which is critical in their management.

New Prognostic Indicators in Pediatric Adrenal Tumors: Neuroblastoma and Adrenal Cortical Tumors, Can We Predict When These Will Behave Badly?   625

Jason A. Jarzembowski

Pediatric adrenal tumors are unique entities with specific diagnostic, prognostic, and therapeutic challenges. The adrenal medulla gives rise to peripheral neuroblastic tumors (pNTs), pathologically defined by their architecture, stromal content, degree of differentiation, and mitotic-karyorrhectic index. Successful risk stratification of pNTs uses patient age, stage, tumor histology, and molecular/genetic aberrations. The adrenal cortex gives rise to adrenocortical tumors (ACTs), which present diagnostic and prognostic challenges. Histologic features that signify poor prognosis in adults can be meaningless in children, who have superior outcomes. The key clinical, pathologic, and molecular findings of pediatric ACTs have yet to be completely identified.

Pediatric Cystic Lung Lesions: Where Are We Now?   643

Nahir Cortes-Santiago and Gail H. Deutsch

Pediatric cystic lung lesions have long been a source of confusion for clinicians, radiologists, and pathologists. They encompass a wide spectrum of entities with variable prognostic implications, including congenital lung malformations, pulmonary neoplasms, and hereditary conditions. As our understanding of the developmental and genetic origins of these conditions has evolved, revised nomenclature and classifications have emerged in an attempt to bring clarity to the origin of these lesions and guide clinical management. This review discusses cystic lung lesions and the current understanding of their etiopathogenesis.

Strategies for the Neonatal Lung Biopsy: Histology to Genetics   657

Jill Lipsett and Megan K. Dishop

Neonatal lung biopsy guides important medical decisions when the diagnosis is not clear from prior clinical assessment, imaging, or genetic testing. Common scenarios that lead to biopsy include severe acute respiratory distress in a term neonate, pulmonary hypertension disproportionate to that expected for gestational age or known cardiac anomalies, and assessment of suspected genetic disorder based on clinical features or genetic variant of unknown significance. The differential diagnosis includes genetic developmental disorders, genetic surfactant disorders, vascular disorders, acquired infection, and meconium aspiration. This article describes pathologic patterns in the neonatal lung and correlation with molecular abnormalities, where appropriate.

Wilms Tumor: Challenges and Newcomers in Prognosis   683

Lauren N. Parsons

Wilms tumor is the most common renal tumor of childhood. It is a biologically and morphologically diverse entity, with ongoing studies contributing to our understanding of the pathobiology of various subgroups of patients with Wilms tumor. The interplay of histologic examination and molecular interrogation is integral in prognostication and direction of therapy. This review provides an overview of some of the challenging aspects and pitfalls in pathologic assessment of Wilms tumor, along with discussion of current and up-and-coming markers of biological behavior with prognostic significance.

Pediatric Renal Tumors: Updates in the Molecular Era   695

Amy L. Treece

Molecular characterization has led to advances in the understanding of pediatric renal tumors, including the association of pediatric cystic nephromas with DICER1 tumor syndrome, the metanephric family of tumors with somatic BRAF mutations, the characterization of ETV6-NTRK3–negative congenital mesoblastic nephromas, the expanded spectrum of gene fusions in translocation renal cell carcinoma, the relationship of clear cell sarcoma of the kidney with other BCOR-altered tumors, and the pathways affected by SMARCB1 alterations in rhabdoid tumors of the kidney. These advances have implications for diagnosis, classification, and treatment of pediatric renal tumors.

Newcomers in Vascular Anomalies   719

Alyaa Al-Ibraheemi

Vascular anomalies are composed of tumors and malformations and with overlapping histologies, thus are often misdiagnosed or labeled with imprecise terminology. Lesions are common and usually diagnosed during infancy or childhood; the estimated prevalence is 4.5%. Vascular tumors rapidly enlarge postnatally and demonstrate endothelial proliferation. Malformations are errors in vascular development with stable endothelial turnover; they are typically named based on the primary vessel that is malformed (capillary, arterial, venous, lymphatic). This article reviews the pathologic and molecular genetic characteristics for select recently described vascular anomalies.

Challenges in the Diagnosis of Pediatric Spindle Cell/Sclerosing Rhabdomyosarcoma   729

Sonja Chen, Erin R. Rudzinski, and Michael A. Arnold

Rhabdomyosarcoma (RMS) is the most common pediatric soft tissue sarcoma, representing approximately 40% of all pediatric soft tissue sarcomas. The spindle cell/sclerosing subtype of RMS (SSRMS) accounts for roughly 5% to 10% of all cases of adult and pediatric RMS. Historically, SSRMS were described as paratesticular tumors with an excellent outcome. However, more recent studies have identified unique molecular subgroups of SSRMS, including those with MYOD1 mutations or VGLL2/NCOA2 fusions, which have widely disparate outcomes. The goal of this article is to better describe the biological heterogeneity of SSRMS, which may allow the pathologist to provide important prognostic information.

Pediatric and Infantile Fibroblastic/Myofibroblastic Tumors in the Molecular Era   739

Jessica L. Davis and Erin R. Rudzinski

Pediatric fibroblastic/myofibroblastic tumors are rare but include a wide variety of benign to malignant tumors. Given their uncommon frequency, they may present as a diagnostic dilemma. This article is focused on using clinical and pathologic clues in conjunction with the increasingly relevant and available molecular techniques to classify, predict prognosis, and/or guide treatment in these tumors.

Round Cell Sarcomas: Newcomers and Diagnostic Approaches   763

Anita Nagy and Gino R. Somers

Undifferentiated sarcomas of soft tissue and bone have been defined as tumors with no identifiable morphologic, immunohistochemical, or molecular features indicating tumor cell origin. In young patients, these tumors frequently have a round or spindle cell morphology. Recently described recurrent translocations within this category have led to the recognition of new molecular subtypes of round cell sarcomas, and several of them have a more aggressive clinical course and less chemosensitivity. Because these "newcomers" are diagnosed based on their molecular characteristics, molecular investigation is key in the diagnosis and optimal treatment of these challenging tumors.

Histopathologic and Molecular Features of Central Nervous System Embryonal Tumors for Integrated Diagnosis Reporting   783

Bonnie L. Cole and Christopher R. Pierson

Embryonal tumors of the pediatric central nervous system are challenging clinically and diagnostically. These tumors are aggressive, and patients often have poor outcomes even with intense therapy. Proper tumor classification is essential to patient care, and this process has undergone significant changes with the World Health Organization recommending histopathologic and molecular features be integrated in diagnostic reporting. This has especially impacted the workup of embryonal tumors because molecular testing has resulted in the identification of clinically relevant tumor subgroups and new entities. This review summarizes recent developments and provides a framework to workup embryonal tumors in diagnostic practice.

Updates in Pediatric Glioma Pathology   801

Melanie H. Hakar and Matthew D. Wood

Gliomas are a diverse group of primary central nervous system tumors with astrocytic, oligodendroglial, and/or ependymal features and are an important cause of morbidity/mortality in pediatric patients. Glioma classification relies on integrating tumor histology with key molecular alterations. This approach can help establish a diagnosis, guide treatment, and determine prognosis. New categories of pediatric glioma have been recognized in recent years, due to increasing application of molecular profiling in brain tumors. The aim of this review is to alert pediatric pathologists to emerging diagnostic concepts in pediatric glioma neuropathology, emphasizing the incorporation of molecular features into diagnostic practice.

SURGICAL PATHOLOGY CLINICS

FORTHCOMING ISSUES

March 2021
Head and Neck Pathology
Justin Bishop, *Editor*

June 2021
Dermatopathology
Michael Tetzlaff, *Editor*

September 2021
Molecular Pathology
Lauren Ritterhouse, *Editor*

RECENT ISSUES

September 2020
Gastrointestinal Pathology
Raul Gonzalez, *Editor*

June 2020
Current Trends in Neuropathology
David M. Meredith, *Editor*

March 2020
Pulmonary Pathology
Kirk D. Jones, *Editor*

SERIES OF RELATED INTEREST

Clinics in Laboratory Medicine
https://www.labmed.theclinics.com/
Medical Clinics
https://www.medical.theclinics.com/

Preface

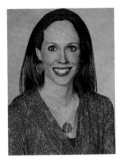

Jessica L. Davis, MD

Editor

Pediatric pathology is a distinct and challenging field, encountering a diversity of pathologic conditions, including developmental anomalies, metabolic diseases, malformations, and a set of neoplasms uniquely germane to infants and children. Recent genetic/molecular discoveries have accelerated our knowledge of developmental biology and pediatric pathology. New advancements encompass, but are not limited to, the clinicopathologic and genetic bases of pediatric enteropathies (Updates in Pediatric Enteropathies: Differential Diagnosis, Testing, and Genetics by Pierre Russo), recently described vascular anomalies with recurrent genetic aberrations (Newcomers in Vascular Anomalies by Alyaa Al-Ibraheemi), and potential targeted therapies in fibroblastic tumors of childhood (Pediatric and Infantile Fibroblastic/Myofibroblastic Tumors in the Molecular Era by Jessica L. Davis and Erin Rudzinski). While some challenges in pediatric pathology may be familiar to those of us in pediatric pathology (eg, pitfalls in Hirschsprung diagnosis, by Samuel Hwang and Raj Kapur;

anaplasia in Wilm tumor, by Amy L. Treece and Lauren Nicole Parsons; the neonatal lung biopsy, by Megan Dishop), these areas of challenge have also seen changes and advancement in recent years. A compressive review of the momentous knowledge collectively gained over the last 60 years since the birth of pediatric pathology as a subspecialty would not be possible within the scope of this text; however, we hope that each of these articles focuses on either a particular challenge in pediatric pathology with recent updates in the field or areas of recent rapid knowledge growth and changes.

Jessica L. Davis, MD
Surgical Pathology
Department of Pathology
Oregon Health & Science University
3181 Southwest Sam Jackson Park Road, L-471
Portland, OR 97239, USA

E-mail address:
davisjes@ohsu.edu

Surgical Pathology 13 (2020) xi
https://doi.org/10.1016/j.path.2020.09.001
1875-9181/20/© 2020 Published by Elsevier Inc.

Advances and Pitfalls in the Diagnosis of Hirschsprung Disease

Samuel Hwang, MD[a,b], Raj P. Kapur, MD, PhD[c,*]

KEYWORDS

- Hirschsprung disease • Aganglionosis • Transition zone pull-through • Choline transporter
- Calretinin

Key points

- Suction biopsies should be obtained routinely from more than 1 site.

- Perform calretinin immunohistochemistry on at least 1 biopsy from every patient; in some situations AChE histochemistry or ChT IHC may be particularly helpful.

- Look for nerve hypertrophy, even if ganglion cells are present.

- Any of the following is a histologic feature of transition zone: partial circumferential aganglionosis, myenteric hypoganglionosis, or submucosal nerve hypertrophy.

- To avoid retained transition zone, advise resection of at least 5 cm of ganglionic bowel and frozen section of the entire proximal resection margin.

ABSTRACT

Surgical pathology for Hirschsprung disease (HSCR) occasionally is difficult, especially for those who encounter the disorder infrequently. This article reviews pathologic features of HSCR, considers various specimens the pathologist is required to evaluate, and discusses useful ancillary tests. Potential diagnostic pitfalls are highlighted, and helpful hints are provided to successfully navigate challenging situations. Finally, the article looks forward to new ancillary tests on the horizon and future topics for HSCR research.

proximal alterations at the transition zone (TZ) between normal and abnormal bowel. These neuroanatomic alterations correlate with intestinal spasticity and chronic bowel obstruction. This article reviews the anatomic findings in HSCR and considers practical surgical pathology, potential diagnostic pitfalls, and anticipated new research developments.

ANATOMIC FINDINGS IN HIRSCHSPRUNG DISEASE

AGANGLIONOSIS

Patients with HSCR lack ganglion cells in the distal rectum and a variable length of contiguous proximal bowel. Aganglionosis results from failure of neural crest-derived neuronal progenitors to completely colonize the gastrointestinal tract. Eighty percent of aganglionic segments are limited

OVERVIEW

Hirschsprung disease (HSCR) is the congenital absence of enteric ganglion cells (aganglionosis) in the distal intestinal tract, with more subtle

---

[a] Department of Pathology, University of Utah, Salt Lake City, UT, USA; [b] Seattle Children's Hospital, University of Washington, OC.8.720 4800, Sand Point Way Northeast, Seattle, WA 98105, USA; [c] Department of Pathology, Seattle Children's Hospital, University of Washington, OC.8.720 4800, Sand Point Way Northeast, Seattle, WA 98105, USA
* Corresponding author.
E-mail address: raj.kapur@seattlechildrens.org

Surgical Pathology 13 (2020) 567–579
https://doi.org/10.1016/j.path.2020.07.001

surgpath.theclinics.com

to the rectosigmoid colon and termed short-segment HSCR (ss-HSCR).[1] Less common subtypes are classified by their proximal extent of involvement: colonic (left colon), long-segment (transverse or right colon), total colonic (ileum), small intestinal (jejunum), and panintestinal (gastric) variants. Very short-segment aganglionosis (vssHSCR), limited to 2 to 3 cm of the distalmost rectum, is important, because a rectal biopsy may be within or adjacent to the TZ, where the presence of ganglion cells and/or calretinin-immunoreactive mucosal neurites may lead to erroneous exclusion of HSCR.[2,3]

The aganglionic segment is devoid of intrinsic ganglia, but mucosal, submucosal, and muscular architecture is preserved. Extrinsic innervation persists in the aganglionic bowel and derives from autonomic ganglia in the pelvis, spinal sensory ganglia, paravertebral sympathetic ganglia, and, in long-segment HSCR, vagal ganglia.[4–6] Extrinsic nerves from pelvic autonomic ganglia ascend in the perirectal connective tissue and aganglionic myenteric plexus and radially penetrate the muscularis interna to reach the submucosa and mucosa[7] (Fig. 1A).

Extrinsic nerves in HSCR are enlarged (hypertrophic) because of an increased content of individual neurites and have immunohistochemical and ultrastructural properties characteristic of nonenteric peripheral nerves. These features include the presence of glucose transporter 1 (GLUT1)-positive perineurium,[8] occasional myelinated fibers,[9] endoneurial collagen,[10] Schwann cells with an antigenically different form of GFAP (compared with enteric glial cells),[11] and peripheral nerve laminin isoforms that are absent in intrinsic nerves[12] (Fig. 2). Hypertrophic nerves are larger in the distal rectum and less pronounced in more proximal left colon, and minimal or nonexistent in aganglionic bowel proximal to the splenic flexure. This trend probably is because of the proximity of the distal rectum to the pelvic autonomic ganglia (a major source of extrinsic innervation).[5] In hematoxylin-and-eosin (H&E)-stained sections, enlarged nerves are most obvious in the myenteric and submucosal plexuses.

Although nerve hypertrophy in the submucosa is usually identified subjectively by an experienced pathologist as conspicuous or crowded large nerves, morphometric measurement is occasionally helpful. In infants younger than 6 months, submucosal nerve diameter is generally less than 40 μm.[13] Although this may be a useful feature of HSCR in this age group, nerve caliber increases

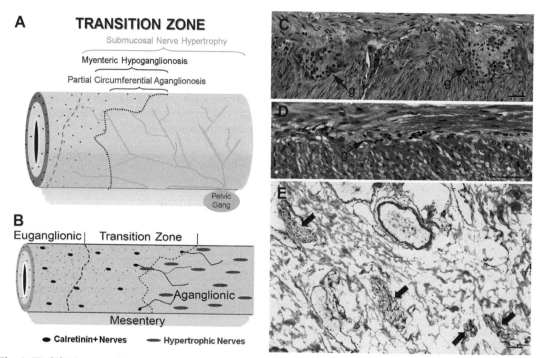

Fig. 1. TZ. (A) Diagram of 3 major histologic features: partial circumferential aganglionosis, myenteric hypoganglionosis, and submucosal nerve hypertrophy. (B) Illustration of distal projections from calretinin-immunoreactive ganglion cells from TZ into the proximal aganglionic segment. In ssHSCR, hypertrophic nerves extend from aganglionic segment into TZ. (C) Euganglionic myenteric plexus. (D) Hypoplastic ganglion in TZ with myenteric hypoganglionosis. (E) Submucosal nerve hypertrophy (arrows) in frozen section. g, ganglion. Scale bars: 40 μm.

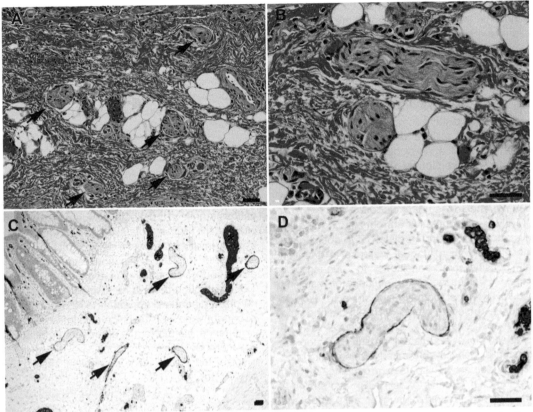

Fig. 2. Submucosal nerve hypertrophy. (*A*, *B*) H&E. (*C*, *D*) Glut-1 immunohistochemistry. Nerves (*arrows*). Blood vessels (*asterisks*). Scale bars: 40 μm.

with age, and the 40 μm rule should not be applied to older patients.[14] One should also be aware that rectal submucosal nerve hypertrophy (SNH) is paradoxically absent or limited to the distal rectum in some patients with long-segment aganglionosis.[5,7,15]

At the interface between ganglionic and proximal aganglionic bowel, intrinsic ganglia project nerves 1 to 2 cm distally into the aganglionic segment, including calretinin-positive mucosal neurites. Distal to these downstream projections, the mucosa of aganglionic bowel is completely devoid of calretinin-immunoreactive innervation[3,16] (**Fig. 1**B).

On rare occasions, the aganglionic segment is discontinuous and contains an intervening skip area of myenteric and/or submucosal ganglion cells.[17,18] Skip areas are most commonly present in the colon with an upstream proximal aganglionic segment that encompasses the appendix/cecum with or without extension into the ileum. With the conventional surgical approach to HSCR disease, skip areas may not be recognized intraoperatively, because leveling biopsies (see below) cease once ganglionic bowel is identified. Therefore, a skip area with retained proximal aganglionic bowel should be considered in any patient whose obstructive symptoms persist after pull-through surgery or diversion. In rare patients, a skip area extends into the distal rectum and produces the same diagnostic challenges as vssHSCR.

TRANSITION ZONE

The TZ is the segment of abnormally innervated bowel immediately proximal to the aganglionic segment.[19,20] Failure to resect the TZ (TZ pull-through, TZPT) is 1 explanation for persistent obstructive symptoms after HSCR surgery.[5] The most widely accepted histologic features of the TZ include partial circumferential aganglionosis (PCAg), myenteric hypoganglionosis (MyHy), and SNH[20] (**Fig. 1**). The presence of one or more of these features is considered diagnostic of TZ and an indication for further surgery.

PCAg is the cross-sectional representation of an irregular interface between ganglionic and aganglionic bowel whereby portions of the ganglionic bowel extend farther distally compared with other portions of the ganglionic circumference. In ssHSCR, PCAg typically occupies a segment less than 3 cm proximal to the circumferentially aganglionic segment.[20] Generally, the ganglionic cells in the submucosal and myenteric plexuses are aligned and overlie each other closely. However, in a significant subset of HSCR cases, this is not so, and there can be deviations of 1 to 2 cm between the submucosal and myenteric ganglion cells. Most often the myenteric ganglion cells extend farther distally compared with the submucosal ganglion cells, and the reverse is rare.[20] Regardless, evaluation of both plexuses in a full-circumference section is ultimately required to exclude PCAg. Conversely, the presence of ganglion cells in a biopsy from a small portion of the circumference does not exclude PCAg.

MyHy is a quantitative abnormality in ganglion cells, most severe in the distal TZ in conjunction with PCAg, with a gradual increase in ganglion cell density that transitions to euganglionic bowel.[21,22] Because of the difficulty of resolving mild MyHy, most pathologists strive to exclude moderate-to-severe cases.[21] This is defined as a contiguous one-eighth circumference of the myenteric plexus populated primarily by hypoplastic ganglia (ganglia composed of single ganglion cells or doublets with sparse surrounding neuropil) (see **Fig. 1**D). Studies of ssHSCR have shown a gradual normalization of ganglion cells within a 5 cm-long segment proximal to the circumferentially aganglionic segment,[20,22] but anecdotal data suggest that greater than 5 cm of MyHy may be more common in patients with lsHSCR.

SNH, which has similar pathogenesis and histology to SNH in aganglionic bowel, is another feature of the TZ[22,23] (see **Fig. 1**E). SNH is predominantly found in the TZ of HSCR involving the left colon (colonic HSCR, ssHSCR, or vssHSCR) because of the proximity of abnormal bowel to the pelvic ganglia. The caliber of submucosal nerves is site- and age-dependent; therefore assessing for SNH in the TZ can be difficult. However, in an infant younger than 1 year, it is extremely unlikely to find nerves larger than 40 μm in the TZ or more than two of these nerves in a single 400x field.[14]

SECONDARY CHANGES

Secondary changes in HSCR, comprised of adaptive changes, injury responses, and inflammatory conditions, are due to chronic obstruction caused by the primary neuroanatomic malformations previously described. The most common secondary change is upstream distension of ganglionic bowel leading to significant dilatation (megacolon) and hypertrophy of the muscularis propria. Other secondary changes include fibrosis in and around the myenteric plexus, eosinophilic inflammation of the plexus or adjacent muscularis propria,[20,24] and HSCR-associated enterocolitis (HAEC).[25] Of these, HAEC is the only finding with proven clinical significance. HAEC can involve the ganglionic or aganglionic bowel in a multifocal patchy distribution, present before or after enterostomy or pull-through surgery, and prove fatal if not recognized and treated promptly.[25]

SURGICAL PATHOLOGY OF HIRSCHSPRUNG DISEASE

Surgical pathology of HSCR is performed at various stages in a patient's clinical course. These include the primary diagnosis performed on biopsies, intraoperative mapping of the colon, examination of the resection specimen, and evaluation of postoperative biopsies to exclude TZPT. Although there is no single accepted/standardized diagnostic approach to HSCR, the most important variable is technical and interpretational experience. No matter the approach, understanding methodological limitations and the ability to resolve diagnostic versus atypical results are paramount.

SUCTION RECTAL BIOPSY

Suction rectal biopsies (SRBs) are commonly used to diagnose aganglionosis, and an adequate biopsy has been shown to have a sensitivity of 97% and a specificity of 99%.[26] Adequacy is operator-dependent and influenced by biopsy size, depth, and location. Suboptimal sampling can be caused by a shallow biopsy or an insufficient amount of submucosa. Reasonable minimum adequacy criteria to exclude ganglion cells are: 2 to 3 mm in greatest dimension, surfaced entirely by colonic mucosa, and approximately 33% or more submucosa. A shallow biopsy increases the risk of excluding submucosal ganglia, many of which are concentrated close to the muscularis propria, as well as hypertrophic submucosal nerves. In a laboratory setting where H&E staining is the sole diagnostic method, it is appropriate to exhaust the block to evaluate as much of the submucosa as possible. If adequacy remains an issue, further sampling (preferably by incisional biopsy) may be warranted to ensure sufficient submucosal sampling.

From a clinical perspective, the location where the biopsy is taken can be problematic. If too low, it may sample the zone of physiologic hypoganglionosis that exists normally near the dentate line (squamocolumnar junction or transitional epithelium).[27] Conversely, a high biopsy may miss vssHSCR. One strategy to mitigate these problems is to obtain multiple biopsies at various levels starting in the distal 1 to 2 cm of the rectum (typically 2 to 3 cm internal to the anal verge of a young infant). Multiple biopsies also provide additional submucosa for examination and topographic information to aid in the diagnosis of vssHSCR.

Once the specimen is processed into formalin-fixed paraffin-embedded (FFPE) tissue, 50 to 75 H&E stained sections (4 to 5 μm thick) are employed in many laboratories to initially assess for ganglion cells. Most sections should consist of one-third or more of submucosa. If these criteria are met and no ganglion cells are identified in the setting of nerve hypertrophy, then the diagnosis is established. When all of these unequivocal findings are not present in the biopsy or atypical findings are identified, additional sections and/or ancillary tests are required.

INCISIONAL BIOPSY

Incisional biopsies are taken under direct visualization of the dentate line such that the precise location is known. In addition, incisional biopsies sample more submucosa plus or minus muscularis propria (full thickness), which is especially important in the setting of an inadequate SRB or a patient older than 1 year of age. SRB tends to sample less submucosa in older patients, because as the patient ages the submucosa becomes more fibrotic (resistant to SRB), and submucosal ganglia are more widely spaced.[28] A major drawback with incisional biopsy is that it requires general anesthesia, which has its own inherent risks and is more time consuming. There is also a risk of hemorrhage or perirectal infection, because full-thickness biopsies are transmural. Incisional biopsies are especially useful in the assessment for vssHSCR and TZPT.[29,30] Compared with SRB, fewer H&E sections are required for incisional biopsies because of greater sampling of the submucosa. In general, 2 slides with 2 ribbons per slide are sufficient to evaluate for aganglionosis and SNH.

ANCILLARY DIAGNOSTIC TESTS

With the advent of ancillary testing, in the form of enzyme histochemistry and/or immunohistochemistry (IHC) (**Fig. 3**), biopsy adequacy concerns and equivocal H&E findings have become less problematic. Ancillary tests highlight changes in mucosal innervation that correlate strongly with aganglionosis and are impossible to visualize by H&E alone.

Acetylcholinesterase (AChE) enzyme histochemistry is one of the earliest methods to be widely applied in the evaluation for HSCR. AChE is expressed in extrinsic cholinergic nerves, and AChE enzyme histochemistry highlights these nerves, which are thicker and more numerous in the mucosa of aganglionic bowel (see **Fig. 3**C, D). This method requires frozen tissue, because enzymatic activity of AChE is lost after FFPE. In laboratories proficient in enzyme histochemistry, frozen section alone is sufficient to diagnose or exclude HSCR.[31] The utility is confined to a single clinical setting, which makes implementation and maintenance of this method unappealing to many laboratories.

An FFPE tissue-based method is calretinin IHC. Calretinin (calbindin 2) is a calcium-binding protein expressed in most submucosal ganglion cells and a minority of myenteric ganglion cells (see **Fig. 3**A, B). Calretinin IHC labels neuronal perikarya and nerve processes and is a marker for intrinsic mucosal innervation. Conversely, mucosa of aganglionic bowel, except within 1 to 2 cm of the TZ, is devoid of calretinin immunostaining. Completely absent calretinin-immunoreactive mucosal innervation is a specific and highly sensitive finding in HSCR.[16,32,33]

Bear in mind several pitfalls when interpreting calretinin IHC. First, calretinin is expressed in mast cells, which extend short processes that may mimic neurites. Focus on staining quality to avoid this mistake; mast cells stain lighter and do not show the beaded pattern of staining of neurite varicosities. Second, some submucosal extrinsic nerves retain calretinin immunoreactivity. Therefore, the complete presence or absence of calretinin immunostaining is a diagnostic finding limited to the mucosa. Calretinin IHC should not be used in seromuscular biopsies to establish the diagnosis of aganglionosis. Third, submucosal ganglia from the TZ send calretinin-immunoreactive mucosal neurites downstream into the 1 to 2 cm proximal portion of the aganglionic bowel (see **Fig. 1**B). In a biopsy from a patient with vssHSCR or a distal skip area, these TZ-derived, calretinin-immunoreactive mucosal nerves should not lead one to erroneously exclude HSCR (**Fig. 4**).[3,18] Rather, calretinin-immunoreactive mucosal nerves in the setting of aganglionosis and unequivocal submucosal nerve hypertrophy should raise concern for vssHSCR or a distal skip area, and may warrant an incisional biopsy. Fourth, certain commercially available calretinin antibodies have been found to lose reactivity to previously frozen tissue.[34] Finally, the diagnostic finding is a negative staining result; therefore it is important to run a positive control, ideally pieces of ganglionic

NORMAL   AGANGLIONIC

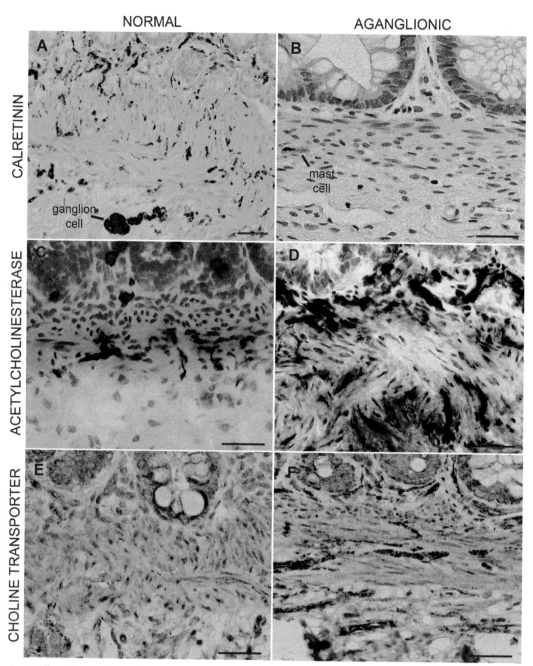

Fig. 3. Ancillary diagnostic methods. (*A, B*) Calretinin immunohistochemistry. (*C, D*) Acetylcholinesterase enzyme histochemistry. (*E, F*) Choline transporter immunohistochemistry. Scale bars: 40 μm.

and aganglionic bowel on the same slide as the patient.

Recently, choline transporter (ChT) has been proposed as a surrogate for AChE. ChT IHC, compared with AChE enzyme histochemistry, is more accessible to laboratories, because it is based on FFPE tissue (see **Fig. 3**E, F). Similar to AChE enzyme histochemistry, ChT immunostaining labels abnormal mucosal nerves in aganglionic bowel.[35] ChT immunostaining may be especially useful in the setting of vssHSCR, where calretinin immunostaining can be misleading. Overall ChT IHC is a promising replacement for AChE enzyme histochemistry, but interpretation of either requires regular practice and experience.

Fig. 4. Rectal biopsy in vssHSCR. (*A*) Unequivocal submucosal nerve hypertrophy. (*B*) Calretinin plus neurites in mucosa. Ganglion cells may or may not be present. Scale bars: 40 μm.

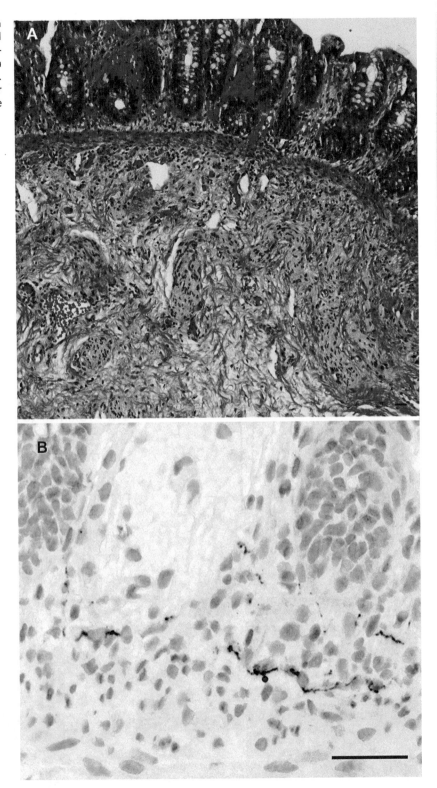

INTRAOPERATIVE CONSULTATIONS

Before bowel resection, an intraoperative mapping procedure is performed by the surgeon to localize the distal-most extent of normal ganglionic bowel (**Fig. 5**). This ensures either the primary pull-through or diverting ostomy is performed proximal to the aganglionic segment and TZ. Multiple sero-muscular or full-thickness leveling biopsies are taken, and careful coordination is needed between the surgeon and pathologist. For either biopsy type, the pathologist should receive at least mus-cularis propria and myenteric plexus in the sample. The specimen should be embedded and frozen so that sections (5–8 μm thick) are perpendicular to the serosal surface and both layers of the muscu-laris propria are sectioned. Frozen sections are stained, typically with H&E (see **Fig. 5**B, C), but some pathologists prefer Romanowsky (Diff-Quik) staining. Diff-Quik stains the cytoplasm of neurons blue, which increases the contrast be-tween ganglion cells and the background colonic tissue[36] (see **Fig. 5**D).

In a well-oriented leveling biopsy, less than 10 sections are usually required to identify ganglion cells. One strategy is to initially cut 2 sections for assessment. If no ganglion cells are present, then another 8 sections should be cut to confirm aganglionosis. A limitation of the biopsy specimen is that the presence or absence of ganglion does not exclude TZ, as only a small portion of the circumference is sampled. In light of this and the fact that the TZ in ssHSCR is typically less than 5 cm, the bowel should be resected at least

A   INTRAOPERATIVE HISTOPATHOLOGY
Excluding Transition Zone

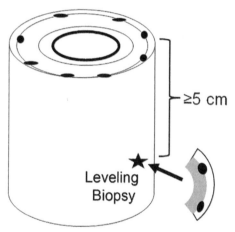

≥5 cm

Leveling Biopsy

Find ganglion cells and make anastomosis **at least 5 cm** proximal to that point

Conduct frozen section examination of donut from proximal margin to assess circumferential distribution of ganglion cells and submucosal nerve hypertrophy

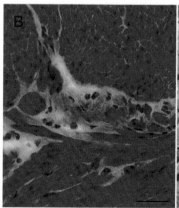
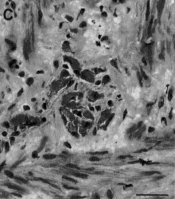
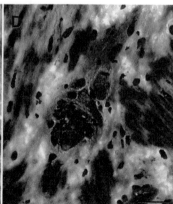

Fig. 5. Intraoperative leveling biopsies to identify ganglionic bowel. (*A*) Recommended approach to leveling bi-opsy and subsequent resection. (*B–D*) Frozen sections of leveling biopsies showing large nerve in aganglionic myenteric plexus (*B*, H&E) and myenteric ganglia with H&E (*C*) and Romanowsky (*D*) stains. Scale bars: 40 μm.

5 cm proximal from a ganglionic biopsy site. Even so, a risk of retained TZ exists.[20,22] Therefore, after the resection site (or ostomy site) has been chosen, a full en face circumferential frozen section (donut) of the proximal margin should be performed to look for features of TZ (**Fig. 6**). Identification of PCAg, MyHy, or SNH should prompt the surgeon to resect more proximal bowel to avoid TZPT. When examining the proximal donut, it may be helpful to divide it into linear segments and align them in the freezing medium. This usually allows all the tissue to fit on the freezing platform and secures proper bowel wall orientation during the embedding process. When cutting the specimen into sectors, carefully mark the relationship between each quadrant to avoid missing TZ features that may span 2 sectors, such as MyHy (one-eighth the myenteric circumference occupied primarily by single ganglia or doublets).

Finding the proximal extent of the aganglionic segment can be arduous and time-consuming. Histologic examination of leveling biopsies requires sectioning and processing multiple levels. Not only can this wear on the patience of everyone involved, it increases the patient's exposure to anesthesia and its associated risks. In an attempt to reduce anesthesia time, it may be tempting to forego taking successive biopsies and jump to an appendiceal biopsy in order to diagnose total colonic aganglionosis, but this strategy is not advised, as an aganglionic appendix does not always correlate with aganglionosis of the remaining colon distal to the appendix. There can be intervening areas of normally ganglionic bowel (skip areas) downstream from the aganglionic appendix not requiring resection. Additionally, post-pull-through severe chronic constipation is sometimes treated with anterograde enemas through an appendicostomy, and appendectomy would deprive the patient of this treatment option.

RESECTION SPECIMENS

The type of specimen the pathologist will receive depends on the surgical procedure (single- or multistage). In a single-stage pull-through, the resection specimen is typically submitted as 1 segment of bowel. A multistage procedure (diverting enterostomy followed later by ostomy take-down and pull-through) will yield separate segments of bowel, one of which will be an ostomy excision. When evaluating the specimen, it is important that the pathologist know the type of procedure performed in order to understand the type of specimen he or she will receive and have correct orientation. This ensures the pathologist can clearly identify the proximal-most margin; in a multistage resection, the proximal margin of the end ostomy takedown is the proximal-most margin and is most representative of the enteric neuroanatomy at the final anastomotic site.

Examination of the resection specimen has 3 major goals: confirm the presence of aganglionosis, exclude the presence of TZ at the proximal margin, and describe the approximate length of aganglionosis (**Fig. 7**). During the gross examination, the relative positions of margins, biopsy sites, and sites where bowel caliber changes should be

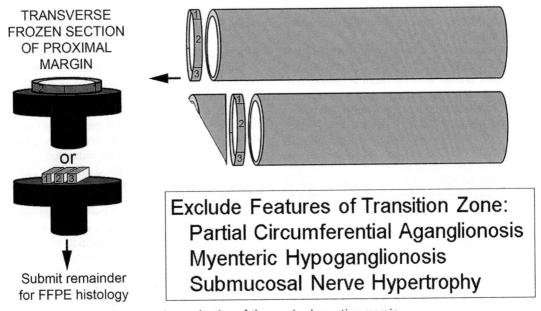

TRANSVERSE
FROZEN SECTION
OF PROXIMAL
MARGIN

or

Submit remainder
for FFPE histology

Exclude Features of Transition Zone:
Partial Circumferential Aganglionosis
Myenteric Hypoganglionosis
Submucosal Nerve Hypertrophy

Fig. 6. Intraoperative frozen section evaluation of the proximal resection margin.

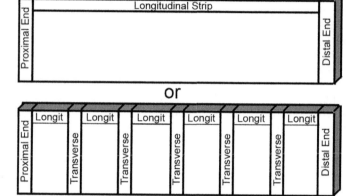

Open lengthwise to evaluate mucosa
Consider overnight fixation of flat specimen to
improve orientation of histologic sections

Minimal goals are to
1.Confirm distal
   aganglionosis
2.Exclude features of
   transition zone at
   proximal margin
3.Document the length
   of the aganglionic
   segment

Fig. 7. Histologic sampling of an HSCR resection.

measured and recorded. This will allow the pathologist to correlate resection pathology to the intraoperative surgical and biopsy findings. Full-circumference en face sections of the distal and proximal margins should be taken to confirm aganglionosis and exclude TZ respectively. A longitudinal strip representing the entire length of the resection specimen is typically obtained to demonstrate a transition point between aganglionic and ganglionic bowel. The section can then be rolled like a placental membrane roll, and processed in a single cassette. If desired, a more refined map of the TZ can be constructed from multiple longitudinal sections from various points along the circumference or multiple closely spaced transverse sections.

Microscopic examination should indicate clearly the distribution of ganglion cells. The presence of TZ features should also be reported along with other histopathologic findings such as the presence of active inflammation, epithelial injury, and other features of colitis that may indicate HSCR-related enterocolitis. Although the presence of eosinophilic infiltrates, ectopic ganglia, muscular hypertrophy, and mitotic activity in the muscularis propria may be noted, the clinical significance of these is unknown and therefore not essential to the report.

POSTOPERATIVE DIAGNOSIS OF TRANSITION ZONE PULL-THROUGH

Postoperative obstructive symptoms are common among HSCR patients. Potential causes of obstruction include strictures, torsion around the anastomotic site, retained aganglionic bowel (secondary to inadequate resection of a long aganglionic segment or retained skip segment with proximal aganglionic bowel), and TZPT. The cause of obstruction is often identified by physical examination or imaging studies. In certain instances, such as retained proximal aganglionic segments in skip segment HSCR, a confirmatory biopsy may be needed. Diagnosis of TZPT relies entirely on histopathology.[37]

The presence of one or more histologic features of TZ at the proximal-most margin of the original resection specimen is the most reliable method of diagnosing TZPT, and therefore the original slides should be reviewed when assessing for TZPT. If the original slides are not available, full-thickness biopsy of the neorectum may be helpful. In addition to assessing for TZPT, full-thickness biopsy can be used to exclude the possibility of retained aganglionic bowel. Biopsies can be taken at the time of anorectal examination under anesthesia.[29,30,38] SRB should be discouraged in this setting, because the patients are usually greater than 1 year of age; additionally, submucosal sampling is limited with this method of biopsy.[28]

In an adequate full-thickness biopsy, the presence of aganglionosis suggests the possibilities of incomplete resection of the proximal aganglionic segment (retained aganglionic segment and TZ), PCAg (TZPT), or a biopsy of retained native rectum below the anastomotic site. The presence of fibrosis, smooth muscle hyperplasia filling the submucosa, or other surgical site change may indicate a biopsy of the anastomotic site, which is considered inadequate to exclude

TZ features. If an incisional biopsy is not sufficiently deep to include the myenteric plexus, SNH is the only TZ feature one can diagnose. In the post-pull-through setting, assessing for SNH alone is complicated by age-related changes in rectal submucosal nerve density and caliber, surgery-related nerve caliber changes, and post-pull-through nerve remodeling of the neorectum.[19,39] Therefore, SNH should be dramatic and unequivocal, if it is to be use as the sole criterion for diagnosis of TZPT and potential repeat surgery. Adjunct testing such as AChE histochemistry or ChT IHC may be helpful in identifying abnormal cholinergic nerves, but research is required to characterize the performance of these stains in this setting. Calretinin immunostaining is generally not helpful in the setting of TZPT, because the mucosa in the TZ and 1 to 2 cm of proximal aganglionic bowel retain calretinin-immunoreactive mucosal innervation.

SUMMARY AND FUTURE DIRECTIONS

Histology is currently the main modality in diagnosing HSCR, and understanding the differences in normal enteric neuroanatomy compared with HSCR is essential. Additionally, having technical proficiency in ancillary testing methods and knowing the limitations of adjunct tests are key elements in assessing for and managing HSCR. Although laboratories that see a low volume of HSCR cases each year may find diagnosing the disease especially challenging, several ancillary tests along with new technologies (such as telemedicine) are available or are in development to aid the pathologist in difficult situations.

A search for simpler or less invasive methods to diagnose HSCR continues. Although AChE-positive innervation is increased in aganglionic bowel, and biochemical quantification is able to identify higher AChE-activity in aganglionic rectal tissue from many patients, the variance in values observed in individual patients limits its diagnostic utility.[40] A reduction in glutamate with increases in gamma aminobutyric acid and 3 peptide markers, detected in 42 patients' sera by mass spectrometry, was reported to be 100% sensitive and specific for HSCR.[41] These potential serologic tests require independent validation and have yet to be widely adopted.

Recently, confocal laser endomicroscopy (CLE) has been proposed as a less invasive diagnostic approach. No tissue sampling is needed, because ganglion cells are directly visualized. In a feasibility study, CLE was found to be 88.4% concordant with traditional H&E methods (n = 69) and to have 78.6% sensitivity and 95.7% specificity.[42] Performance characteristics with CLE are, in part, operator-dependent, and as endoscopists gain technical and interpretational experience, there may be improvement upon these promising preliminary findings.

HSCR is a genetically complex disorder, and specific genetic alterations in more than 20 genes act as susceptibility factors. Although some specific mutations explain syndromic associations with HSCR, mutational analysis has had a limited diagnostic role because of variable penetrance of aganglionosis (even in syndromic presentations).[43] The genetic alterations that lead to HSCR likely also affect poorly understood aspects of enteric neuromuscular biology that are not resolved by standard histopathology, such as neurochemical coding, network circuitry, interstitial cells of Cajal, and smooth muscle physiology. HSCR-associated defects in histologically normal ganglionic bowel may underlie postsurgical dysmotility despite complete resection of the aganglionic segment and TZ. Advancement in the management of HSCR may require comprehensive examination of these complex cellular properties.

DISCLOSURE

The authors have nothing to disclose.

REFERENCES

1. Taguchi T, Obata S, Ieiri S. Current status of Hirschsprung's disease: based on a nationwide survey of Japan. Pediatr Surg Int 2017;33(4):497–504.
2. Meier-Ruge WA, Bruder E, Holschneider AM, et al. Diagnosis and therapy of ultrashort Hirschsprung's disease. Eur J Pediatr Surg 2004;14(6):392–7.
3. Kapur RP. Calretinin-immunoreactive mucosal innervation in very short-segment Hirschsprung disease: a potentially misleading observation. Pediatr Dev Pathol 2014;17(1):28–35.
4. Okamoto E, Satani M, Kuwata K. Histologic and embryologic studies on the innervation of the pelvic viscera in patients with Hirschsprung's disease. Surg Gynecol Obstet 1982;155(6):823–8.
5. Meier-Ruge W, Hunziker O, Tobler HJ, et al. The pathophysiology of aganglionosis of the entire colon (Zuelzer-Wilson syndrome). Morphometric investigations of the extent of sacral parasympathetic innervation of the circular muscles of the aganglionic colon. Beitr Pathol 1972;147(3):228–36.
6. Garrett JR, Howard ER, Nixon HH. Autonomic nerves in rectum and colon in Hirschsprung's disease: a cholinesterase and catecholamine histochemical study. Arch Dis Child 1969;44(235):406–17.

7. Matsuda H, Hirato J, Kuroiwa M, et al. Histopathological and immunohistochemical study of the enteric innervations among various types of aganglionoses including isolated and syndromic Hirschsprung disease. Neuropathology 2006;26(1):8–23.

8. Kakita Y, Oshiro K, O'Briain DS, et al. Selective demonstration of mural nerves in ganglionic and aganglionic colon by immunohistochemistry for glucose transporter-1: prominent extrinsic nerve pattern staining in Hirschsprung disease. Arch Pathol Lab Med 2000;124(9):1314–9.

9. Wedel T, Holschneider AM, Krammer HJ. Ultrastructural features of nerve fascicles and basal lamina abnormalities in Hirschsprung's disease. Eur J Pediatr Surg 1999;9(2):75–82.

10. Baumgarten HG, Holstein AF, Stelzner F. Nervous elements in the human colon of Hirschsprung's disease - with comparative remarks on neuronal profiles in the normal human and monkey colon and sphincter ani internus. Virchows Arch A Pathol Pathol Anat 1973;358(2):113–36.

11. Jessen KR, Thorpe R, Mirsky R. Molecular identity, distribution and heterogeneity of glial fibrillary acidic protein: an immunoblotting and immunohistochemical study of Schwann cells, satellite cells, enteric glia and astrocytes. J Neurocytol 1984;13(2):187–200.

12. Alpy F, Ritié L, Jaubert F, et al. The expression pattern of laminin isoforms in Hirschsprung disease reveals a distal peripheral nerve differentiation. Hum Pathol 2005;36(10):1055–65.

13. Monforte-Muñoz H, Gonzalez-Gomez I, Rowland JM, et al. Increased submucosal nerve trunk caliber in aganglionosis: a "positive" and objective finding in suction biopsies and segmental resections in Hirschsprung's disease. Arch Pathol Lab Med 1998;122(8):721–5.

14. Kapur RP. Submucosal nerve diameter of greater than 40 μm is not a valid diagnostic index of transition zone pull-through. J Pediatr Surg 2016;51(10):1585–91.

15. Narayanan SK, Soundappan SS, Kwan E, et al. Aganglionosis with the absence of hypertrophied nerve fibres predicts disease proximal to rectosigmoid colon. Pediatr Surg Int 2016;32(3):221–6.

16. Kapur RP, Reed RC, Finn LS, et al. Calretinin immunohistochemistry versus acetylcholinesterase histochemistry in the evaluation of suction rectal biopsies for Hirschsprung disease. Pediatr Dev Pathol 2009;12(1):6–15.

17. Kapur RP, Desa DJ, Luquette M, et al. Hypothesis: Pathogenesis of skip areas in long-segment Hirschsprung's disease. Pediatr Pathol Lab Med 1995;15(1):23–37.

18. Coe A, Avansino JR, Kapur RP. Distal rectal skip-segment Hirschsprung disease and the potential for false-negative diagnosis. Pediatr Dev Pathol 2016;19(2):123–31.

19. Kapur RP, Kennedy AJ. Transitional zone pull through: surgical pathology considerations. Semin Pediatr Surg 2012;21(4):291–301.

20. Kapur RP. Histology of the transition zone in Hirschsprung disease. Am J Surg Pathol 2016;40(12):1637–46.

21. Swaminathan M, Kapur RP. Counting myenteric ganglion cells in histologic sections: an empirical approach. Hum Pathol 2010;41(8):1097–108.

22. Kapur RP, Kennedy AJ. Histopathologic delineation of the transition zone in short-segment Hirschsprung disease. Pediatr Dev Pathol 2013;16(4):252–66.

23. Coe A, Collins MH, Lawal T, et al. Reoperation for Hirschsprung disease: pathology of the resected problematic distal pull-through. Pediatr Dev Pathol 2012;15(1):30–8.

24. Lowichik A, Weinberg AG. Eosinophilic infiltration of the enteric neural plexuses in Hirschsprung's disease. Pediatr Pathol Lab Med 1997;17(6):885–91.

25. Teitelbaum DH, Caniano DA, Qualman SJ. The pathophysiology of Hirschsprung's-associated enterocolitis: importance of histologic correlates. J Pediatr Surg 1989;24(12):1271–7.

26. Friedmacher F, Puri P. Rectal suction biopsy for the diagnosis of Hirschsprung's disease: a systematic review of diagnostic accuracy and complications. Pediatr Surg Int 2015;31(9):821–30.

27. Aldridge RT, Campbell PE. Ganglion cell distribution in the normal rectum and anal canal. A basis for the diagnosis of Hirschsprung's disease by anorectal biopsy. J Pediatr Surg 1968;3(4):475–90.

28. Vadva Z, Nurko S, Hehn R, et al. Rectal suction biopsy in patients with previous anorectal surgery for Hirschsprung disease. J Pediatr Gastroenterol Nutr 2017;65(2):173–8.

29. Langer JC, Rollins MD, Levitt M, et al. Guidelines for the management of postoperative obstructive symptoms in children with Hirschsprung disease. Pediatr Surg Int 2017;33(5):523–6.

30. Chumpitazi BP, Nurko S. Defecation disorders in children after surgery for Hirschsprung disease. J Pediatr Gastroenterol Nutr 2011;53(1):75–9.

31. Bagdzevičius R, Gelman S, Gukauskienė L, et al. Application of acetylcholinesterase histochemistry for the diagnosis of Hirschsprung's disease in neonates and infants: a twenty-year experience. Medicina 2011;47(7):374–9.

32. Holland SK, Ramalingam P, Podolsky RH, et al. Calretinin immunostaining as an adjunct in the diagnosis of Hirschsprung disease. Ann Diagn Pathol 2011;15(5):323–8.

33. de Arruda Lourenção PLT, Takegawa BK, Ortolan EVP, et al. A useful panel for the diagnosis of Hirschsprung disease in rectal biopsies: calretinin

immunostaining and acetylcholinesterase histochesmistry. Ann Diagn Pathol 2013;17(4):352–6.

34. Lim KH, Wan WK, Lim TKH, et al. Primary diagnosis of Hirschsprung disease – calretinin immunohistochemistry in rectal suction biopsies, with emphasis on diagnostic pitfalls. World J Pathol 2014;9(3): 14–22.

35. Kapur RP, Raess PW, Hwang S, et al. Choline transporter immunohistochemistry: an effective substitute for acetylcholinesterase histochemistry to diagnose Hirschsprung disease with formalin-fixed paraffin-embedded rectal biopsies. Pediatr Dev Pathol 2017;20(4):308–20.

36. Holland SK, Hessler RB, Reid-Nicholson MD, et al. Utilization of peripherin and S-100 immunohistochemistry in the diagnosis of Hirschsprung disease. Mod Pathol 2010;23(9):1173–9.

37. Kapur RP, Smith C, Ambartsumyan L. Postoperative pullthrough obstruction in Hirschsprung disease: etiologies and diagnosis. Pediatr Dev Pathol 2020; 23(1):40–59.

38. Smith C, Ambartsumyan L, Kapur RP. Surgery, surgical pathology, and postoperative management of patients with Hirschsprung disease. Pediatr Dev Pathol 2020;23(1):23–39.

39. Kapur RP, Arnold MA, Conces MR, et al. Remodeling of rectal innervation after pullthrough surgery for Hirschsprung disease: relevance to criteria for the determination of retained transition zone. Pediatr Dev Pathol 2019;22(4):292–303.

40. Wells FE, Addison GM. Acetylcholinesterase activity in rectal biopsies: an assessment of its diagnostic value in Hirschsprung's disease. J Pediatr Gastroenterol Nutr 1988;5(6):912–9.

41. Wang JX, Qin P, Liu QL, et al. Detection and significance of serum protein marker of Hirschsprung disease. Pediatrics 2007;120(1):e56–60.

42. Shimojima N, Kobayashi M, Kamba S, et al. Visualization of the human enteric nervous system by confocal laser endomicroscopy in Hirschsprung's disease: an alternative to intraoperative histopathological diagnosis? Neurogastroenterol Motil 2020; 32(5):e13805.

43. Amiel J, Sproat-Emison E, Garcia-Barcelo M, et al. Hirschsprung disease, associated syndromes and genetics: a review. J Med Genet 2008;45:1–14.

Updates in Pediatric Congenital Enteropathies
Differential Diagnosis, Testing, and Genetics

Pierre Russo, MD

KEYWORDS

- Enteropathies • Autoimmune enteropathy • Very-early-onset inflammatory bowel disease

---

Key points

- Congenital enteropathies comprise a rare group of genetic disorders characterized by early intestinal failure.
- Autoimmune enteropathy is now recognized to be a heterogeneous group of disorders with a variable age at presentation, from infants to adults, the basis of which is an unregulated T-cell mediated attack on the intestine.
- Very-early onset inflammatory bowel disease (VEO-IBD) represents an emerging group of inflammatory bowel disorders which usually present early infancy and are resistant to conventional therapy.

ABSTRACT

Congenital enteropathies comprise a heterogeneous group of disorders typically resulting in severe diarrhea and intestinal failure. Recent advances in and more widespread application of genetic testing have allowed more accurate diagnosis of these entities as well as identification of new disorders, provided a deeper understanding of intestinal pathophysiology through genotype-phenotype correlations, and permitted the exploration of more specific therapies to diseases that have heretofore been resistant to conventional treatments. The therapeutic armamentarium for these disorders now includes intestinal and hematopoietic stem cell transplantation, specific targeted therapy, such as the use of interleukin-1 receptor antagonists and, in some cases, gene therapy. These considerations are particularly applicable to the group of disorders identified as "very-early onset inflammatory bowel disease" (VEO-IBD), for which a veritable explosion of knowledge has occurred in the last decade. The pathologist plays a crucial role in assisting in the diagnosis of these entities and in ruling out other disorders that enter into the differential diagnosis.

The aim of this article is to present the salient histopathologic features and differential diagnosis of enteropathies of infancy, discuss their diagnostic modalities, highlight their genetic aspects, and briefly discuss relevant therapeutic implications. The author has chosen to divide this article into the following sections: (A) Congenital disorders of intestinal differentiation; (B) Disorders of immunomodulation (including autoimmune enteropathy [AIE] and autoimmune polyendocrine syndrome [APS]); and (C) VEOIBD. Celiac disease, eosinophilic disorders, and infections, more frequently encountered in daily practice, will not be discussed except as they enter into the differential diagnosis because considerable information on these disorders is readily available in reviews and textbooks.

CONGENITAL DISORDERS OF INTESTINAL DIFFERENTIATION

MICROVILLUS INCLUSION DISEASE

Initially described by Davidson and colleagues[1] in 1978, and subsequently recognized worldwide, microvillus inclusion disease (MVID; OMIM #251850) is an autosomal recessive disease

Department of Pathology and Laboratory Medicine, Division of Anatomic Pathology, The University of Pennsylvania School of Medicine, The Children's Hospital of Philadelphia, 324 South 34th Street, Main Building, Philadelphia, PA 19104, USA
E-mail address: russo@email.chop.edu

Surgical Pathology 13 (2020) 581–600
https://doi.org/10.1016/j.path.2020.08.001
1875-9181/20/© 2020 Elsevier Inc. All rights reserved.

characterized by refractory secretory diarrhea usually occurring within the first week of life, although a late-onset form may manifest in the first few months of life. It is the leading cause of neonatal secretory diarrhea and accounts for about 7% of pediatric bowel transplantations worldwide.[2] Geographically, there is a relatively high prevalence of the disorder in the Mediterranean region and in the Navajo population. MVID appears to be a heterogeneous disease with an expanding spectrum of genotypes and phenotypes. Most patients have been found to have mutations in the gene *MYO5B*, located on chromosome 18q21, coding for myosin Vb (MYO5B), which, by interacting with RAB small GTPases (RAB8a, RAB10, RAB11), plays a crucial role in maintaining cell polarity, apical trafficking, and development of microvilli.[3] Several extraintestinal manifestations have been observed in these patients, the most well known a low/normal gamma-glutamyl transferase (GGT) cholestasis observed both before and following intestinal transplantation. More recently, *MYO5B* deficiency has also been demonstrated to be associated with isolated low/normal GGT cholestasis without clinical bowel disease,[4] suggesting an abnormal canalicular organization, resulting in impaired bile acid secretion. These findings are consistent with reports of apical membrane alterations in nonintestinal organs with *MYO5B* mutations, including the stomach, colonic mucosa (despite normal hematoxylin and eosin [H&E] appearance), and aberrant expression of hepatocellular canalicular transporters, such as BSEP and MRP2.[5] Other reported manifestations include obesity, *Pneumocystis jiroveci* pneumonia, renal Fanconi syndrome, hypophosphatemic rickets as well as psychiatric problems, and the relationship of these manifestations with *MYO5B* deficiency is unclear. Whole-exome sequencing (WES) of patients with a milder intestinal phenotype has identified mutations in the gene *STX3* (chromosome 11q12.1; OMIM #600876), coding for syntaxin 3, which also acts as a regulator of cellular protein trafficking.[6,7] Mutations in syntaxin binding protein 2 (*STXB2*, alias *MUNC18-2*, chromosome 19p13.2; OMIM #601717) have also been described in patients with familial hemophagocytic lymphohistiocytosis type 5 who developed a severe enteropathy not responsive to immunomodulation with intestinal histopathologic changes consistent with MVID.[8]

Small bowel biopsies are typically characterized by severe villus atrophy, mild to moderate crypt hyperplasia, and mild to minimal inflammation of the lamina propria (**Fig.** 1A). The surface epithelium may appear atrophic or vacuolated. The diagnosis may be strongly suspected on paraffin-embedded sections by the absence of a distinct brush border using the periodic acid–Schiff (PAS) stain, with the presence of diffuse PAS-positive staining at the apex of the enterocytes (**Fig.** 1B, C). Similar observations are noted using immunohistochemical staining for alkaline phosphatase, anti-CD10, and villin.[9] Similar results using antibodies directed against anti-RAB11a, a small guanosine triphosphatase (GTPase) protein on the surface of recycling endosomes, has provided further evidence that MVID is a disorder of apical plasma membrane recycling.[10] The pathognomonic ultrastructural features include absent or small stubby microvilli, and vesicular structures located toward the apex of the enterocytes containing microvilli and granules containing dense amorphous material (**Fig.** 1D). Microvillus inclusions have also been reported in the colon, gallbladder, and renal tubular epithelium in these patients.[11] A variety of different ultrastructural features has also been noted in patients with this disorder, and finding the "typical" inclusions may require a prolonged search.[12] Patients with MVID are dependent on total parenteral nutrition (TPN), although improved survival may require small bowel transplantation.[13]

CONGENITAL TUFTING ENTEROPATHY (EPITHELIAL DYSPLASIA)

As initially described by Reifen and colleagues,[14] patients with tufting enteropathy also present in the neonatal period with a watery diarrhea. Prenatal history is uneventful, and the disease appears to be inherited in an autosomal recessive fashion, as suggested by the finding of other affected siblings and frequent parental consanguinity. The incidence is estimated at 1/50,000 to 1/100,000 live births in Europe and appears to be more frequent in patients of Arabic origin. The disorder has been linked to biallelic inactivating mutations in the *EPCAM* gene (OMIM #613217), located on chromosome 2p21, coding for the epithelial cell adhesion molecule.[15] This molecule belongs to a family of cell adhesion receptors, associates with tight junction proteins, and is responsible for cell-cell interaction by recruiting actin filaments to sites of contact.[16] Patients with this mutation appear to have disease limited to the gastrointestinal (GI) tract. Monoallelic deletions of the 3′ end of the *EPCAM* gene inactivate the downstream *MSH2* gene, resulting in Lynch syndrome.[17] A second group of patients with congenital tufting enteropathy (CTE) has been described with a syndromic form of the disorder, characterized by choanal and intestinal atresia, punctate keratitis, dermatologic abnormalities, and bone malformations, resulting from mutations in *SPINT2*, encoding Kunitz-type serine protease inhibitor 2 (chromosome 19q13.2; OMIM

Fig.   1. MVID.   (*A*) Duodenal biopsy with to-tal villous atrophy and mild to moderately hy-perplastic crypts without significant inflammation (original   magnification x100). (*B*) PAS stain at higher power shows lack of a well-defined brush border   and   a   diffuse periapical   positivity within the enterocytes (original   magnification x400). (*C*) PAS-positive staining of normal duo-denum by comparison. Note the sharply defined brush   border   (original magnification x400).

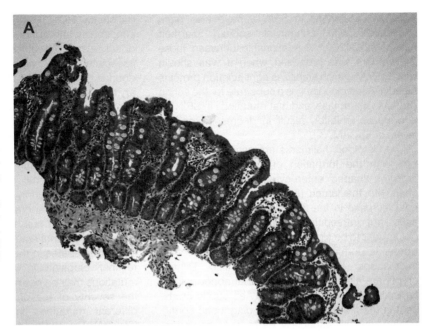

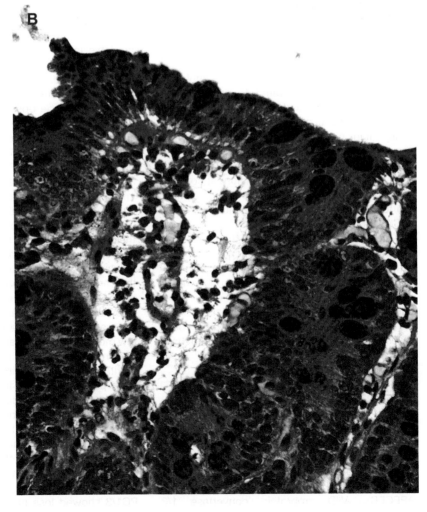

#605124). Mutations in *SPINT2* have also been associated with congenital sodium diarrhea (OMIM #270420).[18] A relationship between these 2 disorders was proposed when it was shown that EpCAM, which stabilizes tight junction proteins claudin-7 and claudin-1, is a substrate for the serine protease matriptase, and that mutations in SPINT2, a protease inhibitor, result in decreased cellular levels of EpCAM.[19]

The histologic hallmarks are severe villus atrophy with the formation of "tufts" of rounded, teardrop-shaped enterocytes, which appear to shed into the lumen (**Fig. 2**A). There may be a mild increase in the lamina propria inflammatory cells, but Intraepithelial lymphocytes (IELs) do not appear to be significantly increased. The brush border is normal by PAS staining, and electron microscopic findings are nonspecific. Dilated crypts are also observed. Epithelial abnormalities typically vary over time and may be subtle or absent in the first biopsy, making diagnostic confirmation difficult, especially early in presentation. Biopsies from patients with congenital sodium diarrhea are reportedly normal, although a few patients have been reported with histologic features suggesting tufting enteropathy.[19] Absence of immunohistochemical staining for MOC31 (an antibody directed against EPCAM) is a useful diagnostic feature in patients with CTE and mutations in the *EPCAM* gene and should be included in the histologic panel of intestinal biopsy evaluation in any infant presenting with prolonged diarrhea (**Fig. 2**B).[18,20] Immunohistochemical staining for EPCAM in patients with *SPINT2* mutations, however, is preserved and similar to normal controls, whereas no change in staining intensity or localization for SPINT2 was seen in patients with either *EPCAM* or *SPINT2* mutations.[18]

In most patients, the severity of the malabsorption and diarrhea makes them dependent on long-term parenteral nutrition, and in some cases, intestinal transplantation is a therapeutic option with or without liver transplantation because of the associated parenteral nutrition–induced cirrhosis. A more indolent clinical course has also been observed with some patients reported to have been eventually weaned off TPN.[21]

ENTEROENDOCRINE CELL DYSGENESIS

Loss of enteroendocrine cells is a relatively recently recognized cause of global malabsorptive diarrhea that encompasses several disorders: enteric anendocrinosis, autoimmune-mediated loss, as in the autoimmune–polyendocrine-candidiasis-ectodermal dystrophy syndrome (APECED), AND proprotein convertase 1/3

deficiency (PC1/3), and patients with X-linked lissencephaly and abnormal genitalia. Enteric anendocrinosis is an autosomal recessive disorder associated with congenital absence of enteroendocrine cells in the small and large bowel secondary to mutations in the *NEUROG3* gene, located on chromosome 10q21.3 (OMIM #610370), required for differentiation of epithelial cells to the endocrine phenotype.[22] Affected patients are characterized by a congenital diarrheal syndrome with profound malabsorption of all nutrients from birth. Patients also typically develop insulin-dependent diabetes, some during infancy and others later in childhood.[22,23] Pancreatic exocrine function is normal. *Neurog3* null mice are devoid of all islet cells and intestinal enteroendocrine cells and succumb to diabetes in the first few days of life.[24] Intestinal biopsies in patients with *NEUROG3* mutations may be normal or reveal villous atrophy, the severity of the changes perhaps related to different mutations in the *NEUROG3* gene23 (**Fig. 3**A). The characteristic absence of enteroendocrine cells in the small bowel and colon is confirmed by immunohistochemistry for chromogranin A (**Fig. 3**B, C). At present, no treatment is available for this disorder. Patients with autoimmune polyglandular syndrome I may have absent or markedly reduced enteroendocrine cells, which may be transient.[25,26] Loss of enteroendocrine cells may also be observed in patients with AIE, along with loss of goblet and Paneth cells.

Homozygous mutations in *PCSK1* (chromosome 5q15; OMIM #162150), which encodes an endoprotease named PC1/3, have been associated with malabsorptive diarrhea, hypoglycemia, impaired adrenal and thyroid function, hypogonadism, and obesity with onset in infancy.[27] PC1/3 is responsible for converting prohormones to their biologically active form. PC1/3 is expressed in gut endocrine cells, in the arcuate and periventricular hypothalamic nuclei, and in the β cells of the pancreas. In addition, 2 heterozygote variants of *PCSK1* have been associated with obesity. In a review of 13 cases, all patients presented with a severe malabsorptive diarrhea within the first few months of life that failed to resolve upon elimination diets and were dependent on parenteral nutrition. Diabetes insipidus, hypogonadism in male patients, adrenal insufficiency, and central hypothyroidism were accompanying clinical manifestations.[28] Intestinal biopsies are either normal or show mild villous atrophy without significant inflammation.[29] In the author's experience with 1 such case, small bowel biopsies showed mild nonspecific changes with retained staining for chromogranin. Only the use of antibody against PC1/3 showed loss of staining.[29] The diagnosis

Fig. 1. (*continued*). (*D*) By electron microscopy, the duodenal surface is characterized by absent or short stubby microvilli and numerous periapical vacuoles in the enterocyte, some of which contain microvilli.

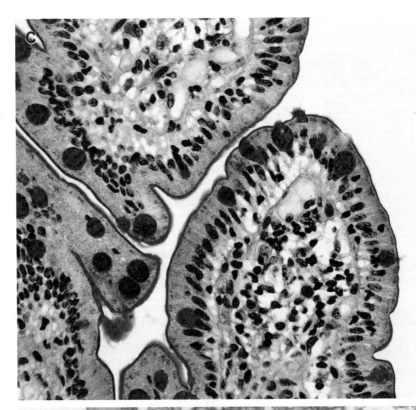

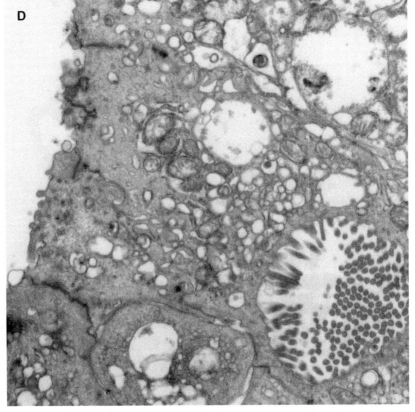

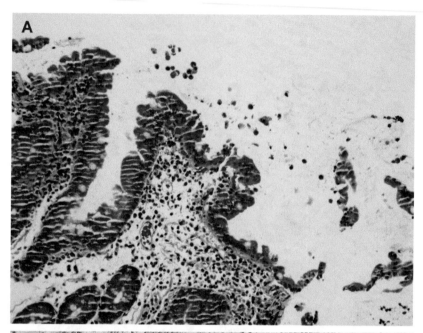

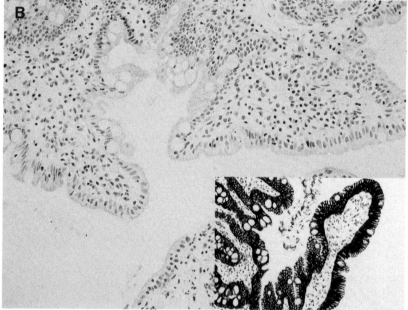

Fig. 2. Tufting enteropathy. (A) The duodenal surface epithelium forms tufts, with shedding of rounded oval-shaped enterocytes (hematoxylin-eosin, original magnification ×200). (B) Immunostaining with an antibody to EpCAM (MOC 31) in a patient with an *EPCAM* mutation shows loss of staining (inset, normal control) [hematoxylin-eosin, original magnification ×200].

is suspected clinically by the combination of malabsorption with endocrinopathies.

X-linked lissencephaly with abnormal genitalia (chromosome Xp21.3; OMIM #3002125) is a rare disorder characterized by lissencephaly, agenesis of the corpus callosum, hypothalamic dysfunction, chronic diarrhea, hypothyroidism, and pancreatic insufficiency.[30] The chronic diarrhea is a major issue in the management of these patients. Intestinal biopsies are essentially normal by H&E, and

chromogranin-staining cells are preserved. More specific hormonal immunostaining reveals a severe decrease in cholecystokinin- and glucose-dependent insulinotropic peptide 1-containing cells.[31]

TRICHO-HEPATO-ENTERIC SYNDROME

Girault and colleagues[32] described a group of patients with dysmorphic features, consisting of

Fig. 3. Enteric anendocrinosis due to *NEUROGEN 3* mutation. (*A*) Partial villous atrophy and mild inflammatory changes (hematoxylin-eosin, original magnification ×200). (*B*) Absence of enteroendocrine cells using chromogranin immunostain (hematoxylin-eosin, original magnification ×200). (*C*) Chromogranin staining in a normal duodenum (hematoxylin-eosin, original magnification ×200).

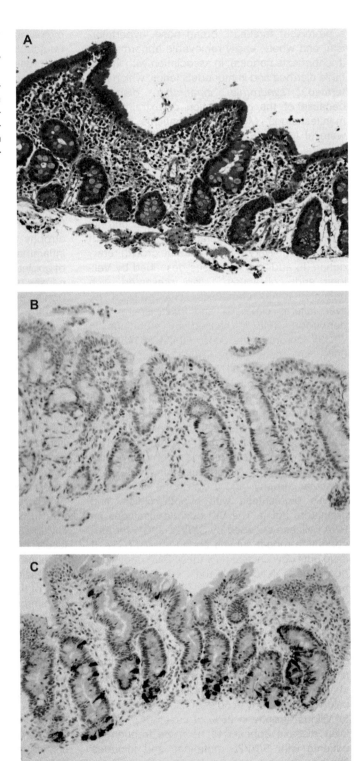

a prominent forehead, broad nose, hypertelorism, and wooly, easily removable abnormal hair (trichorrhexis nodosa), in association with intractable diarrhea and immunodeficiency, which they termed *"syndromic intractable diarrhea,"* because of the constellation of extraintestinal manifestations. Most of the patients reported were of Middle Eastern origin, and there were parental consanguinity and a history of similarly affected siblings. Infants with similar clinical features had been previously reported as the tricho-hepato-enteric syndrome (THE),[33,34] in which hair abnormalities (trichorrhexis nodosa) are seen in association with hypertelorism, chronic diarrhea, and immune defects, and a history of premature delivery with intrauterine growth retardation. In addition, the cases described by Verloes and colleagues[34] also presented with neonatal hemochromatosis, characterized by liver failure, cirrhosis, and multivisceral iron deposition. THE is caused by mutations in *TTC37* (chromosome 5q15; OMIM #614589) in 60% of cases and *SKIV2L* (chromosome 6p21.33; OMIM #600478) in 40% of cases.[35,36] Each gene encodes different subunits of the SKI complex, a highly conserved tetraprotein complex required for exosome-mediated RNA surveillance and essential for cell viability.[35] Other diseases associated with mutations in exosome core proteins include a pontocerebellar hypoplasia with hypomyelination, a spinal muscular atrophy, and a syndrome associating retinitis pigmentosa with hypothyroidism and premature aging. The SKI complex includes an RNA helicase encoded by *SKIV2L* and a tetratricopeptide repeat subunit encoded by *TTC37*. It is up until now unclear how these RNA decay abnormalities lead to the various clinical manifestations.

Intractable diarrhea, hair abnormalities, and facial dysmorphism, characterized by a prominent forehead with a broad nasal root and hypertelorism, are nearly constant clinical features in patients with either mutations (**Fig. 4**A). Histopathology of the small bowel shows normal mucosa in about 25% of cases, mild villous atrophy in 50% of cases, and subtotal villous atrophy in 25% of cases (**Fig. 4**B).[37] Liver disease appears to be more frequent in patients with *SKIV2L* mutations and includes fibrosis, cirrhosis, iron overload, and sometimes hemochromatosis. An initial cholestatic picture has also been reported.[36] The immunodeficiency is not well characterized and is reportedly dominated by low immunoglobulins and poor response to immunization along with platelet abnormalities. Clinical management mainly involves parenteral nutrition and immunoglobulin supplementation. Steroids, immunosuppression, and hematopoietic stem cell transplantation have so far no proven efficacy in this disorder.[38]

DISORDERS OF IMMUNOMODULATION

AUTOIMMUNE ENTEROPATHY

AIE is the most frequent disorder leading to infantile intractable diarrhea. The main diagnostic criteria are severe protracted diarrhea, intestinal biopsy changes generally characterized by villous atrophy with a usually marked crypt-destructive inflammation, often with a decrease or absence of goblet and Paneth cells, and exclusion of other causes of villus atrophy. Circulating gut autoantibodies are a useful but not necessary diagnostic feature. Most cases occur in infancy or the first year of life, although this entity has also been reported in older children, in girls, and even in adults, in whom it may be responsible for a proportion of cases referred to as "refractory sprue." Thus, several clinical types exist and include pediatric and adult forms.[39] Pediatric forms can be subdivided into IPEX, IPEX-like, and secondary forms, such as those associated with a primary immunodeficiency. The most commonly recognized form is the X-linked syndrome of immunodysregulation, polyendocrinopathy, and enteropathy (IPEX syndrome) initially described by Powell and colleagues.[40] This syndrome is due to mutations in the *FOXP3* gene (Xp11.23; OMIM #304790). These mutations result in lower levels of $CD4^+CD25^+$ regulatory T cells with absence or very low levels of FOXP3 protein expression, with consequent impaired suppression of the inflammatory response and extensive autoimmune manifestations.[41] Approximately 50% of patients with otherwise typical manifestations of AIE, including female patients, have no detectable mutations in *FOXP3*, and have been designated IPEX-like. These patients have been found to harbor mutations in a variety of immune regulatory genes, including *STAT5b*, *STAT1*, *CTLA4*, *LRBA*, and others. In some of these patients, the percentage of $CD4^+$ $FOXP3^+$ cells was normal, whereas CD25 expression was absent, suggesting preservation of Treg quantity but abnormal function.[41] There is extensive overlap in the clinical manifestations of IPEX and IPEX-like patients, the most frequent being enteropathy characterized by watery diarrhea, usually starting in the first year of life in IPEX patients, typically a little later in the IPEX-like group. Eczema, exfoliative dermatitis, and autoimmune

Fig. 4. THE syndrome. (*A*) Abnormal hair. Trichorrhexis nodosa of the hair shafts observed on whole mount sections. (*B*) Duodenal biopsy with mild to moderate villous atrophy with crypt hyperplasia (hematoxylin-eosin, original magnification ×100).

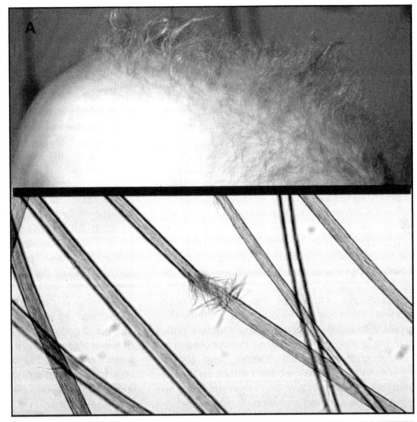

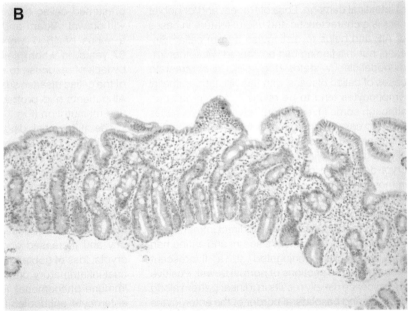

endocrinopathies, most commonly type 1 diabetes, are also common to both groups. Other manifestations include anemia, neutropenia, glomerulonephritis, interstitial nephritis, autoimmune hepatitis, and cardiopulmonary disease, seen in various proportions in patients with different mutated genes.[41] Mortality in earlier reported cases of IPEX has been high. A combination of immunosuppressants has been used in most cases, including steroids, calcineurin inhibitors, and rapamycin, resulting in an overall survival of 65%, whereas hematopoietic stem cell transplantation in selected patients has resulted in similar survival with better disease resolution.[42] Immunosuppression has been used in adults with AIE.[43]

The entire GI tract is often involved in AIE, and the histopathologic findings in duodenal and small bowel biopsies are usually characterized by severe villus atrophy, crypt hyperplasia, and a mixed inflammatory infiltrate of the lamina propria. Marked inflammatory destruction of intestinal crypts with extensive apoptosis is a feature noted in many of the cases, similar to those noted in intestinal graft-versus-host disease, and confirm an abnormal immune-mediated attack against intestinal epithelium[44] (Fig. 5A). However, there appears to be marked variation in the histologic features, with some cases showing milder degrees of intestinal damage. Loss of Paneth and/or goblet cells is a characteristic and useful feature in cases of AIE and helps to distinguish it from celiac disease, but this finding can be shared with other immunodeficiency states (Fig. 5B). In contrast to cases of celiac disease with flat villi, intraepithelial lymphocytes tend to be relatively few in number, although some investigators have reported cases with increased intraepithelial lymphocytes, indistinguishable from celiac disease except for a usually negative celiac serology.[45] A concomitant crypt-destructive colitis and gastritis are present in most cases.

One of the hallmarks of this entity, noted since the first reports of AIE, is the presence of antienterocyte antibodies, detected by indirect immunofluorescence using the patient's serum and antihuman immunoglobulins conjugated to a fluorescent probe on frozen sections of normal bowel. Positive fluorescence usually results in a linear pattern along the apex and basolateral border of the enterocytes (Fig. 5C). The antibodies are predominantly immunoglobulin G (IgG) and have been described as complement fixing,[46] although IgM and IgA have also been described. Antibodies reacting against mucus or goblet cells have also been described, and intestinal biopsies in these cases have shown a marked depletion of goblet cells.[47,48]

The target of the anti–enterocyte antibodies is still a matter of investigation, although a 75- kDa antigen reactive with autoantibody in the sera of patients with the IPEX syndrome has been reported.[49] This protein is expressed in the epithelial cells of the small bowel, colon, and kidney and may play a role in protein-protein interactions in the enterocyte. A 95-kDa antigen identified as villin has also been reported in IPEX patients,[50] and more than 1 antigen is likely involved.

However, the role of these antibodies in the pathogenesis of AIE is debatable because they may represent an epiphenomenon without playing a causative role in mucosal damage. Similar anti–enterocyte antibodies have also been described in adult AIDS patients without digestive symptoms.[51] The specificity of anti–goblet cell antibodies has also been questioned. Anti–goblet cell antibodies have been detected in patients with chronic IBD (Crohn and ulcerative colitis) and their first-degree relatives,[52] and in a series of treated and untreated patients with celiac disease and controls.[53] Furthermore, the usefulness of these antibodies in the diagnosis of AIE in young infants is also probably limited, given that there is little IgG production in the first 3 months of life and that IgG detected in the infant is likely maternal in origin.

In adults, the clinical picture is usually that of presumed celiac disease unresponsive to gluten withdrawal. Akram and colleagues[43] reported on a series of 15 (7 women) patients, aged 42 to 67 years, in whom celiac disease was excluded by lack of response to gluten-free diet or absence of the celiac disease susceptibility HLA genotypes. All patients had protracted diarrhea, weight loss, and malnutrition (Fig. 5D).

The differential diagnosis of AIE includes, in addition to celiac disease and graft-versus-host disease, enterocolitis associated with various immunodeficiency states, in whom histologic features of AIE with circulating autoantibodies may be observed.[54] A high index of suspicion for AIE should be present when there is a severe inflammatory crypt destructive process with villous atrophy and increased apoptosis in the base of the crypts, loss of goblet and Paneth cells, or an intestinal inflammatory process in a patient with autoimmune phenomena. Testing for circulating anti–enterocyte antibodies is useful in the older child and adult but may be of more use limited in the young infant.

AUTOIMMUNE POLYENDOCRINE SYNDROME

APSs include APSs type 1 (APS-1) and type 2 (APS-2), and a third rarer type characterized by

Fig. 5. AIE. (*A*) Duodenal biopsy from a patient with IPEX is characterized by villous atrophy, inflammation, and crypt apoptosis (hematoxylin-eosin, original magnification ×200). (*B*) Duodenal biopsy from an 18-year-old woman with AIE and other autoimmune manifestations shows a some villous atrophy, crypt hyperplasia, mildly increased intraepithelial lymphocytes. Note, however, the total absence of goblet and Paneth cells (hematoxylin-eosin, original magnification ×100).

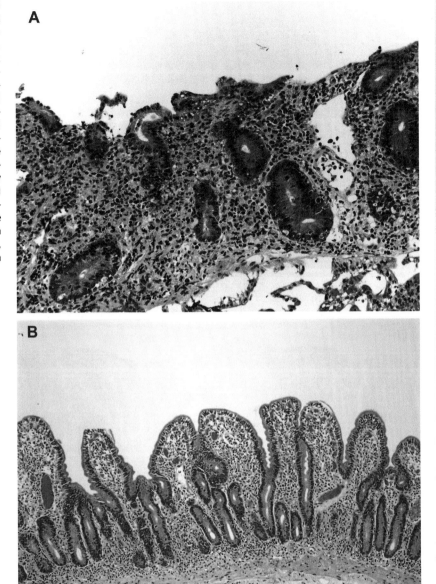

mucocutaneous candidiasis, hypothyroidism, and autoimmune hepatitis caused by mutations in *STAT-1*. APS-2 (OMIM #269200) affects older patients, predominantly women, is associated with HLA-DR 3/4, and is characterized by a triad of major endocrinopathies: type1 diabetes, autoimmune thyroiditis, and Addison disease. GI manifestations include celiac disease and autoimmune gastritis.[55] APS-1, also known as APECED, is an autosomal recessive disorder caused by mutations in the

AutoImmune REgulator gene (*AIRE*, chromosome 21q22.3; OMIM #240300). AIRE is a transcriptional regulator expressed by stromal cells in immune organs. In the thymus, AIRE induces expression peripheral tissue self-antigens and promotes deletion of autoreactive T cells, preventing spontaneous autoimmunity. The clinical diagnosis is defined by the expression of at least two of the classic triad: chronic mucocutaneous candidiasis, chronic hypoparathyroidism, and Addison disease. Other

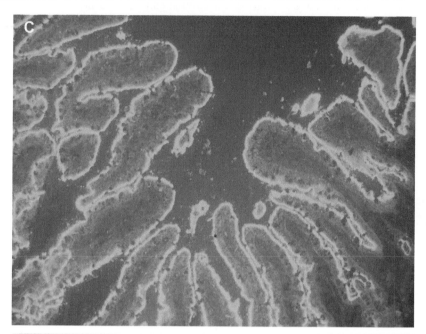

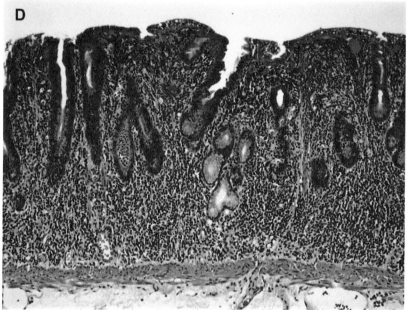

Fig. 5. (*continued*). (*C*) Indirect immunofluorescence using the patient's serum shows diffuse linear staining along the surface of the enterocytes on frozen sections of control duodenum (IF x100). (*D*) Duodenal biopsy from a 36-year-old man initially diagnosed as celiac disease. There is extensive crypt shortening and absence of goblet and Paneth cells (hematoxylin-eosin, original magnification ×200).

manifestations include hypergonadotropic hypogonadism, alopecia, vitiligo, and autoimmune hepatitis. APECED usually manifests before age 5, most typically mucocutaneous candidiasis. Autoimmune gastritis is the most common GI manifestation, resulting in vitamin B12 deficiency (Fig. 6A). Intestinal disease usually manifests with chronic diarrhea and malabsorption consequent to destruction of enteroendocrine cells (Fig. 6B); some patients may present with an AIE associated with circulating anti–enterocyte antibodies (Fig. 6C). Other GI manifestations include celiac disease and lymphangiectasia. Diarrhea may also result from hypocalcemia because of chronic hypoparathyroidism. Autoimmune hepatitis may be asymptomatic or fulminant. Periodic evaluation of liver enzymes is recommended.[56] Salient clinicopathologic features of congenital enteropathies are presented in Table 1.

Fig. 6. APS. (*A*) Chronic gastritis (hematoxylin-eosin, original magnification ×200). (*B*) Absence of enteroendocrine cells in the duodenum with chromogranin immunostain (original magnification ×100). (*C*) Anti–enterocyte antibodies demonstrated in patient serum by indirect immunofluorescence (IF x100).

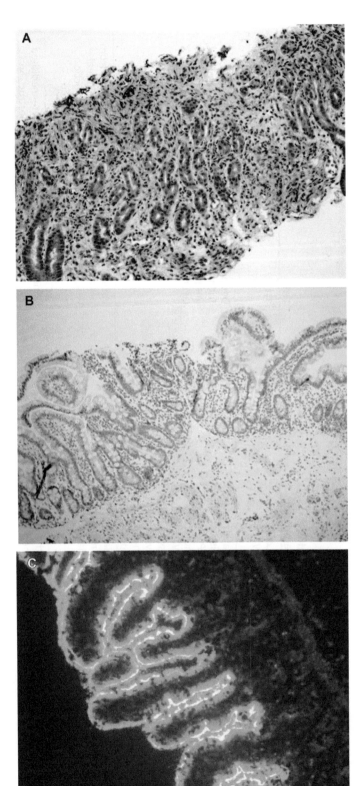

Table 1
Clinicopathologic features of pediatric enteropathies

	MVID	Tufting Enteropathy	Enteroendocrine Dysgenesis	THE	Autoimmune Enteropathy
Genetics	*MYO5B* *STX3* *STXB2*	*EPCAM* *SPINT2*	*NEUROG3*	*TTC37*	*FOXP3* *STAT1, 5B* *CTLA4*
Accompanying disease	Low GGT cholestasis Renal Fanconi hypophosphatemia	Isolated GI disease with *EPCAM* mutations *SPINT2* mutations associated with dysmorphism, choanal and intestinal atresia	Insulin-dependent diabetes	Dysmorphism Trichorrhexis nodosa Immune defects Liver disease	Dermatitis, diabetes, thyroiditis, nephritis, neutropenia
Biopsy features Villous architecture Crypts Lamina propria Inflammation	Atrophy Normal/hyperplastic Minimal	Variable atrophy Normal/hyperplastic Variable	Variable atrophy Normal Variable, usually mild	Variable atrophy Variable Variable, usually mild	Variable atrophy, from severe to minimal Variable destruction Usually marked
Diagnostic histopathologic features	Loss of brush border with apical vacuolization	Epithelial tufts, shedding of epithelial cells Absent MOC31 by IHC in *EPCAM* mutations	Absence of enteroendocrine cells with chromogranin stain	None	Lymphocyte-mediated crypt destruction Crypt apoptotic bodies (variable) Anti–gut autoantibodies
Electron microscopy	Microvillus inclusion vacuoles	Not significant	Not significant	Not significant	Not significant

VERY-EARLY-ONSET INFLAMMATORY BOWEL DISEASE

A diagnosis of IBD is established before 6 years of age in about 15% of pediatric patients, with up to 6% diagnosed at less than 3 years of age. For reasons that are unclear, a marked increase in the occurrence of IBD has occurred in this age group in recent decades.[57] This subgroup of IBD patients, referred to as "very-early-onset inflammatory bowel disease," presents significant differences from IBD occurring in older children and in adults, including more severe clinical disease unresponsive to conventional IBD therapy and a greater proportion of cases featuring an underlying monogenic disorder. Individuals with monogenic disorders may have features not typically associated with IBD, such as nail and hair anomalies, epidermolysis bullosa, and autoimmune hemolytic anemia.[58] They may develop significant problems, such as immunodeficiency, impacting treatment options, and a greater potential for receiving escalated treatment regimens involving extensive surgery and more intensive medical therapies.[58] There is significant overlap with known primary immunodeficiencies, as it is well known that patients with common variable immunodeficiency (CVID), Wiskott-Aldrich syndrome (WAS), and chronic granulomatous disease may present with VEO-IBD.[59,60]

The landmark discovery of mutations involving the anti-inflammatory interleukin-10 (IL-10) cytokine and its receptors IL-10RA and IL10RB, resulting in severe infantile enterocolitis and perianal disease, was the first to demonstrate causal genetic defects in patients with VEO-IBD.[61] The essential role for IL-10 in limiting intestinal inflammation had already been demonstrated by the spontaneous development of severe colitis in IL-10–deficient mice.[62]

Recent advances in molecular technology, such as WES, have allowed the discovery of more than 50 genes and pathways associated with VEO-IBD. These genes are for the most part different from the genetic variants found in genome-wide association studies of IBD in older children and adults.[63] The defects that are associated with VEO-IBD include genes involved in the intestinal epithelial barrier function, phagocyte bacterial killing, T-cell regulation, hyper or autoimmune inflammatory disorders, and function of the adaptive immune system; a partial listing is provided in Box 1 (for a more extensive listing see Table 1 in the review article by Conrad and Kelsen[64]).

Genetic variants associated with dysfunction of the intestinal epithelial barrier can result in severe enteropathy. Mutations in the gene tetratricopeptide repeat domain-7A (TTC7A, chromosome 2p21; OMIM #609332) leads to several phenotypes, including hereditary multiple intestinal atresia syndrome, a disorder initially described in French-Canadian kindreds, as well as different forms of combined immunodeficiency and infantile onset IBD. Histologic findings in the intestines in patients with truncating mutations include complete multifocal atresias found anywhere from the pylorus to the rectum, with a sievelike lumen caused by multiple adhesions and luminal calcifications (Fig. 7).[65] Patients also have a hypoplastic thymus with a paucity of CD4$^+$ and CD8$^+$ T cells and, possibly, early-onset liver disease. TTC7A is expressed by intestinal epithelial cells and localizes at the plasma membrane, where it is responsible for epithelial integrity. It also appears to regulate the cytoskeleton of lymphocytes. Missense mutations are thought to result in hypomorphic variants with a monogenic VEO-IBD rather than intestinal atresias.[66] Patients with truncating mutations and multiple atresias have a high mortality, whereas surviving patients tend to have IBD; no standard of care has been established as of yet in this disorder. Other examples of defects involving epithelial barrier function include mutations in ADAM 17 (which results in impaired release of TNF-α) associating malabsorptive diarrhea with skin and hair abnormalities.[67] Mutations in IKBKG (which encodes NEMO) result in X-linked ectodermal dysplasia and immunodeficiency.[68]

Many defects in adaptive immunity have been associated with severe combined immune deficiency (SCID) and can occur with loss-of-function mutations in recombination activating genes (RAG1 or RAG2), IL-7 receptor (IL7R) causing Omenn syndrome, and the PTEN gene.

Several autoimmune/autoinflammatory diseases have been associated with VEO-IBD, including mutations. These include mutations in NLRC4, the Hermansky-Pudlak syndrome, and X-linked lymphoproliferative syndrome (XIAP). Activating mutations in NLRC4 cause an uncontrolled activation of the inflammasome complex, resulting in hemophagocytic lymphohistiocytosis and a severe panenteritis with increased levels of IL-1 and IL-18, manifesting as early as several months of age (Fig. 8). Loss-of-function mutations of the X-linked inhibitor of apoptosis (XIAP), which regulates NOD2-mediated NF-kB signaling, results in an impaired ability to sense pathogens. In addition, impaired apoptosis results in uncontrolled expansion of T cells, resulting in a hyperinflammatory state because of both the inability to clear pathogens and survival of T cells with excess production of cytokines.

Box 1
Monogenic disorders associated with inflammatory bowel disease-like pathology

Epithelial barrier defects

- Dystrophic Epidermolysis bullosa (EB)

- Kindler syndrome

- X-linked ectodermal dysplasia

- ADAM 17 deficiency

- Familial diarrhea

- Hereditary multiple intestinal atresia (*TTC7A*)

Neutropenia and phagocyte defects

- Chronic granulomatous disease (CGD)

- Glycogen storage disease (GSD) type 1

- Congenital neutropenia

- Leukocyte adhesion deficiency

Hyper and autoinflammatory disorders

- Mevalonate kinase deficiency

- Phospholipase C2 defects

- Familial Mediterranean fever

- Familial macrophage activation syndrome

- X-linked lymphoproliferative syndrome

- Hermansky-Pudlak syndrome

- *NLRC4* gain-of-function mutations

Complex defects in T- and B-cell function (WAS, CVID, SCID)

Defects in regulatory T cells and IL-10 signaling

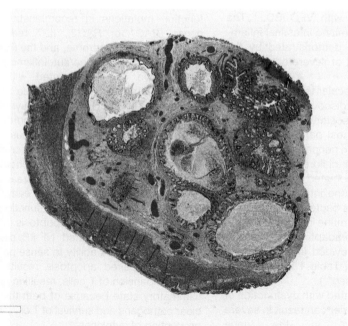

Fig. 7. Hereditary multiple intestinal atresia (*TTC7A* deficiency). Cross-section of the intestinal lumen in a constricted area reveals multiple lumina forming a "sieve-like" arrangement (hematoxylin-eosin, original magnification ×40).

Fig. 8. VEO-IBD with activation mutation in *NLRC4*. (*A*) The duodenal biopsy is characterized by villous atrophy with extensive inflammatory crypt destruction (hematoxylin-eosin, original magnification ×100). (*B*) Marked active chronic colitis is also noted (hematoxylin-eosin, original magnification ×100). (*C*) Mucosal eosinophilia with eosinophil microabscesses (hematoxylin-eosin, original magnification ×400).

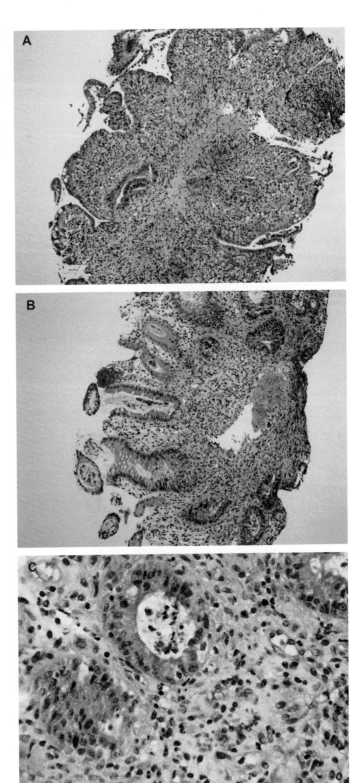

As conventional therapy for IBD is largely ineffective in these children, treatment depends on establishment of the proper diagnosis using either VEO-IBD–specific gene panels or WES, and the application of more targeted therapies. Other than age of onset and associated clinical manifestations, histologic features that are observed more frequently in VEO-IBD as compared with older-onset IBD include increased crypt apoptosis, involvement of the small bowel with villous blunting, and mucosal eosinophils, in association with more crypt and mucosal abnormalities than would be expected for an allergic cause.[69]

REFERENCES

1. Davidson GP, Cutz E, Hamilton JR, et al. Familial enteropathy: a syndrome of protracted diarrhea from birth, failure to thrive, and hypoplastic villus atrophy. Gastroenterology 1978;75(5):783–90.
2. van der Velde KJ, Dhekne HS, Swertz MA, et al. An overview and online registry of microvillus inclusion disease patients and their MYO5B mutations. Hum Mutat 2013;34(12):1597–605.
3. Jin Y, Sultana A, Gandhi P, et al. Myosin V transports secretory vesicles via a Rab GTPase cascade and interaction with the exocyst complex. Dev Cell 2011;21(6):1156–70.
4. Gonzales E, Taylor SA, Davit-Spraul A, et al. MYO5B mutations cause cholestasis with normal serum gamma-glutamyl transferase activity in children without microvillous inclusion disease. Hepatology 2017;65(1):164–73.
5. Schlegel C, Weis VG, Knowles BC, et al. Apical membrane alterations in non-intestinal organs in microvillus inclusion disease. Dig Dis Sci 2018; 63(2):356–65.
6. Wiegerinck CL, Janecke AR, Schneeberger K, et al. Loss of syntaxin 3 causes variant microvillus inclusion disease. Gastroenterology 2014;147(1):65–8.e10.
7. Alsaleem BMR, Ahmed ABM, Fageeh MA. Microvillus inclusion disease variant in an infant with intractable diarrhea. Case Rep Gastroenterol 2017; 11(3):647–51.
8. Stepensky P, Bartram J, Barth TF, et al. Persistent defective membrane trafficking in epithelial cells of patients with familial hemophagocytic lymphohistiocytosis type 5 due to STXBP2/MUNC18-2 mutations. Pediatr Blood Cancer 2013;60(7): 1215–22.
9. Shillingford NM, Calicchio ML, Teot LA, et al. Villin immunohistochemistry is a reliable method for diagnosing microvillus inclusion disease. Am J Surg Pathol 2015;39(2):245–50.
10. Talmon G, Holzapfel M, DiMaio DJ, et al. Rab11 is a useful tool for the diagnosis of microvillous inclusion disease. Int J Surg Pathol 2011;20(3):252.
11. Cutz E, Sherman PM, Davidson GP. Enteropathies associated with protracted diarrhea of infancy: clinicopathological features, cellular and molecular mechanisms. Pediatr Pathol Lab Med 1997;17(3):335–68.
12. Iancu TC, Mahajnah M, Manov I, et al. The liver in congenital disorders of glycosylation: ultrastructural features. Ultrastruct Pathol 2007;31(3):189–97.
13. Halac U, Lacaille F, Joly F, et al. Microvillous inclusion disease: how to improve the prognosis of a severe congenital enterocyte disorder. J Pediatr Gastroenterol Nutr 2011;52(4):460–5.
14. Reifen RM, Cutz E, Griffiths AM, et al. Tufting enteropathy: a newly recognized clinicopathological entity associated with refractory diarrhea in infants. J Pediatr Gastroenterol Nutr 1994;18(3):379–85.
15. Sivagnanam M, Mueller JL, Lee H, et al. Identification of EpCAM as the gene for congenital tufting enteropathy. Gastroenterology 2008;135(2):429–37.
16. Carpenter G, Red Brewer M. EpCAM: another surface-to-nucleus missile. Cancer Cell 2009;15(3): 165–6.
17. Red Brewer SJ, Mueller JL, Okamoto K, et al. EPCAM mutation update: variants associated with congenital tufting enteropathy and Lynch syndrome. Hum Mutat 2019;40(2):142–61.
18. Salomon J, Goulet O, Canioni D, et al. Genetic characterization of congenital tufting enteropathy: epcam associated phenotype and involvement of SPINT2 in the syndromic form. Hum Genet 2014; 133(3):299–310.
19. Holt-Danborg L, Vodopiutz J, Nonboe AW, et al. SPINT2 (HAI-2) missense variants identified in congenital sodium diarrhea/tufting enteropathy affect the ability of HAI-2 to inhibit prostasin but not matriptase. Hum Mol Genet 2019;28(5):828–41.
20. Ranganathan S, Schmitt LA, Sindhi R. Tufting enteropathy revisited: the utility of MOC31 (EpCAM) immunohistochemistry in diagnosis. Am J Surg Pathol 2014;38(2):265–72.
21. Lemale J, Coulomb A, Dubern B, et al. Intractable diarrhea with tufting enteropathy: a favorable outcome is possible. J Pediatr Gastroenterol Nutr 2011;52(6):734–9.
22. Wang J, Cortina G, Wu SV, et al. Mutant neurogenin-3 in congenital malabsorptive diarrhea. N Engl J Med 2006;355(3):270–80.
23. Pinney SE, Oliver-Krasinski J, Ernst L, et al. Neonatal diabetes and congenital malabsorptive diarrhea attributable to a novel mutation in the human neurogenin-3 gene coding sequence. J Clin Endocrinol Metab 2011;96(7):1960–5.
24. Bjerknes M, Cheng H. Neurogenin 3 and the enteroendocrine cell lineage in the adult mouse small intestinal epithelium. Dev Biol 2006;300(2):722–35.
25. Posovszky C, Lahr G, von Schnurbein J, et al. Loss of enteroendocrine cells in autoimmune-polyendocrine-candidiasis-ectodermal-dystrophy

(APECED) syndrome with gastrointestinal dysfunction. J Clin Endocrinol Metab 2012;97(2):E292–300.

26. Hogenauer C, Meyer RL, Netto GJ, et al. Malabsorption due to cholecystokinin deficiency in a patient with autoimmune polyglandular syndrome type I. N Engl J Med 2001;344(4):270–4.

27. Stijnen P, Ramos-Molina B, O'Rahilly S, et al. PCSK1 mutations and human endocrinopathies: from obesity to gastrointestinal disorders. Endocr Rev 2016;37(4):347–71.

28. Martin MG, Lindberg I, Solorzano-Vargas RS, et al. Congenital proprotein convertase 1/3 deficiency causes malabsorptive diarrhea and other endocrinopathies in a pediatric cohort. Gastroenterology 2013;145(1):138–48.

29. Bandsma RH, Sokollik C, Chami R, et al. From diarrhea to obesity in prohormone convertase 1/3 deficiency: age-dependent clinical, pathologic, and enteroendocrine characteristics. J Clin Gastroenterol 2013;47(10):834–43.

30. Coman D, Fullston T, Shoubridge C, et al. X-linked lissencephaly with absent corpus callosum and abnormal genitalia: an evolving multisystem syndrome with severe congenital intestinal diarrhea disease. Child Neurol Open 2017;4, 2329048X17738625.

31. Terry NA, Lee RA, Walp ER, et al. Dysgenesis of enteroendocrine cells in Aristaless-Related Homeobox polyalanine expansion mutations. J Pediatr Gastroenterol Nutr 2015;60(2):192–9.

32. Girault D, Goulet O, Le Deist F, et al. Intractable infant diarrhea associated with phenotypic abnormalities and immunodeficiency. J Pediatr 1994;125(1):36–42.

33. Stankler L, Lloyd D, Pollitt RJ, et al. Unexplained diarrhoea and failure to thrive in 2 siblings with unusual facies and abnormal scalp hair shafts: a new syndrome. Arch Dis Child 1982;57(3):212–6.

34. Verloes A, Lombet J, Lambert Y, et al. Tricho-hepato-enteric syndrome: further delineation of a distinct syndrome with neonatal hemochromatosis phenotype, intractable diarrhea, and hair anomalies. Am J Med Genet 1997;68(4):391–5.

35. Fabre A, Martinez-Vinson C, Roquelaure B, et al. Novel mutations in TTC37 associated with tricho-hepato-enteric syndrome. Hum Mutat 2011;32(3):277–81.

36. Bourgeois P, Esteve C, Chaix C, et al. Tricho-hepato-enteric syndrome mutation update: mutations spectrum of TTC37 and SKIV2L, clinical analysis and future prospects. Hum Mutat 2018;39(6):774–89.

37. Fabre A, Breton A, Coste ME, et al. Syndromic (phenotypic) diarrhoea of infancy/tricho-hepato-enteric syndrome. Arch Dis Child 2014;99(1):35–8.

38. Fabre A, Bourgeois P, Coste ME, et al. Management of syndromic diarrhea/tricho-hepato-enteric

syndrome: a review of the literature. Intractable Rare Dis Res 2017;6(3):152–7.

39. Umetsu SE, Brown I, Langner C, et al. Autoimmune enteropathies. Virchows Arch 2018;472(1):55–66.

40. Powell BR, Buist NR, Stenzel P. An X-linked syndrome of diarrhea, polyendocrinopathy, and fatal infection in infancy. J Pediatr 1982;100(5):731–7.

41. Gambineri E, Ciullini Mannurita S, Hagin D, et al. Clinical, immunological, and molecular heterogeneity of 173 patients with the phenotype of immune dysregulation, polyendocrinopathy, enteropathy, X-linked (IPEX) syndrome. Front Immunol 2018;9:2411.

42. Barzaghi F, Amaya Hernandez LC, Neven B, et al. Long-term follow-up of IPEX syndrome patients after different therapeutic strategies: an international multicenter retrospective study. J Allergy Clin Immunol 2018;141(3):1036–1049 e5.

43. Akram S, Murray JA, Pardi DS, et al. Adult autoimmune enteropathy: Mayo Clinic Rochester experience. Clin Gastroenterol Hepatol 2007;5(11):1282–90, [quiz: 1245].

44. Patey-Mariaud de Serre N, Canioni D, Ganousse S, et al. Digestive histopathological presentation of IPEX syndrome. Mod Pathol 2009;22(1):95–102.

45. Masia R, Peyton S, Lauwers GY, et al. Gastrointestinal biopsy findings of autoimmune enteropathy: a review of 25 cases. Am J Surg Pathol 2014;38(10):1319–29.

46. Mirakian R, Richardson A, Milla PJ, et al. Protracted diarrhoea of infancy: evidence in support of an autoimmune variant. Br Med J (Clin Res Ed) 1986;293(6555):1132–6.

47. Moore L, Xu X, Davidson G, et al. Autoimmune enteropathy with anti-goblet cell antibodies. Hum Pathol 1995;26(10):1162–8.

48. Rogahn D, Smith CP, Thomas A. Autoimmune enteropathy with goblet-cell antibodies. J R Soc Med 1999;92(6):311–2.

49. Kobayashi I, Imamura K, Yamada M, et al. A 75-kD autoantigen recognized by sera from patients with X-linked autoimmune enteropathy associated with nephropathy. Clin Exp Immunol 1998;111(3):527–31.

50. Kobayashi I, Kubota M, Yamada M, et al. Autoantibodies to villin occur frequently in IPEX, a severe immune dysregulation, syndrome caused by mutation of FOXP3. Clin Immunol 2011;141(1):83.

51. Martin-Villa JM, Camblor S, Costa R, et al. Gut epithelial cell autoantibodies in AIDS pathogenesis. Lancet 1993;342(8867):380.

52. Folwaczny C, Noehl N, Tschöp K, et al. Goblet cell autoantibodies in patients with inflammatory bowel disease and their first-degree relatives. Gastroenterology 1997;113(1):101–6.

53. Biagi F, Bianchi PI, Trotta L, et al. Anti-goblet cell antibodies for the diagnosis of autoimmune enteropathy? Am J Gastroenterol 2009;104(12):3112.

54. Singhi AD, Goyal A, Davison JM, et al. Pediatric autoimmune enteropathy: an entity frequently associated with immunodeficiency disorders. Mod Pathol 2014;27(4):543–53.

55. Husebye ES, Anderson MS, Kampe O. Autoimmune polyendocrine syndromes. N Engl J Med 2018; 378(26):2543–4.

56. Capalbo D, Improda N, Esposito A, et al. Autoimmune polyendocrinopathy-candidiasis-ectodermal dystrophy from the pediatric perspective. J Endocrinol Invest 2013;36(10):903–12.

57. Benchimol EI, Manuel DG, Guttmann A, et al. Changing age demographics of inflammatory bowel disease in Ontario, Canada: a population-based cohort study of epidemiology trends. Inflamm Bowel Dis 2014;20(10):1761–9.

58. Ashton JJ, Andreoletti G, Coelho T, et al. Identification of variants in genes associated with single-gene inflammatory bowel disease by whole-exome sequencing. Inflamm Bowel Dis 2016;22(10): 2317–27.

59. Glocker E, Grimbacher B. Inflammatory bowel disease: is it a primary immunodeficiency? Cell Mol Life Sci 2012;69(1):41–8.

60. Cannioto Z, Berti I, Martelossi S, et al. IBD and IBD mimicking enterocolitis in children younger than 2 years of age. Eur J Pediatr 2009;168(2): 149–55.

61. Glocker EO, Kotlarz D, Boztug K, et al. Inflammatory bowel disease and mutations affecting the interleukin-10 receptor. N Engl J Med 2009; 361(21):2033–45.

62. Kuhn R, Löhler J, Rennick D, et al. Interleukin-10-deficient mice develop chronic enterocolitis. Cell 1993;75(2):263–74.

63. Jostins L, Ripke S, Weersma RK, et al. Host-microbe interactions have shaped the genetic architecture of inflammatory bowel disease. Nature 2012; 491(7422):119–24.

64. Conrad MA, Kelsen JR. Genomic and immunologic drivers of very early-onset inflammatory bowel disease. Pediatr Dev Pathol 2019;22(3):183–93.

65. Fernandez I, Patey N, Marchand V, et al. Multiple intestinal atresia with combined immune deficiency related to TTC7A defect is a multiorgan pathology: study of a French-Canadian-based cohort. Medicine (Baltimore) 2014;93(29):e327.

66. Jardine S, Dhingani N, Muise AM. TTC7A: steward of intestinal health. Cell Mol Gastroenterol Hepatol 2019;7(3):555–70.

67. Blaydon DC, Biancheri P, Di WL, et al. Inflammatory skin and bowel disease linked to ADAM17 deletion. N Engl J Med 2011;365(16):1502–8.

68. Karamchandani-Patel G, Hanson EP, Saltzman R, et al. Congenital alterations of NEMO glutamic acid 223 result in hypohidrotic ectodermal dysplasia and immunodeficiency with normal serum IgG levels. Ann Allergy Asthma Immunol 2011;107(1): 50–6.

69. Conrad MA, Carreon CK, Dawany N, et al. Distinct histopathological features at diagnosis of very early onset inflammatory bowel disease. J Crohns Colitis 2019;13(5):615–25.

Pediatric Liver Tumors
Updates in Classification

Soo-Jin Cho, MD, PhD

KEYWORDS

- Hepatoblastoma • Hepatocellular neoplasm • NOS • Hepatocellular carcinoma
- Fibrolamellar carcinoma

Key points

- Accurate classification of pediatric hepatocellular neoplasms is critical in the clinical management of these patients, yet owing to overlapping morphologic features, can be challenging.
- Understanding and recognizing the diverse clinical settings in which pediatric hepatocellular neoplasms arise play an important role in diagnosis in conjunction with the pathologic findings.
- Owing to their overall rarity, large-scale studies of pediatric hepatocellular neoplasms have been lacking, but the establishment of international collaborative trials holds promise for furthering our understanding of tumor biology and its correlation with histology.

ABSTRACT

Malignant primary liver tumors are rare in children. Yet a wide histologic spectrum is seen, particularly in hepatoblastoma, the most common malignant liver tumor in children. Furthermore, there can be significant morphologic overlap with hepatocellular carcinoma, the second most common pediatric liver malignancy, and tumors with hybrid features of hepatoblastoma and hepatocellular carcinoma are also reported (currently placed in the provisional category of malignant hepatocellular neoplasm, not otherwise specified). This review provides detailed morphologic descriptions and updates in the evolving clinical context of these tumors, and presents recent molecular advances that may further help in accurate classification of these tumors, which is critical in their management.

INTRODUCTION

Malignant primary liver tumors are rare in children, accounting for approximately 1% to 2% of pediatric solid tumors. Hepatoblastoma (HB) is the most common malignant liver tumor, accounting for approximately 70% to 80% of hepatic malignancies overall and 90% of tumors in children aged 5 years or younger. Hepatocellular carcinoma (HCC) is the second most common and accounts for approximately 20% to 30% of hepatic malignancies.[1] More recent studies have focused on HB, with international collaborative studies allowing for better characterization, risk stratification, and treatment of these rare tumors. Larger studies of pediatric HCC are lacking, but the inclusion of HCC in the ongoing prospective international trial (Pediatric Hepatic International Tumors Trial [PHITT]) holds promise for additional information and data that may be used to further stratify and treat this challenging group of tumors.

Department of Pathology, University of California San Francisco, 1825 4th Street Room M2369, Box 4066, San Francisco, CA 94143, USA
E-mail address: soo-jin.cho@ucsf.edu

Surgical Pathology 13 (2020) 601–623
https://doi.org/10.1016/j.path.2020.09.002

Although primary liver tumors in children encompass many other entities, this review focuses on the hepatocellular neoplasms, including HB, the still-provisional category of malignant hepatocellular neoplasm, not otherwise specified (HCN-NOS), and HCC, including the fibrolamellar type.

HEPATOBLASTOMA

HB most frequently occurs in children younger than 5 years of age and can be congenital. The overall incidence seems to be increasing worldwide,[2] possibly related to increases in premature births and low birth weight babies and their survival, as well as early detection and better imaging modalities. In the United States, the incidence of HB has increased from 1.89 per 1,000,000 in 2000 to 2.16 per 1,000,000 in 2015, according to review of the Surveillance, Epidemiology, and End Results cancer registries.[3] There has been a disproportionate increase in incidence in males, with a male:female ratio of approximately 2:1 in recent studies.[3]

Most cases are sporadic and occur in livers without background chronic liver disease. However, HB can be associated with many genetic syndromes (summarized in **Table 1**).[4] Other reported associations include prematurity and low birth weight, as noted elsewhere in this article.[5–8]

Table 1
Conditions associated with development of HB and hepatocellular carcinoma (HCC) in children

HB	Genetic syndromes	Beckwith–Wiedemann syndrome Familial adenomatous polyposis Trisomy 18 Trisomy 13 Simpson–Golabi–Behmel syndrome Sotos syndrome Prader–Willi syndrome Kabuki syndrome Neurofibromatosis type 1 Fanconi anemia Tyrosinemia type 1 Noonan syndrome DiGeorge syndrome Wolf–Hirschhorn syndrome Li–Fraumeni syndrome FGFR3 mutation

HCC	Inherited liver disease	Tyrosinemia type 1
		Glycogen storage disease (types 1 and 3)
		Progressive familial intrahepatic cholestasis (PFIC types 2, 3, and 4)
		  BSEP deficiency
		  MDR3 deficiency
		  TJP2 deficiency
		Alagille syndrome
		Alpha-1-antitrypsin deficiency
		Mitochondrial respiratory chain disorders
		Fanconi–Bickel syndrome
		Ataxia–telangiectasia
		Fanconi anemia
		Familial adenomatous polyposis
		Neurofibromatosis type 1

	Noninherited liver disease	Biliary atresia
		Vascular liver disease
		  Congenital portosystemic shunt (Abernethy malformation)
		  Hepatic venous outflow obstruction/Budd–Chiari syndrome
		  Congenital heart disease with or without a Fontan operation[77]
		Hepatitis B infection

GROSS FEATURES

HB is typically a single, well-circumscribed, lobu-lated mass, often surrounded by a variable pseu-docapsule. The gross appearance may be heterogeneous, with variation in color from tan to green, with bile production by tumors. After ther-apy, a pseudocapsule may be more evident and areas of necrosis, hemorrhage, and fibrosis can be seen, along with cystic change. Gritty areas of calcification or osteoid formation may be appreciated.

MICROSCOPIC FEATURES

The current classification of HB follows the consensus recommendations published in 2014 by Lopez-Terrada and colleagues.[9] HB may be composed entirely of epithelial components (epithelial HB) or may also have mesenchymal components (mixed epithelial-mesenchymal HB). Epithelial HB patterns recapitulate the various stages of fetal liver development, from primitive/undifferentiated (small cell undifferentiated [SCU] pattern) to embryonic (embryonal pattern) to differ-entiated (fetal pattern). These various patterns are discussed in more detail elsewhere in this article, from most differentiated to least differentiated, along with mixed epithelial-mesenchymal HB. Of note, although these entities are presented as discrete patterns, the cytomorphologic features lie on a spectrum and many tumors demonstration zonation, with transition from undifferentiated pat-terns to embryonal to crowded fetal to well-differentiated (WD) fetal pattern tumor cells.

Epithelial Hepatoblastoma: Well-Differentiated (Mitotically Inactive) Fetal Pattern

Tumor cells of the WD fetal pattern are character-ized by uniform, small, round nuclei, inconspic-uous nucleoli, and abundant granular eosinophilic to clear cytoplasm, arranged in thin trabeculae (1–2 cells thick) (Fig. 1A–D). By defini-tion, mitotic activity is low, at 2 or fewer mitoses per 10 high-power fields. On low-power examina-tion, a characteristic light–dark pattern is seen, owing to alternating areas of cells with clear or eosinophilic cytoplasm, respectively. Admixed areas of extramedullary hematopoiesis may be seen.

Immunohistochemistry is not typically neces-sary for diagnosis of this pattern, but may be help-ful in the assessment of small biopsies or to delineate the various epithelial HB patterns (Ta-ble 2). A WD fetal pattern usually shows diffuse but weak cytoplasmic (pericanalicular) staining for glypican-3 (GPC3), which contrasts with the diffuse, coarse, granular staining seen in the embryonal pattern. Beta-catenin (BCAT) staining is most often membranous and may only show rare nuclear positivity. Glutamine synthetase shows strong, diffuse cytoplasmic positivity.

A diagnosis of pure fetal HB is reserved for cases in which the entire tumor is composed of WD fetal pattern only.[9] By definition, this requires examination of the entire tumor; thus, this diag-nosis cannot be made on biopsy samples and this designation does not apply to tumors after treatment. Determination of pure fetal HB is impor-tant because patients with such tumors have excellent outcomes. In the current PHITT protocol, patients with pure WD fetal HB are placed in the very low-risk category and treated with upfront surgery and do not receive additional chemo-therapy if completely resected.[10]

Epithelial Hepatoblastoma: Crowded (Mitotically Active) Fetal Pattern

Compared with WD fetal, crowded fetal tumor cells show increased nuclear-to-cytoplasmic ra-tios, lending a crowded appearance of the cells on low-power examination, with visible nucleoli, and more uniformly dense, eosinophilic cytoplasm that leads to loss of the light–dark appearance characteristic of WD fetal (Fig. 1E, F). By definition, mitotic activity is increased compared with WD fetal, at more than 2 mitoses per 10 high-power fields. Extramedullary hematopoiesis may be seen more frequently than in WD fetal pattern.

Immunohistochemically, crowded fetal tumor cells, similar to embryonal pattern tumor cells, show diffuse, coarse, granular cytoplasmic posi-tivity for GPC3. Increased numbers of nuclei posi-tive for BCAT are seen compared with WD fetal (see Table 2).

Epithelial Hepatoblastoma: Embryonal Pattern

The embryonal pattern is the most common in HB and characterized by tumor cells with high nuclear-to-cytoplasmic ratios and enlarged, angu-lated to oval nuclei that seem to mold to each other owing to scant cytoplasm (Fig. 1G–J). Rosette for-mation may be seen, resembling glandular struc-tures. Serpentine and microcystic patterns with myxoid change have also been described. Mitoses are frequent as well as areas of necrosis.

As noted elsewhere in this article, the various epithelial patterns lie on a spectrum and even within embryonal pattern HB, morphology and immunophenotype can show a range, with some tumor cells that seem to be better differentiated than others. Immunophenotypically, embryonal

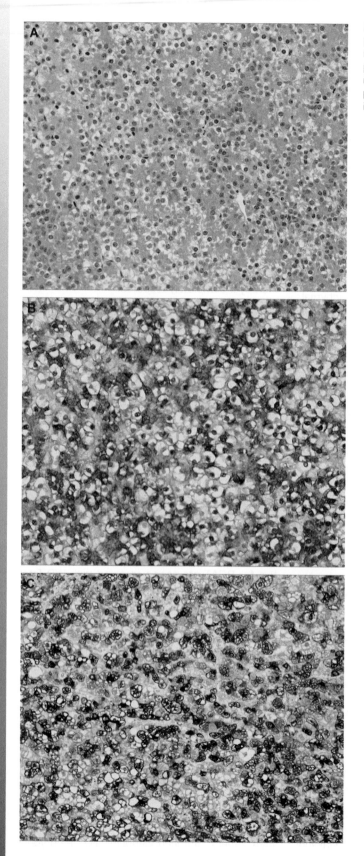

Fig. 1. Epithelial HB. (A) WD fetal pattern, hematoxylin-eosin (original magnification x100). (B) WD fetal pattern, beta-catenin (BCAT; original magnification x100). (C) WD fetal pattern, glutamine synthetase (GS; original magnification x100).

Fig. 1. (continued). (D) WD fetal pattern, glypican-3 (GPC3; original magnification x200). (E) Crowded fetal pattern, hematoxylin-eosin (original magnification x100). (F) Crowded fetal pattern, BCAT (original magnification x100).

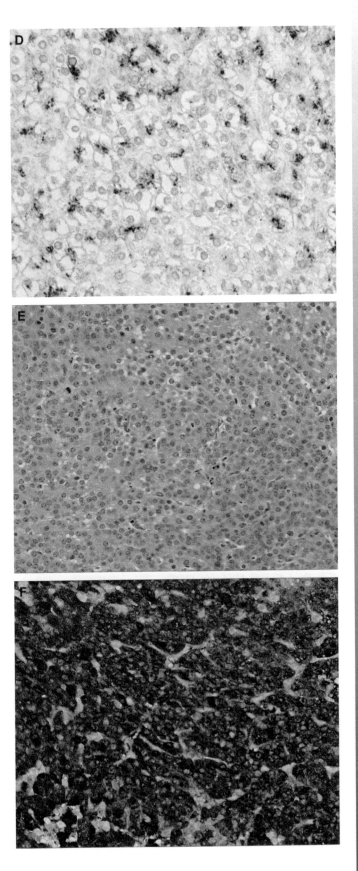

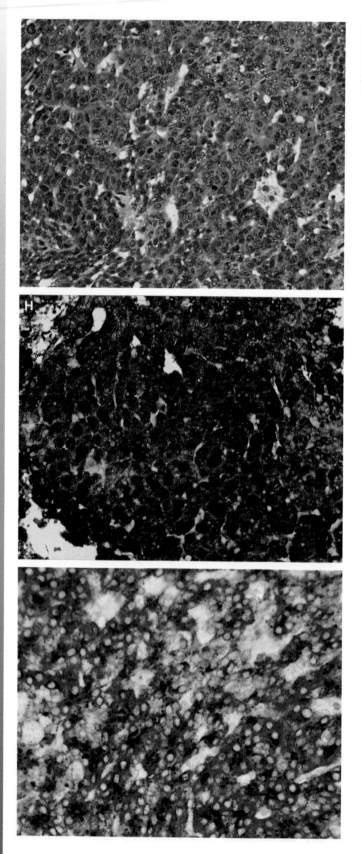

Fig. 1. (continued). (G) Embryonal pattern, hematoxylin-eosin (original magnification x100). (H) Embryonal pattern, BCAT (original magnification x100). (I) Embryonal pattern, GPC3 (original magnification x100).

Fig. 1. (*continued*). (J) Embryonal pattern, SALL4 (original magnification x200). (K) Small cell undifferentiated (SCU) pattern, present as small nests surrounded by embryonal and crowded fetal pattern tumor cells (hematoxylin-eosin, original magnification x40). (L) SCU pattern with strong, diffuse nuclear and cytoplasmic positivity for BCAT (original magnification x40).

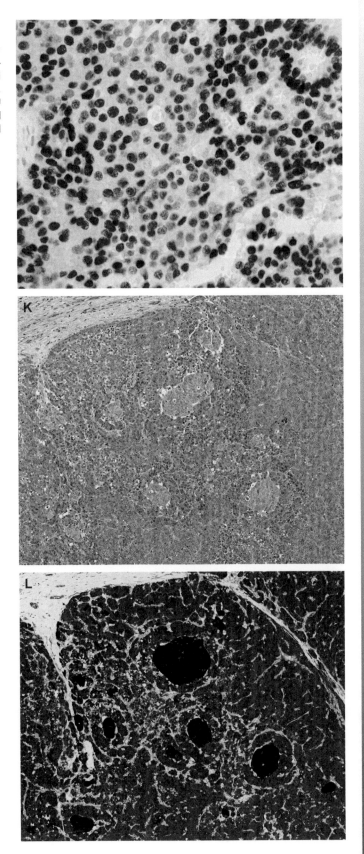

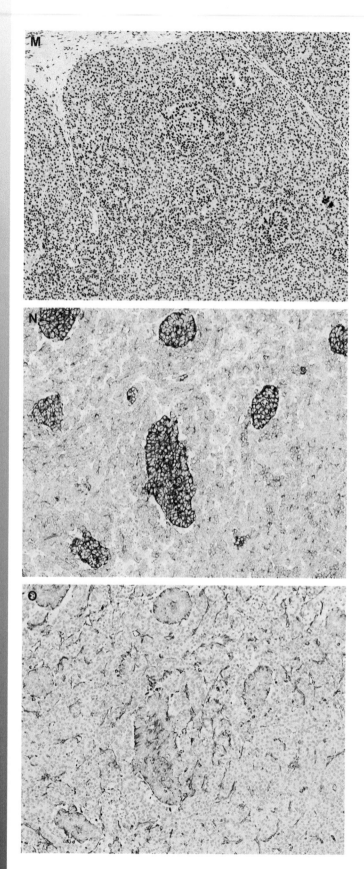

Fig. 1. (continued). (M) SCU pattern showing intact nuclear expression of INI-1 (original magnification x40). (N) SCU pattern showing strong, diffuse expression of CK19 (original magnification x40). (O) SCU pattern showing patchy vimentin expression (original magnification x40).

HB typically shows diffuse, strong, coarse cytoplasmic staining for GPC3 with diffusely nuclear staining for BCAT. However, glutamine synthetase expression can be variable, depending on the degree of differentiation, and may be negative.

Epithelial Hepatoblastoma: Small Cell Undifferentiated Pattern

This pattern is perhaps one of the most controversial owing to an evolving understanding of the significance of this pattern in the prognosis of HB (Fig. 1K–O). Prior studies have demonstrated that tumors with a predominantly SCU pattern harbor alterations in the SMARCB1 gene, leading to loss of nuclear expression of INI-1. Cytomorphology ranges from small round blue cells to those with frank rhabdoid morphology, including enlarged, eccentric nuclei, prominent nucleoli, and eosinophilic cytoplasmic inclusions. These morphologic findings as well as aggressive behavior of SCU HB have allowed for these tumors to now be classified as malignant rhabdoid tumors and receive appropriately directed therapy.

In most HB, SCU is present as a minor component. Although SCU is classified as an epithelial pattern in the 2014 consensus classification, it has entirely overlapping morphologic and immunophenotypic features with the blastemal pattern of HB, which experts have variously considered to be a mesenchymal component[9] or undifferentiated/primitive component that is perhaps best considered neither epithelial nor mesenchymal HB.

Both SCU and blastemal patterns generally demonstrate cells with rounded to ovoid nuclei with stippled chromatin, inconspicuous nucleoli, and scant lightly eosinophilic cytoplasm. SCU tends to occur as scattered nests and sheets surrounded by other epithelial patterns, namely, embryonal, and is typically poorly cohesive. Frank rhabdoid morphology has been reported, with cells demonstrating enlarged, eccentric nuclei with prominent nucleoli, and eosinophilic cytoplasmic globules. When other mesenchymal tumor components are present, the primitive tumor cell component may be more readily recognizable as blastemal (Fig. 2A), with gradual transition from the more spindled primitive-appearing tumor cells to more differentiated tumor cells associated with matrix production (eg, osteoid). In the absence of obvious mesenchymal components (ie, in a small biopsy sample), blastemal tumor cells may be recognized by their more haphazard distribution and association with various epithelial patterns, including WD fetal. Mitotic activity can be variable in both SCU and blastemal tumor cells and

necrosis is not seen. SCU tends to respond to chemotherapy and may not be identified in post-treatment resection specimens. In contrast, blastemal components may persist or evolve into mixed epithelial–mesenchymal HB, even in cases where a mesenchymal tumor component was not identified in the pretreatment biopsy.

Both SCU and blastemal tumor cells demonstrate coexpression of cytokeratins and vimentin, with strong, diffuse nuclear expression of BCAT. Both patterns are negative for glutamine synthetase, GPC3, and SALL4 expression. Nuclear expression of INI-1 is retained in both SCU and blastemal patterns.

An SCU pattern thus has overlapping morphologic as well as immunophenotypic features with blastemal pattern HB and, as other experts in the field have noted, it may be impossible in some cases to distinguish between the 2 patterns.[11]

Pleomorphic Pattern

Pleomorphic pattern tumor cells may resemble crowded fetal or embryonal patterns at first glance, but show increased nuclear pleomorphism with prominent nucleoli and bizarre, multinucleated forms present. It is more commonly seen in post-treatment resection specimens, but can be the predominant pattern in metastatic disease. This pattern has morphologic overlap with HCN-NOS as well as HCC. Although immunohistochemical stains are not helpful in the distinction from HCN-NOS, they may be helpful in distinguishing pleomorphic pattern HB from HCC given the strong, diffuse staining for BCAT (nuclear) and glutamine synthetase in pleomorphic HB.

Macrotrabecular Pattern

The macrotrabecular pattern is unique in that it is the only architectural pattern and is not based on cytomorphology. It is currently defined, following the 2014 consensus classification,[9] as HB arranged in trabeculae of 5 or more cells in thickness, which was modified from the original definition requiring 20 or more cells in thickness.[12] Although initially thought to be an unfavorable histologic pattern, the significance remains to be clarified given the architectural overlap with HCC and HCN-NOS, which may have resulted in previous misclassification of tumors.

Other Epithelial Patterns

Some tumors may show ductular morphology and differentiation, as demonstrated by immunohistochemical staining for CK7 and CK19, in a pattern designated cholangioblastic. In post-treatment resection specimens, BCAT may be further helpful

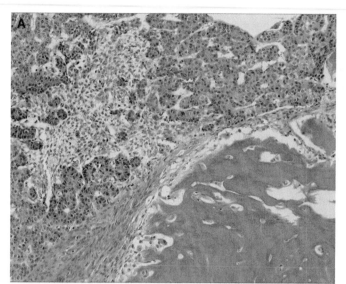

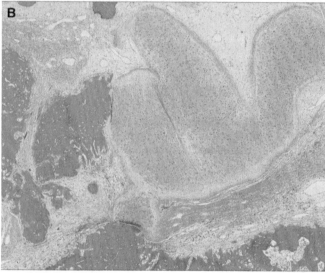

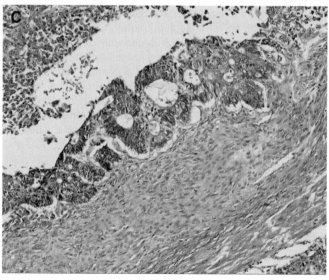

Fig. 2. Mixed epithelial-mesenchymal HB. (*A*) Blastemal pattern tumor cells are surrounded by embryonal and fetal pattern tumor cells (*upper left*) with adjacent tumor osteoid (*lower right*) (hematoxylin-eosin, original magnification x40). (*B*) This post-treatment tumor shows extensive osteoid with focal areas of cartilage. Fibrosis and hemosiderin deposition are also seen (*lower right*) (hematoxylin-eosin, original magnification x40). (*C*) This teratoid HB demonstrates primitive neuroepithelium (middle). Focal melanin pigment was also seen elsewhere (not pictured) (hematoxylin-eosin, original magnification x40).

in distinguishing ductular reaction (no nuclear BCAT staining) that may occur at the periphery of the tumor from cholangioblastic pattern (positive for nuclear BCAT staining).

Glandular (eg, intestinal) and squamous differentiation may be seen in some tumors, more commonly in mixed epithelial-mesenchymal HB (discussed elsewhere in this article), but may also be seen in epithelial HB. Thus, these components alone are not sufficient for a designation of mixed epithelial-mesenchymal HB with teratoid features (discussed elsewhere in this article).

Mixed Epithelial–Mesenchymal Hepatoblastoma

The term *mixed epithelial HB* refers to tumor composed entirely of a mixture of multiple epithelial patterns of HB. This term should not be confused with mixed epithelial-mesenchymal HB, also referred to as *mixed HB* (**Fig. 2**),[9] in which mesenchymal components are present in addition to epithelial components.

The mesenchymal components are present in varying proportions with respect to the epithelial components. The most common mesenchymal components include osteoid formation and cartilaginous differentiation; less commonly, skeletal muscle differentiation, fat, and spindle cell components can be present. Although once thought to represent post-treatment metaplastic change, it is now known that these mesenchymal components are integral parts of the tumor that are not induced by chemotherapy. Immunohistochemical staining of the mesenchymal components demonstrate nuclear BCAT expression. The mesenchymal components may also stain for markers that further support the cell lineage (eg, myogenin and desmin in tumor cells with skeletal muscle differentiation; SATB2 in osteoid producing tumor cells).

In addition to having mesenchymal components, as discussed elsewhere in this article, teratoid HB (or mixed HB with teratoid features) requires the presence of tumor components showing neural or neuroectodermal differentiation. Teratoid components could include mature brain and primitive neuroepithelial areas, as well as cells producing melanin or retinal pigment. The minimum amount of such components necessary for the diagnosis of teratoid HB has not been defined. Glandular and squamous tumor components can be seen in teratoid HB, but in the absence of a neural/neuroectodermal component, are insufficient for a designation of teratoid HB (discussed elsewhere in this article). Rarely, neuroendocrine differentiation as well as areas of endodermal

sinus (yolk sac)-like glands may also be seen in the epithelial components.

MOLECULAR PATHOLOGY FEATURES

In a recent study, Sumazin and colleagues[13] reported the results of a comprehensive genomic analysis of the largest set of clinically annotated HBs to date. This study confirmed that HBs have few coding mutations with a low somatic mutation rate, similar to results in other pediatric tumors.[14] Mutations and deletions in CTNNB1 were found in 90% of HBs tested; other Wnt pathway alterations, including 1 patient with a germline APC mutation, were noted. This study also delineated 3 prognosis-predictive HB molecular subtypes with differential expression of hepatic stem/progenitor markers (LIN28B, SALL4, and AFP) as well as developmental (HNF1A and NOTCH1), metabolic (NFE2L2), and cancer-related pathways (TP53 and TERT). Cairo and colleagues[15] also identified 2 prognostically relevant groups of HBs characterized by a 16-gene signature. More recently, the same group found epigenetic alterations in HB that could be used to define 3 molecular risk stratification categories.[16]

These and future studies of tumor biology (PHITT), combined with histologic correlation, hold promise for more precise risk stratification and treatment of patients with HB.

DIFFERENTIAL DIAGNOSIS

With the exception of pure fetal HB (discussed elsewhere in this article), HB is generally a histologically heterogeneous tumor with a mixture of patterns seen in various proportions, a feature that can be helpful in distinguishing from other hepatocellular neoplasms, including HCN-NOS and HCC. Although focal areas within HB can resemble or raise the possibility of HCN-NOS or HCC, the finding of more primitive components (ie, embryonal pattern) admixed with more differentiated components or mesenchymal components are key diagnostic features that distinguish HB. Immunohistochemistry can also be a helpful adjunct (see **Table 2**).

Hepatocellular Neoplasm, Not Otherwise Specified

Although HCN-NOS is currently a provisional category or diagnosis, as proposed in the 2014 consensus, it deserves further mention, particularly in the differential diagnosis with HB as well as HCC. Tumors currently placed in this category were first reported as transitional liver cell tumors by Prokurat and colleagues[17] in a report

Table 2
Immunohistochemistry in pediatric hepatocellular neoplasms

	HB				HCN-NOS	HCC, Fibrolamellar	HCC, Conventional
	WD Fetal	**Embryonal**	**SCU**	**Blastemal**			
BCAT	Mb (rarely Nuc)	Nuc	Nuc	Nuc	Nuc/Cy/ Mb	Mb/Cyto	Mb/Cyto (rarely Nuc)
Glutamine synthetase	+++	Variable	–	–	++ patchy	–	Variable +/–
GPC3	+	+++	–	–	+/++ patchy	Variable +/–	Variable +/–
SALL4	+/–	++	–	–	+/++	ND	+/–
CK7/CK19	+/–	–	+	+	ND	++/+++	+/–
Vimentin	–	–	+	+	–	–	–
INI-1	Retained	Retained	Retained	Retained	Retained	Retained	Retained

Abbreviation: ND, no data.

Data from Lopez-Terrada D, Alaggio R, de Davila MT, et al. Towards an international pediatric liver tumor consensus classification: proceedings of the Los Angeles COG liver tumors symposium. Mod Pathol 2014;27(3):472–91; and Ranganathan S, Lopez-Terrada D, Alaggio R. Hepatoblastoma and pediatric hepatocellular carcinoma: an update. Pediatr Dev Pathol 2020;23(2):79–95.

describing the clinicopathologic features in 7 older children and adolescents. A subsequent study described clinicopathologic features of tumors in 11 additional children, occurring in a similar age range (4–15 years) and with similar histologic features.[18] The tumors are histologically heterogeneous and may have cells that resemble crowded fetal HB to areas with increased pleomorphism and macrotrabecular architecture that resemble HCC. Some tumors may have an admixture of HB- and HCC-like areas. Staining for BCAT is variable, with a mixed pattern of membranous/cytoplasmic/nuclear staining seen, but importantly, nuclear staining is more frequent than in HCC. GPC3 and SALL4 positivity can also be seen. In all reported cases, tumors arose in livers without background chronic disease. Based on limited clinical information available, these tumors seem to be associated with high serum alpha-fetoprotein (AFP) levels, behave aggressively and are associated with poor outcome. Given that these tumors in the current PHITT are treated as high-risk HB rather than HCC, distinction from HCC is important and immunohistochemistry, including BCAT, may be helpful.

Based on these hybrid histologic features of both HB and HCC, these tumors were thought to represent tumors that were transitional between HB and HCC. Given the incomplete understanding of the biology of these tumors, the provisional category of HCN-NOS was proposed; subsequent studies in a limited number of cases have shown *CTNNB1* mutations, as seen in HB, and additional mutations such as *TERT* promoter mutations, as

seen in HCC.[13,19] It remains to be determined whether it may be more appropriate to rename this category of tumors as HB with HCC features.

DIAGNOSIS

The initial presentation of HB is most often of an abdominal mass, which may be discovered by those caring for the child. Some children may present with signs and symptoms of an acute abdomen owing to acute intratumoral hemorrhage or tumor rupture, which may be spontaneous or traumatic. Other presenting signs and symptoms are nonspecific and can include abdominal pain, weight loss, anorexia, nausea, and vomiting. Serum AFP is typically markedly elevated (in the thousands to millions of nanograms per milliliter range), whereas liver enzymes are generally within normal range. Thrombocytosis is seen in 50% to 80% of patients.[20]

Imaging studies are critical in the diagnosis as well as risk stratification of HB by providing the PRETEXT stage.[21,22] Ultrasound examination is used in the primary assessment of pediatric abdominal masses, including HB, but computed tomography scan or MRI is necessary to confirm the diagnosis. Currently, there is no defined role for PET/computed tomography scan in assessment of pediatric liver tumors.

PROGNOSIS

In the current Children's Oncology Group trial (AHEP1531), which is part of the PHITT, the only histologic pattern of significance is that of pure

WD fetal; histologic classification of the tumor otherwise does not affect the risk stratification or treatment, including SCU pattern. As noted elsewhere in this article, it is now well-established that tumors with a predominant small cell morphology and loss of nuclear expression of INI-1 should be classified as malignant rhabdoid tumors rather than HB.[23,24] However, the data are less clear with regard to the significance of the SCU pattern when it is a minor component of the tumor. Furthermore, it is unclear what proportion of the tumor must consist of the SCU pattern to alter prognosis, if at all. In the previous Children's Oncology Group trial (AHEP0731), even a small or minor component of SCU pattern could place the patient in a higher risk group. Some studies have shown adverse outcomes, even when SCU is present as a minor component,[25] but this is not a consistent finding[26] and the overall number of cases was small. The data from AHEP0731 are forthcoming and may further elucidate the significance of the SCU pattern. Although the designation of SCU versus blastemal does not currently affect patient management, consistent classification will allow for more accurate data collection and hence prognostication. Molecular biology studies may further help to delineate differences in SCU versus blastemal, if any.

The post-treatment effects in HB include necrosis, fibrosis, hemorrhage, and hemosiderin deposition, as well as microcystic change and peliosis-like changes. Increased osteoid may be seen in mixed HB. Some investigators have suggested maturation or differentiation after treatment may lead to better outcomes, but this finding, as well as the prognostic significance of other post-treatment effects has not been validated in larger studies.

Given the overall rarity of HB, comprehensive evaluation of outcomes to determine prognosis has required analysis of pooled data from multiple global consortia, leading to the formation of the Children's Hepatic tumors International Collaboration (CHIC). The risk stratification scheme used in the PHITT is based on the CHIC analysis.[10] Poor prognostic factors based on the CHIC analysis include age 8 years or older (≥3 years in patients with PRETEXT IV disease), serum AFP of less than 100 ng/dL at diagnosis, a high PRETEXT stage (III or IV), and presence of PRETEXT annotation factors (including metastatic disease, macrovascular involvement of all hepatic veins or portal bifurcation, contiguous extrahepatic tumor, multifocal tumor, and spontaneous rupture). In addition, other studies have suggested that microscopic vascular invasion outside of the tumor boundaries and positive margin status after resection may be associated with worse outcome.[27]

HEPATOCELLULAR CARCINOMA

HCCs in children are histologically identical to those occurring in adults and follow classification and grading as proposed in the World Health Organization Digestive System Tumors histologic classification [5th ed] (Fig. 3). Tumors are thus graded as well, moderately, and poorly differentiated. Subtypes that occur in the pediatric age range, as reported in the Surveillance, Epidemiology, and End Results registry, include conventional (73%), fibrolamellar (25%), and clear cell (2%).[28] Given that fibrolamellar HCC represents a significant portion of pediatric HCC but has distinct clinicopathologic features from conventional HCC, features specific to fibrolamellar HCC will be noted separately in each subheading.

Despite recent advances, including the availability of vaccination against hepatitis B virus, hepatitis B remains the most common cause of pediatric HCC worldwide. In North America and Europe, pediatric HCC occurs in 2 distinct settings: (1) in patients with background liver disease, including inherited liver disease, biliary atresia, or vascular liver disease, and usually occurring in cirrhotic livers, often presenting within the first few years of life (see Table 1) or (2) sporadic or de novo tumors occurring in normal livers, typically in children greater than 10 years of age and presenting at an advanced stage with unresectable or metastatic disease.[29,30] The relative proportions differ by region and series, but the overall incidence seems to be decreasing slightly owing to universal vaccination against hepatitis B, improvement in medical therapies for inherited liver disease (such as nitisinone for tyrosinemia), and early transplantation in patients with inherited liver disease.[29]

While accounting for a significant proportion of HCC presenting in children, fibrolamellar HCC also affects young adults, with a median age of presentation at 25 years.[31] (Figs. 4 and 5).

GROSS FEATURES

HCCs are variably light tan to yellow or green, depending on their fat content and the degree of bile production. HCCs occurring in patients with underlying liver disease tend to be multifocal and small, with the vast majority less than 3 cm in size.[32,33] Tumors occurring in patients without background liver disease are typically unifocal and larger (5–12 cm),[34] some with associated satellite nodules and macroscopic vascular invasion.

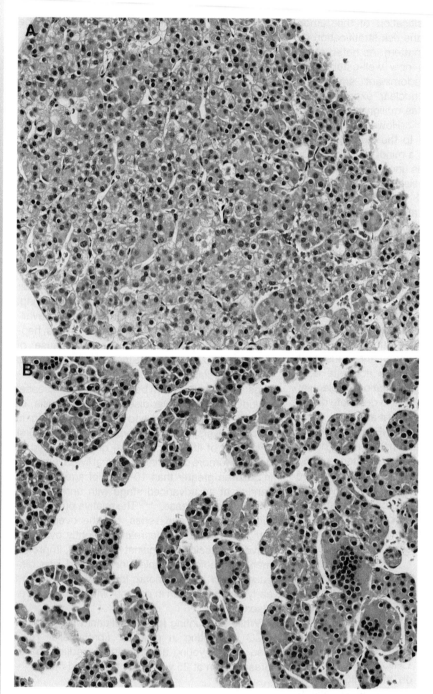

Fig. 3. Malignant HCN-NOS in a 15-year-old boy. (A) Tumor cells resemble crowded fetal pattern HB (hematoxylin-eosin, original magnification x100). (B) Other areas of the same tumor show macrotrabecular architecture with multinucleated tumor cells (hematoxylin-eosin, original magnification x100).

Some tumors may have a pseudocapsule, particularly those occurring in a background of cirrhosis.

Fibrolamellar HCC almost always occurs in a noncirrhotic liver and is usually solitary and large (9–14 cm) with cut sections revealing a central scar in approximately 70% of cases.[35,36] Gross vascular invasion is seen in approximately 25% of cases.[36]

MICROSCOPIC FEATURES

As noted elsewhere in this article, pediatric HCCs are histologically identical to those occurring in adults and diagnostic criteria for malignancy, as well as premalignant lesions are the same. A full description of HCC classification, grading, and diagnostic criteria is beyond the scope of this

Fig. 3. (*continued*). (C) All tumor cells show strong, diffuse cytoplasmic and nuclear staining for BCAT (original magnification x100). (D) Tumor cells also show strong, diffuse nuclear expression of GS (original magnification x40).

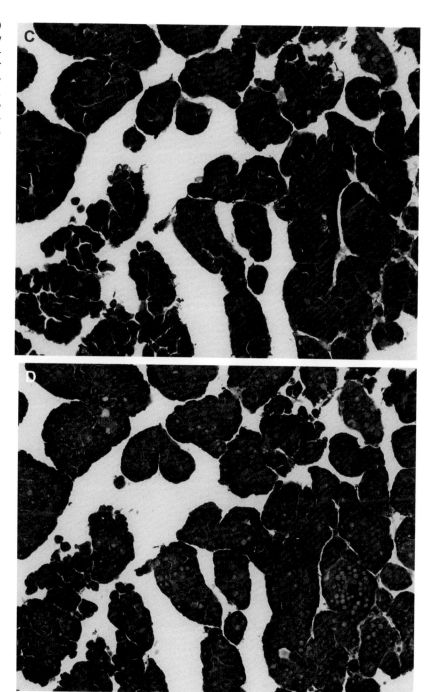

review. The reader is directed to the World Health Organization 5th edition Digestive System Tumors[37] and excellent recent reviews.[38,39]

However, several features are unique or distinct from those seen in adult HCCs, and include:

- HCC occurring in the setting of tyrosinemia is reported to show solid architecture with diffuse clear cell change and multiple nodules of different grades.[40]
- Premalignant lesions (ie, dysplastic foci and dysplastic nodules) are rare in pediatric

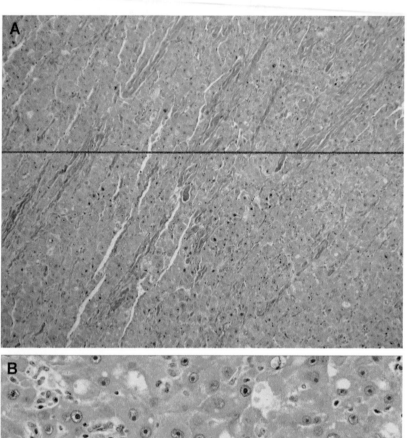

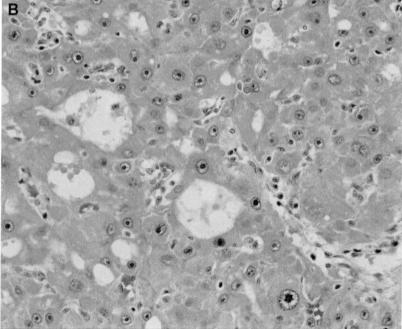

Fig. 4. Fibrolamellar HCC. (A) Tumor cells are arranged in trabeculae with intervening parallel fibrous bands (hematoxylin-eosin, original magnification x20). (B) Tumor demonstrating pseudoglandular architecture with rare cells containing cytoplasmic hyaline globules (center) (hematoxylin-eosin, original magnification x200).

HCC, but have been reported in patients with tyrosinemia[40] and TJP2 deficiency.[41,42]

• Compared with adult HCC, pediatric HCC more shows more frequent expression GPC3, EpCAM, and CK19.[33]

Fibrolamellar HCC shows characteristic morphology, with large, polygonal cells demonstrating vesicular nuclei, prominent nucleoli, and abundant granular, eosinophilic cytoplasm. Ultrastructural evaluation has shown abundant mitochondria,[43] lysosomes,[43] and/or endosome cytoplasmic accumulations.[44] Tumor cells are present in a dense, fibrous stroma that is, classically arranged in a parallel or layered

Fig. 4. (*continued*). (C) Some tumor cells also contain cytoplasmic pale bodies (hematoxylin-eosin, original magnification x400). (D) Tumor cells express markers of hepatocellular differentiation, including arginase-1 (original magnification x200).

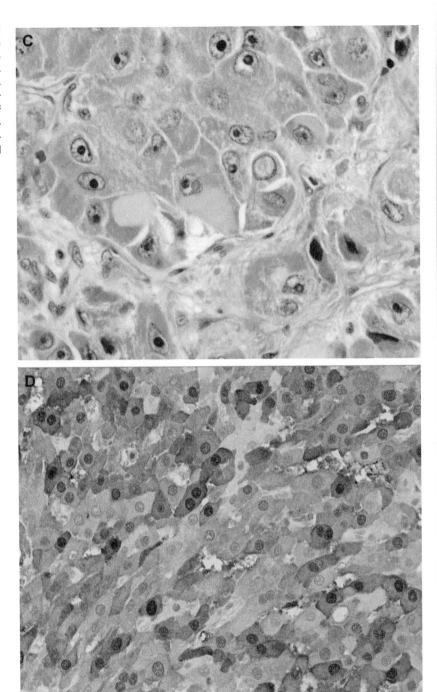

fashion (lamellar), although a more haphazard arrangement is commonly seen. Other features frequently seen (50%), although not pathognomonic or specific for fibrolamellar HCC, include cytoplasmic pale bodies and hyaline bodies. Calcifications and bile production may be seen. Areas of pseudoglandular arrangement with mucin production can mimic adenocarcinoma; solid as well as peliotic patterns have also been described. Immunohistochemically, almost all cases of fibrolamellar HCC demonstrate strong, diffuse expression of CK7 and may show expression of CD68 owing to the abundant lysosomes.[45] Although characteristic of fibrolamellar HCC, this

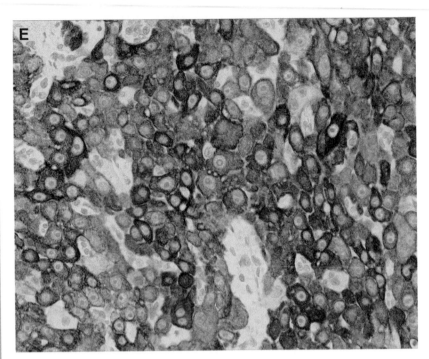

Fig. 4. (continued). (E) Tumor cells show strong, diffuse nuclear staining for CK7 (original magnification x200).

immunophenotype is not specific. Other positive immunohistochemical stains include alpha-1-antitrypsin and EpCAM[46] and rarely neuroendocrine markers[47]; liver fatty acid binding protein expression may be absent.[48]

MOLECULAR PATHOLOGY FEATURES

Owing to the overall rarity of pediatric HCC, large-scale molecular studies are lacking and molecular alterations have largely been inferred from studies of adult HCCs. The most comprehensive study of pediatric HCC to date used multiple modalities and confirmed that some alterations seen in adult HCCs are also present in pediatric HCC, including alterations in Wnt pathway genes (ie, intragenic deletions of CTNNB1 [most common] as well as inversion of APC and somatic mutation of AMER1) and telomerase pathway genes (ie, activation of TERT or mutations in ATRX).[40] TP53 were present, but less commonly seen than in adult HCCs. Of note, molecular alterations in tumors arising in children with underlying liver disease were distinct from those arising sporadically and lacked obvious oncogenic drivers.[40]

Molecularly, fibrolamellar HCC is distinct from conventional HCC and lacks commonly reported alterations, including in TP53 and CTNNB1. Instead, in the vast majority of cases, tumorigenesis is driven by increased activity of PRKACA owing to a 400-kb deletion of chromosome 19

that results in a DNAJB1–PRKACA fusion and consequent PRKACA expression and protein kinase A activity.[49] The fusion transcript is sufficient to induce liver tumors morphologically similar to fibrolamellar HCC in mice.[50] The fusion can be detected by reverse transcriptase polymerase chain reaction, next-generation sequencing methodologies, and fluorescence in situ hybridization. The clinically validated fluorescence in situ hybridization test has a reported sensitivity of 97% and specificity of 100% for fibrolamellar HCC in the context of a primary hepatic neoplasm.[45] However, the same fusion has been reported in pancreatobiliary neoplasms (albeit rare in children).[51] Rare cases that lack the fusion may demonstrate mutations in PRKAR1A, which results in loss of expression of PARKAR1A detectable by immunohistochemistry and consequent gain of function of PRKACA. The majority of such cases occur in patients with Carney complex (60%–70% with germline mutation in PRKAR1A).[52]

DIFFERENTIAL DIAGNOSIS

As noted elsewhere in this article, differentiating HCC from HCN-NOS and HB is critical for patient care and yet overlapping histologic features can make this process difficult. Clinical features and presentation can be helpful; tumors presenting in young children (<5 years of age) with mesenchymal components or less differentiated

Fig. 5. Moderately differentiated HCC (9.5 cm) in a 9-year-old girl with history of Abernethy malformation. (A) Tumor cells demonstrate pleomorphic nuclei with prominent nucleoli and Mallory hyaline (hematoxylin-eosin, original magnification x100). (B) The tumor shows extensive loss of the reticulin framework (original magnification x40). (C) Tumor cells are strongly and diffusely positive for GS, consistent with BCAT activation (original magnification x40).

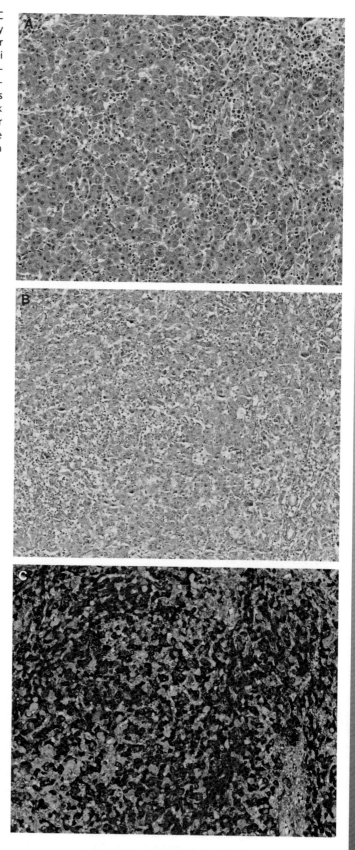

components (ie, embryonal pattern) would favor HB. Immunohistochemistry can be helpful (see **Table 2**).

The differential diagnosis of HCC also includes hepatocellular adenomas (HCAs), which also follow the recent molecular classification of adult HCAs.[53] The distinction between WD HCC and HCA may be aided by immunohistochemistry (eg, GPC3 expression favors HCC) and a reticulin stain, which may help to identify areas of decrease or loss of the reticulin framework in HCC. BCAT-mutated HCAs also occur in children with an increased risk of malignant transformation.

DIAGNOSIS

Common signs and symptoms of HCC are nonspecific and include abdominal pain, mass, and distention, as well as fatigue and weight loss. Patients with chronic liver disease may present with signs and symptoms of end-stage liver disease. However, up to one-third of tumors are asymptomatic and discovered on surveillance imaging for chronic liver disease or as incidental masses in explanted livers.[54,55] Serum AFP level is elevated in greater than two-thirds of patients. Of note, however, children with tyrosinemia may have very high AFP values owing to liver regeneration alone, so an elevated AFP does not always indicate malignancy. Ultrasound examination is useful to detect tumors in the setting of chronic liver disease, but a contrast-enhanced computed tomography scan or MRI is necessary to confirm the diagnosis.

Patients with fibrolamellar HCC present with similar nonspecific clinical findings, and rarely may present with gynecomastia, recurrent deep vein thrombosis, Budd–Chiari syndrome, nonbacterial thrombotic endocarditis, fulminant liver failure, or encephalopathy.[56–58] Other uncommon clinical features include increased serum neurotensin as well as serum transcobalamin I (haptocorrin).[59] Unlike conventional HCCs, no elevation in serum AFP is seen. Almost all cases arise in livers without underlying disease. Imaging studies may detect calcification in approximately one-half of the cases and a central scar is seen in approximately two-thirds of these patients.[35,60,61]

PROGNOSIS

Although the TNM staging system following the American Joint Committee on Cancer's Cancer Staging Manual (8th edition) could be applied to fibrolamellar and conventional pediatric HCC, it is not a universally accepted system and most international groups, including those participating in the PHITT, use the PRETEXT system, which is well-established in the staging of HB.

The overall prognosis of pediatric HCC is poor with a reported 5-year survival of less than 30% (range, 17%–28%).[28,62,63] The most important prognostic factor for fibrolamellar as well as conventional HCC seems to be tumor resectability, with poor prognostic factors, including lymphovascular invasion, extrahepatic tumor, and metastatic disease.[63–71] Unlike conventional HCC, however, lymph node metastasis in fibrolamellar HCC is common and does not seem to be an adverse prognostic indicator.[72,73] In addition to lymphatic spread, peritoneal spread is common in fibrolamellar HCC. There is limited benefit from chemotherapy for both fibrolamellar and conventional HCC. Liver transplantation in children with nonmetastatic disease can be beneficial, even in children who fall beyond Milan criteria.[74–76]

SUMMARY

Malignant hepatocellular neoplasms of the liver occurring in the pediatric setting pose significant challenges owing to their wide morphologic spectrum and yet overall rarity. The classification of these tumors continues to evolve as we gain more experience in their pathologic evaluation, including ancillary testing. Given the inclusion of not only HB but also HCN-NOS and HCC in the ongoing international trial, PHITT, the classification and management of these tumors are likely to undergo further refinement, particularly as we gain a better understanding of their biology.

DISCLOSURE

The author has nothing to disclose.

REFERENCES

1. Darbari A, Sabin KM, Shapiro CN, et al. Epidemiology of primary hepatic malignancies in U.S. children. Hepatology 2003;38(3):560–6.
2. Hubbard AK, Spector LG, Fortuna G, et al. Trends in International Incidence of Pediatric Cancers in Children Under 5 Years of Age: 1988-2012. JNCI Cancer Spectr 2019;3(1):pkz007.
3. Feng J, Polychronidis G, Heger U, et al. Incidence trends and survival prediction of hepatoblastoma in children: a population-based study. Cancer Commun (Lond) 2019;39(1):62.
4. Suchy FJ, Sokol RJ, Balistreri WF, editors. Liver diseaase in children. 4th edition. Cambridge: Cambridge University Press; 2014.
5. Spector LG, Birch J. The epidemiology of hepatoblastoma. Pediatr Blood Cancer 2012;59(5):776–9.

6. Spector LG, Feusner JH, Ross JA. Hepatoblastoma and low birth weight. Pediatr Blood Cancer 2004; 43(6):706.

7. Spector LG, Johnson KJ, Soler JT, et al. Perinatal risk factors for hepatoblastoma. Br J Cancer 2008; 98(9):1570–3.

8. Spector LG, Puumala SE, Carozza SE, et al. Cancer risk among children with very low birth weights. Pediatrics 2009;124(1):96–104.

9. Lopez-Terrada D, Alaggio R, de Davila MT, et al. Towards an international pediatric liver tumor consensus classification: proceedings of the Los Angeles COG liver tumors symposium. Mod Pathol 2014;27(3):472–91.

10. Meyers RL, Maibach R, Hiyama E, et al. Risk-stratified staging in paediatric hepatoblastoma: a unified analysis from the Children's Hepatic tumors International Collaboration. Lancet Oncol 2017;18(1): 122–31.

11. Ranganathan S, Lopez-Terrada D, Alaggio R. Hepatoblastoma and pediatric hepatocellular carcinoma: an update. Pediatr Dev Pathol 2020;23(2):79–95.

12. Gonzalez-Crussi F, Upton MP, Maurer HS. Hepatoblastoma. Attempt at characterization of histologic subtypes. Am J Surg Pathol 1982;6(7):599–612.

13. Sumazin P, Chen Y, Trevino LR, et al. Genomic analysis of hepatoblastoma identifies distinct molecular and prognostic subgroups. Hepatology 2017;65(1): 104–21.

14. Grobner SN, Worst BC, Weischenfeldt J, et al. The landscape of genomic alterations across childhood cancers. Nature 2018;555(7696):321–7.

15. Cairo S, Armengol C, De Reynies A, et al. Hepatic stem-like phenotype and interplay of Wnt/beta-catenin and Myc signaling in aggressive childhood liver cancer. Cancer Cell 2008;14(6):471–84.

16. Carrillo-Reixach J, Torrens L, Simon-Coma M, et al. Epigenetic footprint enables molecular risk stratification of hepatoblastoma with clinical implications. J Hepatol 2020;73(2):328–41.

17. Prokurat A, Kluge P, Kosciesza A, et al. Transitional liver cell tumors (TLCT) in older children and adolescents: a novel group of aggressive hepatic tumors expressing beta-catenin. Med Pediatr Oncol 2002; 39(5):510–8.

18. Zhou S, Venkatramani R, Gupta S, et al. Hepatocellular malignant neoplasm, NOS: a clinicopathological study of 11 cases from a single institution. Histopathology 2017;71(5):813–22.

19. Eichenmuller M, Trippel F, Kreuder M, et al. The genomic landscape of hepatoblastoma and their progenies with HCC-like features. J Hepatol 2014; 61(6):1312–20.

20. Hadzic N, Finegold MJ. Liver neoplasia in children. Clin Liver Dis 2011;15(2):443–62, vii-x.

21. Schooler GR, Squires JH, Alazraki A, et al. Pediatric hepatoblastoma, hepatocellular carcinoma, and other hepatic neoplasms: consensus imaging recommendations from American College of Radiology Pediatric Liver Reporting and Data System (LI-RADS) Working Group. Radiology 2020;296(3): 493–7.

22. Towbin AJ, Meyers RL, Woodley H, et al. 2017 PRETEXT: radiologic staging system for primary hepatic malignancies of childhood revised for the Paediatric Hepatic International Tumour Trial (PHITT). Pediatr Radiol 2018;48(4):536–54.

23. Trobaugh-Lotrario AD, Tomlinson GE, Finegold MJ, et al. Small cell undifferentiated variant of hepatoblastoma: adverse clinical and molecular features similar to rhabdoid tumors. Pediatr Blood Cancer 2009;52(3):328–34.

24. Vokuhl C, Oyen F, Haberle B, et al. Small cell undifferentiated (SCUD) hepatoblastomas: all malignant rhabdoid tumors? Genes Chromosomes Cancer 2016;55(12):925–31.

25. Haas JE, Feusner JH, Finegold MJ. Small cell undifferentiated histology in hepatoblastoma may be unfavorable. Cancer 2001;92(12):3130–4.

26. Zhou S, Gomulia E, Mascarenhas L, et al. Is INI1-retained small cell undifferentiated histology in hepatoblastoma unfavorable? Hum Pathol 2015;46(4): 620–4.

27. Wang LL, Filippi RZ, Zurakowski D, et al. Effects of neoadjuvant chemotherapy on hepatoblastoma: a morphologic and immunohistochemical study. Am J Surg Pathol 2010;34(3):287–99.

28. Allan BJ, Wang B, Davis JS, et al. A review of 218 pediatric cases of hepatocellular carcinoma. J Pediatr Surg 2014;49(1):166–71, [discussion: 171].

29. Hadzic N, Quaglia A, Portmann B, et al. Hepatocellular carcinoma in biliary atresia: King's College Hospital experience. J Pediatr 2011;159(4):617–22.e1.

30. O'Neill AF, Hanto DW, Katzenstein HM. Cause and effect: the etiology of pediatric hepatocellular carcinoma and the role for liver transplantation. Pediatr Transplant 2016;20(7):878–9.

31. Torbenson M. Review of the clinicopathologic features of fibrolamellar carcinoma. Adv Anat Pathol 2007;14(3):217–23.

32. Knisely AS, Strautnieks SS, Meier Y, et al. Hepatocellular carcinoma in ten children under five years of age with bile salt export pump deficiency. Hepatology 2006;44(2):478–86.

33. Zen Y, Vara R, Portmann B, et al. Childhood hepatocellular carcinoma: a clinicopathological study of 12 cases with special reference to EpCAM. Histopathology 2014;64(5):671–82.

34. Vinayak R, Cruz RJ Jr, Ranganathan S, et al. Pediatric liver transplantation for hepatocellular cancer and rare liver malignancies: US multicenter and single-center experience (1981-2015). Liver Transpl 2017;23(12):1577–88.

35. Ichikawa T, Federle MP, Grazioli L, et al. Fibrolamel- lar hepatocellular carcinoma: imaging and patho- logic findings in 31 recent cases. Radiology 1999; 213(2):352–61.

36. Pinna AD, Iwatsuki S, Lee RG, et al. Treatment of fi- brolamellar hepatoma with subtotal hepatectomy or transplantation. Hepatology 1997;26(4):877–83.

37. Board WCoTE, editor. WHO classification of diges- tive system tumours. 5th edition. Lyon (France): In- ternational Agency for Research on Cancer; 2019. No. 1.

38. El Jabbour T, Lagana SM, Lee H. Update on hepato- cellular carcinoma: pathologists' review. World J Gastroenterol 2019;25(14):1653–65.

39. Torbenson MS. Morphologic subtypes of hepatocel- lular carcinoma. Gastroenterol Clin North Am 2017; 46(2):365–91.

40. Haines K, Sarabia SF, Alvarez KR, et al. Character- ization of pediatric hepatocellular carcinoma reveals genomic heterogeneity and diverse signaling pathway activation. Pediatr Blood Cancer 2019; 66(7):e27745.

41. Kelly D, Sharif K, Brown RM, et al. Hepatocellular carcinoma in children. Clin Liver Dis 2015;19(2): 433–47.

42. Vij M, Shanmugam NP, Reddy MS, et al. Paediatric hepatocellular carcinoma in tight junction protein 2 (TJP2) deficiency. Virchows Arch 2017;471(5): 679–83.

43. Farhi DC, Shikes RH, Silverberg SG. Ultrastructure of fibrolamellar oncocytic hepatoma. Cancer 1982; 50(4):702–9.

44. Ross HM, Daniel HD, Vivekanandan P, et al. Fibrola- mellar carcinomas are positive for CD68. Mod Pathol 2011;24(3):390–5.

45. Graham RP, Yeh MM, Lam-Himlin D, et al. Molecular testing for the clinical diagnosis of fibrolamellar car- cinoma. Mod Pathol 2018;31(1):141–9.

46. Ward SC, Huang J, Tickoo SK, et al. Fibrolamellar carcinoma of the liver exhibits immunohistochemical evidence of both hepatocyte and bile duct differen- tiation. Mod Pathol 2010;23(9):1180–90.

47. Wang JH, Dhillon AP, Sankey EA, et al. 'Neuroendo- crine' differentiation in primary neoplasms of the liver. J Pathol 1991;163(1):61–7.

48. Graham RP, Terracciano LM, Meves A, et al. Hepatic adenomas with synchronous or metachronous fibro- lamellar carcinomas: both are characterized by LFABP loss. Mod Pathol 2016;29(6):607–15.

49. Honeyman JN, Simon EP, Robine N, et al. Detection of a recurrent DNAJB1-PRKACA chimeric transcript in fibrolamellar hepatocellular carcinoma. Science 2014;343(6174):1010–4.

50. Engelholm LH, Riaz A, Serra D, et al. CRISPR/Cas9 engineering of adult mouse liver demonstrates that the dnajb1-prkaca gene fusion is sufficient to induce tumors resembling fibrolamellar

hepatocellular carcinoma. Gastroenterology 2017; 153(6):1662–73.e0.

51. Vyas M, Hechtman JF, Zhang Y, et al. DNAJB1- PRKACA fusions occur in oncocytic pancreatic and biliary neoplasms and are not specific for fibro- lamellar hepatocellular carcinoma. Mod Pathol 2020; 33(4):648–56.

52. Graham RP, Lackner C, Terracciano L, et al. Fibrola- mellar carcinoma in the Carney complex: PRKAR1A loss instead of the classic DNAJB1-PRKACA fusion. Hepatology 2018;68(4):1441–7.

53. Nault JC, Paradis V, Cherqui D, et al. Molecular clas- sification of hepatocellular adenoma in clinical prac- tice. J Hepatol 2017;67(5):1074–83.

54. Khanna R, Verma SK. Pediatric hepatocellular carci- noma. World J Gastroenterol 2018;24(35):3980–99.

55. Mogul DB, Ling SC, Murray KF, et al. Characteristics of hepatitis B virus-associated hepatocellular carci- noma in children: a multi-center study. J Pediatr Gastroenterol Nutr 2018;67(4):437–40.

56. Lamberts R, Nitsche R, de Vivie RE, et al. Budd- Chiari syndrome as the primary manifestation of a fi- brolamellar hepatocellular carcinoma. Digestion 1992;53(3–4):200–9.

57. McCloskey JJ, Germain-Lee EL, Perman JA, et al. Gynecomastia as a presenting sign of fibrolamellar carcinoma of the liver. Pediatrics 1988;82(3):379–82.

58. Sethi S, Tageja N, Singh J, et al. Hyperammonemic encephalopathy: a rare presentation of fibrolamellar hepatocellular carcinoma. Am J Med Sci 2009; 338(6):522–4.

59. Graham RP, Torbenson MS. Fibrolamellar carci- noma: a histologically unique tumor with unique mo- lecular findings. Semin Diagn Pathol 2017;34(2): 146–52.

60. Blachar A, Federle MP, Ferris JV, et al. Radiologists' performance in the diagnosis of liver tumors with central scars by using specific CT criteria. Radiology 2002;223(2):532–9.

61. Friedman AC, Lichtenstein JE, Goodman Z, et al. Fi- brolamellar hepatocellular carcinoma. Radiology 1985;157(3):583–7.

62. Czauderna P. Adult type vs. Childhood hepatocellu- lar carcinoma–are they the same or different lesions? Biology, natural history, prognosis, and treatment. Med Pediatr Oncol 2002;39(5):519–23.

63. Murawski M, Weeda VB, Maibach R, et al. Hepato- cellular carcinoma in children: does modified plat- inum- and doxorubicin-based chemotherapy increase tumor resectability and change outcome? lessons learned from the SIOPEL 2 and 3 Studies. J Clin Oncol 2016;34(10):1050–6.

64. Baumann U, Adam R, Duvoux C, et al. Survival of children after liver transplantation for hepatocellular carcinoma. Liver Transpl 2018;24(2):246–55.

65. Czauderna P, Mackinlay G, Perilongo G, et al. Hepa- tocellular carcinoma in children: results of the first

prospective study of the International Society of Pediatric Oncology group. J Clin Oncol 2002;20(12): 2798–804.

66. Ezekian B, Mulvihill MS, Schroder PM, et al. Improved contemporary outcomes of liver transplantation for pediatric hepatoblastoma and hepatocellular carcinoma. Pediatr Transplant 2018;22(8): e13305.

67. Kaseb AO, Shama M, Sahin IH, et al. Prognostic indicators and treatment outcome in 94 cases of fibrolamellar hepatocellular carcinoma. Oncology 2013; 85(4):197–203.

68. Katzenstein HM, Krailo MD, Malogolowkin MH, et al. Fibrolamellar hepatocellular carcinoma in children and adolescents. Cancer 2003;97(8):2006–12.

69. McAteer JP, Goldin AB, Healey PJ, et al. Surgical treatment of primary liver tumors in children: outcomes analysis of resection and transplantation in the SEER database. Pediatr Transplant 2013;17(8): 744–50.

70. Weeda VB, Murawski M, McCabe AJ, et al. Fibrolamellar variant of hepatocellular carcinoma does not have a better survival than conventional hepatocellular carcinoma–results and treatment recommendations from the Childhood Liver Tumour Strategy Group (SIOPEL) experience. Eur J Cancer 2013; 49(12):2698–704.

71. Ziogas IA, Benedetti DJ, Matsuoka LK, et al. Surgical management of pediatric hepatocellular carcinoma: an analysis of the National Cancer Database. J Pediatr Surg 2020. https://doi.org/10. 1016/j.jpedsurg.2020.06.013.

72. Stipa F, Yoon SS, Liau KH, et al. Outcome of patients with fibrolamellar hepatocellular carcinoma. Cancer 2006;106(6):1331–8.

73. Yamashita S, Vauthey JN, Kaseb AO, et al. Prognosis of fibrolamellar carcinoma compared to noncirrhotic conventional hepatocellular carcinoma. J Gastrointest Surg 2016;20(10):1725–31.

74. Beaunoyer M, Vanatta JM, Ogihara M, et al. Outcomes of transplantation in children with primary hepatic malignancy. Pediatr Transplant 2007;11(6):655–60.

75. D'Souza AM, Shah R, Gupta A, et al. Surgical management of children and adolescents with upfront completely resected hepatocellular carcinoma. Pediatr Blood Cancer 2018;65(11):e27293.

76. Mazzaferro V, Regalia E, Doci R, et al. Liver transplantation for the treatment of small hepatocellular carcinomas in patients with cirrhosis. N Engl J Med 1996;334(11):693–9.

77. Komatsu H, Inui A, Kishiki K, et al. Liver disease secondary to congenital heart disease in children. Expert Rev Gastroenterol Hepatol 2019;13(7): 651–66.

New Prognostic Indicators in Pediatric Adrenal Tumors

Neuroblastoma and Adrenal Cortical Tumors, Can We Predict When These Will Behave Badly?

Jason A. Jarzembowski, MD, PhD[a,b,*]

KEYWORDS

- Neuroblastoma • Ganglioneuroblastoma • Ganglioneuroma • Adrenocortical adenoma
- Adrenocortical carcinoma • *MYCN* • *ALK* • *TP53*

Key points

- Peripheral neuroblastic tumors (pNTs) are categorized according to their stromal content, degree of differentiation, architecture, mitotic-karyorrhectic index, and age via the International Neuroblastoma Pathology Committee (INPC) classification.

- The prognosis of patients with pNTs depends most heavily on INPC classification, age, International Neuroblastoma Risk Group stage, *MYCN* amplification status, ploidy, and loss of heterozygosity at 1p and 11q.

- Children with adrenocortical tumors have a better prognosis than adults even when so-called malignant pathologic features are present. Tumor size greater than 5 cm and weight greater than 100 g, higher clinical stage and venous invasion, and increased mitotic rate portend a worse prognosis.

- *TP53* mutations are common in pediatric adrenocortical tumors and, although not prognostically useful, could suggest an underlying tumor predisposition syndrome.

ABSTRACT

Pediatric adrenal tumors are unique entities with specific diagnostic, prognostic, and therapeutic challenges. The adrenal medulla gives rise to peripheral neuroblastic tumors (pNTs), pathologically defined by their architecture, stromal content, degree of differentiation, and mitotic-karyorrhectic index. Successful risk stratification of pNTs uses patient age, stage, tumor histology, and molecular/genetic aberrations. The adrenal cortex gives rise to adrenocortical tumors (ACTs), which present diagnostic and prognostic challenges. Histologic features that signify poor prognosis in adults can be meaningless in children, who have superior outcomes. The key clinical, pathologic, and molecular findings of pediatric ACTs have yet to be completely identified.

OVERVIEW

Pediatric adrenal tumors represent a spectrum of disease; therefore, it is critical to identify which tumors will behave badly and require early aggressive treatment, and which will be indolent, with simple resection effecting a cure. The quest for prognostic factors for pediatric adrenal tumors

[a] Department of Pathology, Medical College of Wisconsin, Milwaukee, WI, USA; [b] Pathology and Laboratory Medicine, Children's Wisconsin, Milwaukee, WI, USA
* Department of Pathology, Children's Wisconsin, MS #701, 9000 West Wisconsin Avenue, Milwaukee, WI 53226.
E-mail address: jjarzemb@mcw.edu

Surgical Pathology 13 (2020) 625–641
https://doi.org/10.1016/j.path.2020.08.002

has been a long and winding journey through a host of clinical, pathologic, and molecular genetic variables, and although there have been some victories en route, the ultimate destination yet lies beyond the horizon.

NEUROBLASTIC TUMORS

INTRODUCTION

Peripheral neuroblastic tumors (pNTs): neuroblastomas, ganglioneuroblastomas, and ganglioneuromas, are the most common extracranial solid tumors in children, with a frequency of roughly 7 to 10 per million and about 650 new cases in the United States annually.[1,2] The relative frequency of these tumors has allowed extensive refinement of the diagnostic and prognostic methods used to guide therapy, and the advancement of this knowledge over the past several decades has led to better outcomes for these patients.[3] The heterogeneity of the diverse spectrum of pNTs can be captured by a combination of clinical, pathologic, and genetic factors, which in turn explains the heterogeneity of their behavior.

CLINICAL PRESENTATION

Most patients with a pNT present before the age of 5 years with a palpable abdominal mass; subsequent imaging often reveals a retroperitoneal mass with calcifications.[4] The anatomic distribution of pNTs reflects their origin from neural crest cells and sympathetic nervous system constituents, within the adrenal medulla and paravertebrally in the thoracic, abdominal, or cervical regions. Other "classic" (but rare) presentations include opsoclonus-myoclonus, periorbital ecchymoses, Horner syndrome, and intractable diarrhea. Several constitutional genotypes confer a predisposition to pNTs, including *ALK* and *PHOX2B* mutations, and pNTs may also be associated with neurofibromatosis, Beckwith-Wiedemann syndrome, Hirschsprung disease, and Turner syndrome.[5] Although the risk of tumor development is higher in these conditions, the resulting pNTs vary in terms of prognosis.

PATHOLOGIC DIAGNOSIS

pNTs are composed of both neuroblastic cells and Schwannian stroma, the types and amount of which are key to proper classification.[6,7] These groupings, in turn, help predict tumor behavior and patient outcome.

The neuroblastic component of a pNT can show a wide range of differentiation from primitive small round blue cells to mature ganglion cells (**Fig. 1**).

Undifferentiated/poorly differentiated neuroblasts have small round to oval nuclei with fine, speckled, "salt-and-pepper" chromatin and scant amphophilic cytoplasm. In contrast, mature ganglion cells have eccentrically located, large, round nuclei with a single large central nucleolus, vesicular chromatin, and abundant amphophilic to eosinophilic cytoplasm. Neuroblasts are often polygonal and fit together with a "paving stone" appearance. By immunohistochemistry, these cells are positive for NB84, neuron-specific enolase, PGP9.5, PHOX2B, synaptophysin, and tyrosine hydroxylase.[7,8] Neuroblasts are often embedded in variable amounts of fibrillary eosinophilic neuropil and may also form Homer Wright rosettes with central neuropil. The degree of neuroblastic differentiation for a pNT is categorized as undifferentiated (no neuropil or ganglionic features; diagnosis relies on ancillary studies), poorly differentiated (some neuropil and/or ganglionic features present), or differentiating (>5% of cells show ganglionic features), defined by the presence of neuropil and ganglionic features (see **Fig. 3**).

Schwann cells are long and spindled with small wiry or comma-shaped nuclei and modest amounts of clear to lightly eosinophilic cytoplasm. The cells are immunohistochemically positive for S100 protein. It is important to correctly distinguish between Schwannian stroma and neuropil. Per the International Neuroblastoma Pathology Committee (INPC) classification, pNTs with less than 50% Schwannian stroma are called neuroblastomas (see **Fig. 1A–C**), and those with more than 50% stroma are deemed ganglioneuroblastoma, intermixed (see **Fig. 1D**), or ganglioneuroma (see **Fig. 1E**); the exception to this is the ganglioneuroblastoma, nodular (GNBn), which is defined by its architecture rather than its exact composition (see **Fig. 1F; Fig. 2**). Ganglioneuroma is distinguished from ganglioneuroblastoma by its lack of immature neuroblasts and neuropil.

CLINICAL PREDICTORS OF PROGNOSIS

Age

It has long been clear that younger children with pNTs fare better than older ones, and most current treatment protocols take this into account. For example, the INPC classification uses 1-year, 18-month, and 5-year cutoff points in its algorithm, and the current International Neuroblastoma Risk Group (INRG) risk group stratification system uses 12- and 18-month cutoffs.[6,9] Age appears to be a continuous variable in terms of its utility as a prognostic factor; although a breakpoint needs to be established somewhere, there is no significant difference in risk for a 546 day old and

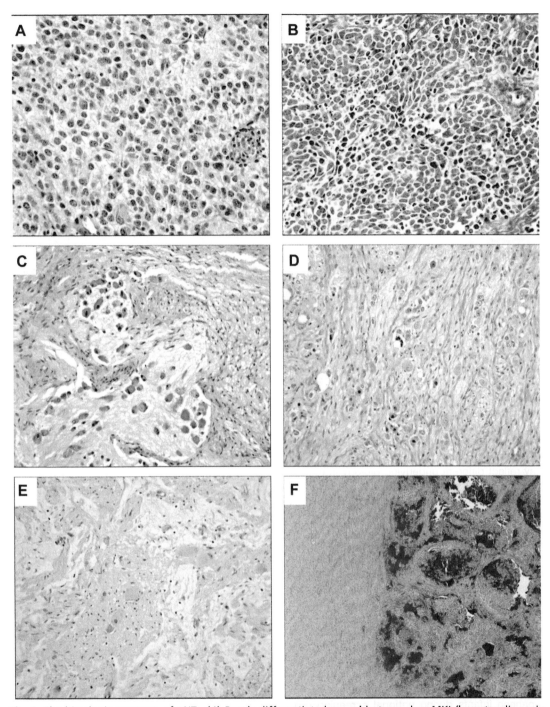

Fig. 1. The histologic spectrum of pNTs. (*A*) Poorly differentiated neuroblastoma, low MKI (hematoxylin-eosin, original magnification ×200). (*B*) Poorly differentiated neuroblastoma, high MKI (hematoxylin-eosin, original magnification ×200). (*C*) Differentiating neuroblastoma, low MKI (hematoxylin-eosin, original magnification ×200). (*D*) Ganglioneuroblastoma, intermixed (hematoxylin-eosin, original magnification ×200). (*E*) Ganglioneuroma (hematoxylin-eosin, original magnification ×200). (*F*) Ganglioneuroblastoma, nodular. Note ganglioneuromatous component on left, and poorly differentiated neuroblastic nodule on right (hematoxylin-eosin, original magnification ×10).

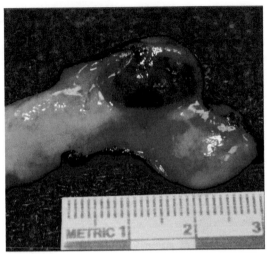
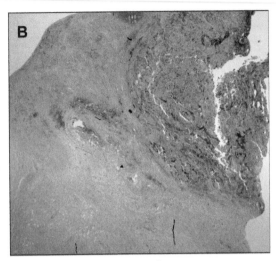

Fig. 2. GNBn. (*A*) Gross specimen shows a 1.6-cm hemorrhagic nodule within otherwise homogenous tan parenchyma. (*B*) Microscopically, the nodule (*upper right*) showed poorly differentiated neuroblastoma and the remainder of the tumor was ganglioneuromatous (hematoxylin-eosin, original magnification ×10). ([*A*] *Courtesy of* Kyle Kopidlansky, PA(ASCP).)

a 548 day old with similar tumors. One study showed an 83.0% 5-year event-free survival for children less than 1 year of age compared with 67.9% for 12 to 18 month olds and 38.3% for children older than 18 months, and numerous other studies show similar findings.[10–12]

The precise reason for the age dependence of prognosis in children with pNTs is unclear but may reflect different underlying biology in tumors of young versus older patients.[13,14] The best evidence for this is the spontaneous regression of many tumors in infants, a phenomenon that seems to occur less frequently with age. In 1963, Beckwith and Perrin[15] observed clustered neuroblasts with mitotic activity and invasive growth patterns within the adrenal medulla of infants at autopsy; these lesions were present at a much higher rate than the incidence of pNTs and were not seen in older children. They postulated that these "neuroblastomas in situ" underwent involution or delayed maturation in most cases and only rarely progressed to clinically apparent neoplasia. This hypothesis is also consistent with the high detection rate of elevated urinary catecholamines in Japanese infants during national screening programs, most of whom did not actually have evidence of a pNT.[16] Finally, the spontaneous regression of the tumors in infants with stage MS neuroblastoma would seem to be another example of this biologic behavior. Thus, pNTs in younger children may represent something more akin to delayed maturation/differentiation instead of neoplasia, thus accounting for the superior outcomes in this cohort.

Stage

Since 2009, the International Neuroblastoma Response Group Staging System (INRGSS) has been used for pNTs.[9] This system replaced the International Neuroblastoma Staging System (INSS), which had some shortcomings around its complexity and its postsurgical basis. The INRGSS, on the other hand, is based on pre-surgical/pre-treatment imaging studies, clinical presentation, and patient age and is summarized in Table 2 here: https://ascopubs.org/doi/full/10.1200/JCO.2008.16.6876.

Patients with higher INRGSS stages have worse prognoses. In the initial paper proposing this system, patients with stage L1 had a 90% 5-year event-free survival compared with 78% for stage L2 patients; overall survival was likewise significantly higher with lower stage.[9] For stage M INRGSS patients, 1 study found an event-free survival rate of 54.8%.[17] Stage MS disease is known to have special characteristics, including very young patient age, absence of adverse molecular features, and a high frequency of spontaneous regression.[14] One study demonstrated that in similarly aged children, stage 4S (MS) patients had markedly better 5-year event-free and overall survival than stage 4 patients (77% and 84% vs 64% and 69%).[18]

The utility of stage as a prognostic factor emphasizes the importance of correct and thorough pathologic evaluation of bone marrow specimens when assessing for stage M disease. The INRG and others have published recommended approaches to this workup, which include ensuring adequate lengths of trabecular bone in the biopsy and adequate cellularity in the aspirate, using at least 2 different antibodies for immunohistochemical detection, reporting the area or percentage of metastatic involvement, and using molecular methods to detect minimal residual disease.[19–24]

PATHOLOGIC PREDICTORS OF PROGNOSIS

Gross Examination

Many of the important gross findings in other cancers, tumor size, resection margins, and vascular invasion, do not affect staging and are of little prognostic significance in pNTs.[7] The primary objective in gross evaluation is detection of well-demarcated nodules within the tumor parenchyma that define a GNBn.[7,25] These nodules may appear hemorrhagic or simply darker than the surrounding tumor and are usually well demarcated but unencapsulated (see **Fig. 2**). GNBn may have a worse prognosis than a homogenous ganglioneuroblastoma, intermixed, depending on the composition of the tumor nodule (as described in later discussion). Needle core biopsies of a GNBn may be deceiving, because either the ganglioneuromatous component or the neuroblastic component, or both may be sampled, thus affecting prognostication.[26,27]

Histologic Examination

pNTs are classified according to their architecture, stromal content, and degree of differentiation of the tumor cells as described above, but several additional factors also contribute to the assignment of "favorable" or "unfavorable" histology, age and mitotic-karyorrhectic index (MKI).[6]

MKI is determined by counting the number of mitotic or apoptotic figures seen in 5000 tumor cells. In theory, the MKI reflects the proliferative and apoptotic rates of the tumor; both are usually higher in aggressive neoplasms than in indolent ones. Determination of an accurate MKI is dependent on several factors.[6,7] First, the MKI should be representative across the entire tumor, so multiple representative fields (not "hot spots") must be counted on each slide. Second, areas of necrosis should be avoided. Third, a cell should only be considered apoptotic if it shows nuclear pyknosis/karyorrhexis; cells with eosinophilic cytoplasm alone do not qualify.

pNTs are categorized as low MKI (<100/5000 cells or <2%), intermediate MKI (100–200/5000 cells or 2%–4%), or high MKI (>200/5000 cells or >4%). Attempts to circumvent the 5000-cell denominator have demonstrated variable success; there is no perfect substitute for performing a true 5000-cell count. This requirement does, however, limit one's ability to obtain a reliable MKI on a small biopsy or a focus of bone marrow involvement.

This histologic information, amount of Schwannian stroma, degree of differentiation, MKI, along with the patient's age, is the basis of INPC classification of pNTs (**Fig. 3**).[6,25] The INPC classification is by itself a remarkably powerful predictor of prognosis. In the initial paper defining the system, patients with favorable histology tumors had 85% overall survival, whereas those with unfavorable histology tumors had only 40% overall survival.[6] In a more recent study validating the age cutoffs, for patients greater than 18 months old, the event-free and overall survival rates for favorable histology tumors were 90.6% and 95.0%, and for unfavorable histology tumors were 31.7% and 38.4%.[28] There are concerns about the confounding presence of age twice within the clinical risk-stratification algorithm (once as part of the INPC system and once as a clinical variable), which have recently generated a newly proposed 4-category system based on age, degree of differentiation, and MKI.[29] Although this approach is more statistically sound, it may oversimplify pathologic classification, and more data and experience will be needed to determine its utility.

MOLECULAR/GENETIC PREDICTORS OF PROGNOSIS

MYCN

The most significant molecular factor in pNT prognosis is *MYCN*, a protooncogene and transcription factor that drives cellular proliferation.[30] *MYCN* is amplified in about 20% of pNTs, as defined by a 4-fold increase in *MYCN* signal over the centromeric probe on a fluorescence in situ hybridization assay; this can occur via linear amplification within homogenously staining regions or as extrachromosomal double minutes.[31] *MYCN* amplification correlates strongly with undifferentiated or poorly differentiated histology as well as with high MKI, and nuclear hypertrophy or "bull's-eye" nucleoli.[32] As such, *MYCN*-amplified tumors usually have unfavorable histology and a poor prognosis; 1 recent study showed that amplification was associated with a 19.6-fold higher risk for children under 18 months and a 3-fold higher risk for older children.[33] However, a small subset of *MYCN*-amplified tumors does not express the N-myc protein and has favorable histologic features and a good outcome; hence, morphology can trump genetics in these cases.[34]

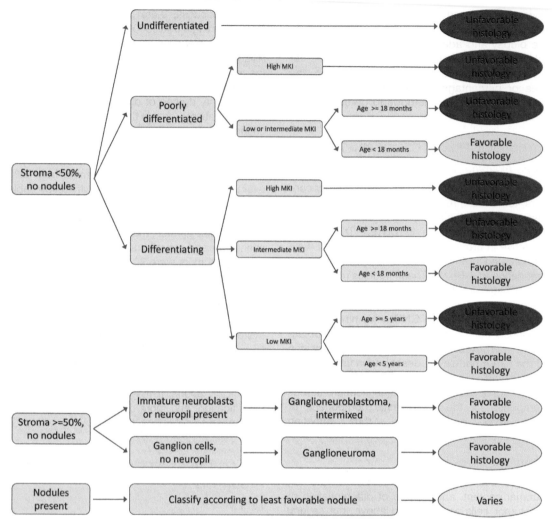

Fig. 3. The International Neuroblastoma Pathology Classification. (*Adapted from* Peuchmaur M, d'Amore ES, Joshi VV, et al. Revision of the International Neuroblastoma Pathology Classification: confirmation of favorable and unfavorable prognostic subsets in ganglioneuroblastoma, nodular. Cancer. 2003;98(10):2274-2281; with permission.)

MYCC

Another subset of neuroblastomas has unfavorable histology with nucleolar hypertrophy, undifferentiated neuroblasts, and high MKI, but does not show *MYCN* amplification or express N-myc protein.[35] Instead, these tumors often express C-myc protein and have poor prognosis, similar to *MYCN*-amplified ones. Immunohistochemistry for C-myc is currently the best way to identify this subset of cases.

ALK

Approximately 20% of pNTs have amplification of *ALK*, a tyrosine kinase receptor gene, and another 5% to 10% have activating point mutations within

the kinase domain.[36] Dysregulated ALK activity leads to increased cell proliferation and portends a worse prognosis.[37] *ALK* acts synergistically with *MYCN*, such that upregulation of both is frequently seen in high-risk neuroblastomas. Identification of *ALK* aberrations is important for prognostication as well as therapy; tumors with constitutive ALK activity may respond to specific tyrosine kinase inhibitors.[38]

Telomeric Maintenance

Telomeres, the repetitive DNA sequences capping the ends of chromosomes, cannot be completely replicated in each mitotic cycle in normal cells; they continually shorten and eventually drive a cell into senescence. Some pNTs upregulate the alternate lengthening of telomeres (ALT) pathway, which uses homologous recombination to overcome this imposed mortality.[39] Rearrangements of telomerase reverse transcriptase (TERT), the catalytic subunit of the telomerase complex, occur in 20% to 30% of high-risk neuroblastomas and are associated with aggressive tumor behavior.[40] Alpha thalassemia/mental retardation syndrome X-linked (*ATRX*), which also participates in ALT, is preferentially overexpressed in pNTs of older children and is associated with a poor prognosis.[41]

Structural Chromosomal Alterations

Several large-scale chromosomal aberrations have prognostic value in pNTs. Diploid or near-diploid neuroblastomas have a worse prognosis than hyperdiploid ones, and this is incorporated into current risk-stratification systems.[42] However, many ganglioneuroblastomas and nearly all ganglioneuromas have diploid DNA content; this does not change their usual favorable prognosis.[43] Segmental chromosomal gains and losses are common in pNTs, with deletion of 1p, deletion of 11q, and gain of 17q associated with aggressive behavior.[42]

Other Molecular/Genetic Alterations

The neurotrophin receptors (TrkA, B, and C [NTRK1-3]) are tyrosine kinases involved in pNT growth and differentiation.[44] TrkA is highly expressed in favorable tumors; it binds nerve growth factor and stimulates neuroblast differentiation. TrkC binds neurotrophin-3 and its expression mirrors TrkA. TrkB is overexpressed in MYCN-amplified tumors; its ligand, brain-derived neurotrophic factor, is produced by the tumor cells and drives an autocrine loop of proliferation.

One study showed that upregulation of *ARID1A* and *ARID1B*, which are involved in chromatin remodeling, was associated with a poor prognosis.[45] Recent attention has focused on the development of gene expression signatures that could be useful for identification of minimal residual disease as well as for identifying biologic risk.[46,47] Some proposed candidates have been shown to be independent predictors of survival.

SUMMARY

Pathologic evaluation plays a major role in the diagnosis, prognosis, and treatment selection for patients with pNTs. This information is then combined with the results of molecular testing to form the foundation for risk stratification. The 2 major algorithms include similar factors: Children's Oncology Group uses age, INSS stage, histology, *MYCN* status, ploidy, and loss of heterozygosity at 1p and 11q to assign patients to one of 3 groups;

the INRG uses INRGSS stage, histology, *MYCN* status, ploidy, and loss of heterozygosity at 11q and places patients in one of 4 categories (Please see **figure 2** here https://ascopubs.org/doi/10.1200/JCO.2008.16.6785).[48,49] The risk grouping helps establish a prognosis and treatment options for the patient. Although great strides have been made in the understanding of pNTs, a constant search is on for better prognostic factors that will help identify those patients in need of novel or more aggressive therapies.

CLINICS CARE POINTS

- Peripheral neuroblastic tumors are diagnosed according to their stromal content, degree of differentiation, and architecture.
- The International Neuroblastoma Pathology Committee classification assigns peripheral neuroblastic tumors favorable or unfavorable histology based on diagnosis, mitotic-karyorrhectic index, and age.
- Overall, patient prognosis depends most heavily on INPC classification, age, stage, *MYCN* amplification status, ploidy, and loss of heterozygosity at 1p and 11q.
- Other genetic aberrations, such as *ALK* mutations/amplification, *TERT*, *ATRX*, and *TRK*, may also be useful in prognostication.

ADRENOCORTICAL TUMORS

INTRODUCTION

Adrenocortical tumors (ACTs) are rare in children (0.1–0.4 per million depending on age) with a female preponderance of 2- to 4-fold.[50,51] Most pediatric ACTs are hormonally active (unlike their adult counterparts), stemming from the function of their cells of origin in the zona fasciculata (glucocorticoids), zona reticularis (androgens), and the provisional/fetal cortex (dehydroepiandrosterone). Many of the genes that drive adrenal development are, unsurprisingly, dysregulated in pediatric ACTs (discussed later). Importantly, children with ACTs have markedly better prognoses than adults with the same clinicopathologic features. Based on common morphologic classification schemes for adult ACTs, the vast majority (usually >90%) of pediatric ACTs would be called adrenocortical carcinomas (ACCs), but this is clearly incorrect based on the high rates of event-free and overall survival in these patients.[52–57] These findings have led to speculation that pediatric ACTs arise from the developing adrenal gland, whereas adult ACTs may arise from mature cortical cells.[54,57] This theory in turn raises the possibility that spontaneous regression and/or maturation may account for the better clinical outcome of ACTs in children. However, because adult ACTs represent most of these tumors, most studies have focused on older patients. Thus, much about pediatric ACTs remains poorly understood, especially the distinction between adrenocortical adenomas (ACAs) and ACCs, and prognostic factors.

CLINICAL PRESENTATION

Children with ACTs primarily exhibit virilization with or without Cushing syndrome; a minority have feminization or isolated Cushing syndrome.[53,58] Aldosterone-secreting tumors (Conn syndrome) are rare in children, although hypertension can be a common symptom of an ACT from either aldosterone or cortisol production.[58] Occasionally, patients have nonsecreting tumors and instead present with abdominal pain, fever, or a palpable mass. True "incidentalomas" are less common in children than adults perhaps because they are less likely to undergo imaging for other reasons.

PATHOLOGIC DIAGNOSIS

ACTs have similar gross and microscopic appearances in children and adults. These tumors are usually unilateral and encapsulated (or at least well circumscribed), and their relationship to the native adrenal gland is evident. Pediatric ACTs can range from 1 to 20 cm and 10 to 2500 g and are usually in the yellow-tan-brown color spectrum, but rarely may be pigmented ("black" adenomas) because of abundant lipofuscin within the cells.[53,54] Cystic change may be seen, and frank necrosis may raise suspicion of malignancy (see later discussion).

Histologically, the tumor cells typically resemble the cortical layer from which they arose and are characterized by cytologically bland round to polygonal cells with clear or lightly eosinophilic, vacuolated cytoplasm and bland nuclei with vesicular chromatin and single small nucleoli (Fig. 4). A wide variety of growth patterns have been described, including diffuse/solid, alveolar, tubular, fibrohyaline, and yolk sac-like. Mitotic activity can vary considerably and, along with cytoatypia, may be prognostic factors (discussed later). Fibrosis, necrosis, hemorrhage, and calcification can all be seen to varying degrees. By immunohistochemistry, the tumor cells are usually positive for vimentin, inhibin, melan A, synaptophysin, and calretinin and variably reactive for cytokeratins; they are negative for S100 and chromogranin.[59,60] Several distinct ACT variants have been described, including oncocytic, myxoid, sarcomatoid, and pediatric; the significance of the first 3 variants is unknown.[54,61]

CLINICAL PREDICTORS OF PROGNOSIS

Age

As described above, with ACTs have a substantially better prognosis that adults with similar stage, histology, and other features. In addition, multiple studies have shown that younger children with ACTs had longer overall survival than older ones.[57,62–64] Although the precise age cutoff varied by study, most were between 3 and 7 years old. This variation has been interpreted by some investigators as further evidence that "pediatric" and "adult" ACTs are biologically distinct tumors with different origins and behaviors.

Stage

Multiple groups have established that stage is an important prognostic factor for pediatric ACTs. In 1 study, outcome correlated with tumor stage using a novel system (stage 1: complete excision/tumor <200 cm^3; stage 2: microscopic residual disease/tumor >200 cm^3/abnormal hormone levels postoperatively; stage 3: gross residual tumor; stage 4: metastatic disease). Overall survival was greater than 90% for children with stage 1 ACTs, and almost 0% for those with stage 4 ACTs; children with stage 2 and 3 tumors had variable prognosis.[58] A subsequent series using the current American Joint Committee on Cancer (AJCC) staging system (T1: tumor <5 cm without local invasion; T2: tumor >5 cm without local invasion; T3: local invasion; T4: involvement of adjacent organs) similarly showed survival of all the T1 patients and none of the T4 patients.[65,66] Although the AJCC staging system potentially confounds tumor size and spread, both have been shown to be independent prognostic factors via multivariate analyses. Recurrence is also a negative prognostic factor and is associated with low overall survival despite additional surgeries to reestablish local control.[58]

PATHOLOGIC PREDICTORS OF PROGNOSIS

Gross Examination

Most analyses of pediatric ACTs have identified size as a clear prognostic factor, and many groups have included it in their staging systems as described above.[53,65,67,68] The definition of favorable versus unfavorable size varies between studies: although 5 cm was a typical linear breakpoint, the weight cutoff used varied from 50 g to 500 g. Although increased size generally portends a worse prognosis, individual patients and tumors

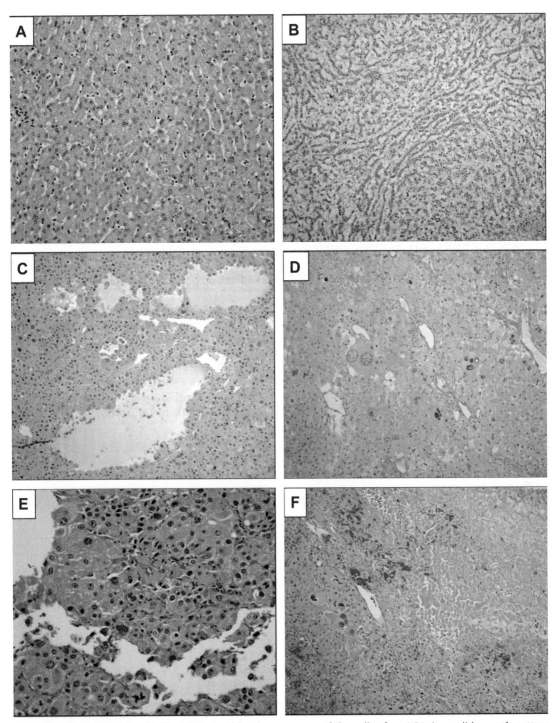

Fig. 4. Histologic features of ACTs. (*A*) Typical bland appearance of the cells of an ACA, in a solid growth pattern (hematoxylin-eosin, original magnification ×200). (*B*) Trabecular growth pattern (hematoxylin-eosin, original magnification ×100). (*C*) Cystic change (hematoxylin-eosin, original magnification ×100). (*D*) Moderate cellular pleomorphism (hematoxylin-eosin, original magnification ×100). (*E*) Geographic necrosis (*upper right*) (hematoxylin-eosin, original magnification ×400). (*F*) Increased number of mitotic figures (*arrows*) (hematoxylin-eosin, original magnification ×100). Histologic features (*D*) through (*F*) have been associated with malignant potential and worse prognosis.

may display unexpected behavior. In the AFIP study, although their proposed cutoff of 400 g was statistically significant, there was a malignant 24-g tumor and a benign one that weighed more than 2 kg; therefore, size must be considered in the context of other clinicopathologic factors.[53]

Histologic Examination

One of the best known forays into morphologic prognostication of ACTs was a study of 43 adult ACTs by Weiss[52] that considered 9 features: nuclear grade (using the Fuhrman system for renal cell carcinoma), mitotic rate (per 50 high-powered fields), atypical mitoses, character of cytoplasm (degree of vacuolization or clearing), architecture of tumor cells, necrosis, invasion of venous structures, invasion of sinusoidal structures, and invasion of tumor capsule. He found that the 3 most useful factors in designating an ACT as an ACC were high mitotic rate (>5 per 50 high-powered fields), the presence of atypical mitoses, and venous invasion. No single criterion could dichotomize these ACTs into benign and malignant, and he proposed a scoring system based on specific values for each of the 9 morphologic features (Table 1). A subsequent paper using some of the same ACC cases demonstrated that mitotic rate was the key

prognostic factor for distinguishing high- and low-risk ACCs; this paper was limited to ACTs called carcinomas by the above criteria, and only included adult patients.[69] Thus, although it seemed like prognosis could be somewhat predicted by morphology, the applicability to pediatric tumors was unknown.

A decade later, Wieneke and colleagues[53] analyzed 83 pediatric ACTs in an attempt to address this gap. They applied the Weiss criteria for adult ACTs to their pediatric group and although many of the features were associated with poor prognosis in univariate analysis, multivariate analysis revealed that only 3 predictors of malignant behavior remained: invasion of the vena cava, tumor necrosis, and high mitotic activity. There was substantial overlap in scoring between patients with benign-behaving tumors (0 and 7 adverse histologic features) and those with metastatic disease (1 and 9 features). The dilemma was succinctly stated by the investigators: "Only 31% of histologically malignant tumors behaved in a clinically malignant fashion."[53] The investigators proposed a 3-tier classification with 0 to 2 points = benign, 3 points = intermediate risk, and 4 points or more = malignant. Another group subsequently applied the Wieneke criteria to a cohort of 13 pediatric ACTs and found that all 7

Table 1
Pathologic features predictive of malignant behavior in adrenocortical tumors

	Hough et al,[55] 1979	Weiss,[52] 1984	Wieneke et al,[53] 2003	van Slooten et al,[56] 1985
Group studied	Adult & pediatric	Adult	Pediatric	Adult
Size		>10 cm	>10.5 cm	
Mass	>100 g	>250 g	>400 g	>150 g
Vascular invasion	X	X	X	X
Capsular invasion		X	X	
Nuclear atypia		X	X	X
Mitoses	>1 per 10 hpf	>5 per 50 hpf or atypical mitoses	>15 per 20 hpf or atypical mitoses	>2 per 10 hpf
Necrosis	X	X	X	Plus other "regressive" changes
Fibrous bands	X			
Diffuse growth pattern	X	X		X
Other			Soft tissue invasion	

Data from Refs.[52,53,55,56]

patients with tumors categorized as benign or intermediate had excellent long-term survival, whereas 4 of 6 patients with tumors deemed malignant behaved as such.[70] A later paper from Das and colleagues[71] showed similar findings in their pediatric ACT cohort. Thus, although the authors might be able to identify the clearly benign ACTs based on morphology, some morphologically malignant tumors have pleasantly unexpected benign clinical courses.

Immunohistochemical and Special Staining

Ki67

Ki67 (MIB-1), an indicator of cell proliferation, has been investigated as a prognostic marker in ACTs in part because of the utility of mitotic counts in the previously described morphologic classifications for adult and pediatric ACTs (**Fig. 5**). Immunohistochemical staining for Ki67 appears useful in predicting the behavior of adult and pediatric ACTs, with cutoff values of 5% to 15% depending on the study.[63,72] One group found that the 3-year event-free survival for patients with Ki-67 index ≥15% was 48.5% compared with 96.2% for patients with a Ki-67 index less than 15%.[63]

Other markers

Several studies have assessed the utility of reticulin staining, in addition to the Weiss score, for distinguishing between ACA and ACC.[73,74] Although nearly all ACC but only rare ACA had disruption of the reticulin network, this method has not been validated for pediatric ACTs. High numbers of tumor-infiltrating CD8+ cytotoxic T lymphocytes correlated with better prognosis in 1 study of pediatric ACC.[75] Although decreased expression of class II HLA

antigens has been shown to be a negative prognostic factor in adult ACTs, there are conflicting reports of its expression in pediatric tumors.[76,77] These and other potential biomarkers will require further investigation before their true prognostic utility is known.

MOLECULAR/GENETIC PREDICTORS OF PROGNOSIS

TP53

The p.R337H mutation, a specific TP53 germline mutation, underlies a Li-Fraumeni-like cancer predisposition syndrome in which affected children have an increased risk of breast, brain, and soft tissue cancers in addition to ACT, which is often the first manifestation.[78] A Children's Oncology Group study found *TP53* mutations in 50% of pediatric ACTs, some of which were p.R337H cases, and only 5% of which were canonical hot-spot mutations.[79] Unfortunately, *TP53* status does not appear to correlate with behavior in pediatric ACTs, despite being a proven negative prognostic factor in adult ACTs.[80–82] One possible exception is the coexistence of *TP53* and *ATRX* mutations, which appeared in 1 study to be associated with a dismal prognosis.[83]

IGF-II and IGF-IR

ACTs occur at greater frequency in patients with Beckwith-Wiedemann syndrome, which is associated with epigenetic alterations at the 11p15 locus. One of the key regulatory genes present in this region and regulated at least in part by imprinting is insulin-like growth factor II (*IGF-II*), which is expressed from the paternal allele.[84]

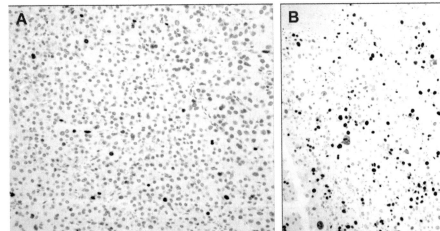

Fig. 5. Ki67 proliferation index as a prognostic factor. Immunohistochemistry for Ki67 on an ACA (hematoxylin-eosin, original magnification ×200) (*A*) and an ACC (hematoxylin-eosin, original magnification ×200) (*B*). Note the markedly higher percentage of positive cells in (*B*), a tumor that was already metastatic at the time of diagnosis, than in (*A*), a localized tumor that was definitively treated by surgical resection alone.

IGF-II signals through its receptor, IGF-IR, to stimulate proliferation through the mitogen-activated protein kinase pathway and to inhibit apoptosis through the phosphoinositol-3-kinase pathway. Most pediatric ACTs (60%–100% of cases, depending on the study) have loss of heterozygosity at 11p15 and associated elevated IGF-II expression, as much as 18-fold higher than normal adrenal glands.[85–87] Furthermore, 1 study of pediatric and adult ACTs showed increased methylation of *IGF-II* regulatory regions in ACC, suggesting upregulated transcription.[88] Neither LOH at 11p15 nor IGF-II overexpression portends poor prognosis in pediatric ACTs, even though the latter is known to be associated with malignant behavior in adult ACTs.[72,85,89,90] However, *IGF-IR* messenger RNA was 3- to -fold higher in pediatric ACC than ACA, and IGF-IR levels were an independent predictor of metastases.[91,92] IGF-I-R levels were similar between adult ACC and ACA.

SF-1

Multiple genomic studies of pediatric ACTs have shown gains of all or part of chromosome 9q, especially 9q34.[93,94] Steroidogenic factor 1 (SF-1) is located near this region (9q33.3) and plays an essential role in adrenal gland development and maintenance. Knockout mice lacking SF-1 have adrenal hypoplasia, and SF-1 is required for contralateral compensatory adrenal growth following unilateral adrenalectomy.[95] SF-1 gene amplification and nuclear expression were found in a large fraction of pediatric ACTs (47% and 56%, respectively) but in only a minority of adult ACTs (10% and 29%).[96] SF-1 expression appeared to correlate with steroid production by the tumor.[97] However, SF-1 levels were similar between pediatric ACAs and ACCs; nonetheless, 1 study showed that expression correlated with prognosis in adult ACCs.[96–98]

Genomic Alterations

West and colleagues[86] found increased *IGF-II* and decreased *KCNQ1* and *CDKN1C* expression in pediatric ACTs compared with normal adrenal cortex. All 3 genes map to the 11p15 locus, with *IGF-II* normally expressed from the paternal allele and *KCNQ1* and *CDKN1C* both expressed from the maternal allele; this suggests that imprinting and methylation may be important in tumorigenesis and echoes the *IGF-II* results described above. They also found decreased expression of class II HLA genes in ACCs versus ACAs, although as mentioned previously, this result has not panned out at the protein expression level in all studies.[77]

SNP analysis of pediatric ACTs (not differentiating between benign and malignant) showed frequent chromosomal abnormalities, including loss of 4q34, gain of 9q33-q34 and 19p, and loss of heterozygosity of chromosome 17 and 11p15; the involvement of 11p15 corresponds well with the above findings.[99] ACTs with *TP53* aberrations tended to have more chromosomal gains and losses than those with wild-type *TP53*. Another group performed network analysis on preexisting gene expression data, comparing pediatric ACCs to normal adrenal glands, and found upregulation of IGF-II as well as 4 novel hubs: *CDK1*, *CCNB1*, *CDC20*, and *BUB1B*.[100] As noted in later discussion, although expression of β -catenin itself has not been shown to be a prognostic factor, other members of the *CCNB1* network may be so.

Aneuploidy was a common finding in pediatric ACTs but did not discriminate between ACA and ACCs.[101] Loss of heterozygosity for 9p21 that was also associated with loss of p16 expression was seen in adult ACC, but not ACA.[102]

Other Markers

Early data for some other proposed markers of malignancy and/or poor prognosis have recently been published. In 1 study of pediatric ACTs, increased cytoplasmic membrane expression of GLUT-1, a key component of the glycolytic pathway, correlated with a greater Weiss score as well as shorter disease-free and overall survival.[103] High expression of YAP-1, a member of the Wnt/β-catenin signaling pathway, was associated with poor outcome, despite the fact that β-catenin expression itself did not correlate with prognosis.[104,105] *SHH* was upregulated in adult ACCs but downregulated in pediatric ones, but neither finding correlated with outcome.[106] The microRNA biogenesis pathway was investigated as a potential marker for ACT behavior, but 2 groups found drastically different relationships between *DICER1* and *TARBP2* levels and prognosis in adult ACTs; furthermore, adrenal tumors are not a consistent finding in the *DICER1*-pleuropulmonary blastoma familial tumor predisposition syndrome.[107–109] ACTs seen in the setting of McCune-Albright syndrome are usually associated with GNAS-activating mutations, but most of these patients have hyperplasia and not adenomas.[110]

Most of these studies were limited by, unsurprisingly, low case numbers and lack of a true definition of malignancy (most used Wieneke criteria), but nonetheless represent the forefront of efforts to find new ways to classify and treat pediatric ACTs.

SUMMARY

Can it be predicted when pediatric ACTs will behave badly? Not for certain, not for everyone, not yet. Some criteria, patient age, tumor size, tumor stage, and mitotic rate, can assist pathologists and their clinical colleagues in distinguishing obviously benign from obviously malignant cases. However, it is the borderline cases and the outlier cases that have historically posed the most trouble for physicians and patients alike. Better prognostic factors must be identified to ensure that patients are managed appropriately. The best opportunity for this lies within the realm of genetics, but much more work lies ahead to reach this important goal.

CLINICS CARE POINTS

- Children with adrenocortical tumors have a better prognosis than adults even when malignant pathologic features are present, and younger children fare better than older ones.
- Gross pathologic features, such as size greater than 5 cm and weight greater than 100 g, as well as higher clinical stage and venous invasion, portend a worse prognosis.
- Histopathologic features are generally inadequate at predicting behavior, although mitotic rate (or Ki67 immunohistochemical staining) and microscopic evidence of invasive growth suggest malignancy.
- *TP53* mutations are common in pediatric ACTs and, although not prognostically useful, could suggest an underlying tumor predisposition syndrome.

DISCLOSURE

None.

REFERENCES

1. Siegel DA, King J, Tai E, et al. Cancer incidence rates and trends among children and adolescents in the United States, 2001-2009. Pediatrics 2014; 134(4):e945–55.
2. Ward E, DeSantis C, Robbins A, et al. Childhood and adolescent cancer statistics, 2014. CA Cancer J Clin 2014;64(2):83–103.
3. Pinto NR, Applebaum MA, Volchenboum SL, et al. Advances in risk classification and treatment strategies for neuroblastoma. J Clin Oncol 2015;33(27): 3008–17.
4. Sharma R, Mer J, Lion A, et al. Clinical presentation, evaluation, and management of neuroblastoma. Pediatr Rev 2018;39(4):194–203.
5. Barr EK, Applebaum MA. Genetic predisposition to neuroblastoma. Children (Basel) 2018;5(9):119.
6. Shimada H, Ambros IM, Dehner LP, et al. The international neuroblastoma pathology classification (the Shimada system). Cancer 1999;86(2):364–72.
7. Jarzembowski JA, Rudzinski E, Shimada H. College of American Pathologists: protocol for the examination of specimens from patients with neuroblastoma. 2014.
8. Picarsic J, Reyes-Múgica M. Phenotype and immunophenotype of the most common pediatric tumors. Appl Immunohistochem Mol Morphol 2015; 23(5):313–26.
9. Monclair T, Brodeur GM, Ambros PF, et al, INRG Task Force. The International Neuroblastoma Risk Group (INRG) staging system: an INRG Task Force report. J Clin Oncol 2009;27(2):298–303.
10. Moroz V, Machin D, Faldum A, et al. Changes over three decades in outcome and the prognostic influence of age-at-diagnosis in young patients with neuroblastoma: a report from the International Neuroblastoma Risk Group Project. Eur J Cancer 2011; 47(4):561–71.
11. London WB, Castleberry RP, Matthay KK, et al. Evidence for an age cutoff greater than 365 days for neuroblastoma risk group stratification in the Children's Oncology Group. J Clin Oncol 2005;23(27): 6459–65.
12. Schmidt ML, Lal A, Seeger RC, et al. Favorable prognosis for patients 12 to 18 months of age with stage 4 nonamplified MYCN neuroblastoma: a Children's Cancer Group Study. J Clin Oncol 2005;23(27):6474–80.
13. Brodeur GM, Bagatell R. Mechanisms of neuroblastoma regression. Nat Rev Clin Oncol 2014; 11(12):704–13.
14. Brodeur GM. Spontaneous regression of neuroblastoma. Cell Tissue Res 2018;372(2):277–86.
15. Beckwith JB, Perrin EV. In situ neuroblastomas: a contribution to the natural history of neural crest tumors. Am J Pathol 1963;43(6):1089–104.
16. Sawada T. Past and future of neuroblastoma screening in Japan. Am J Pediatr Hematol Oncol 1992;14(4):320–6.
17. Naranjo A, Irwin MS, Hogarty MD, et al. Statistical framework in support of a revised Children's Oncology Group neuroblastoma risk classification system. JCO Clin Cancer Inform 2018;2:1–15.
18. Taggart DR, London WB, Schmidt ML, et al. Prognostic value of the stage 4S metastatic pattern and tumor biology in patients with metastatic neuroblastoma diagnosed between birth and 18 months of age. J Clin Oncol 2011; 29(33):4358–64.
19. Burchill SA, Beiske K, Shimada H, et al. Recommendations for the standardization of bone marrow disease assessment and reporting in children with

neuroblastoma on behalf of the International Neuroblastoma Response Criteria Bone Marrow Working Group. Cancer 2017;123(7):1095–105.

20. Beiske K, Burchill SA, Cheung IY, et al. Consensus criteria for sensitive detection of minimal neuroblastoma cells in bone marrow, blood and stem cell preparations by immunocytology and QRT-PCR: recommendations by the International Neuroblastoma Risk Group Task Force. Br J Cancer 2009; 100(10):1627–37.

21. Parsons LN, Gheorghe G, Yan K, et al. Improving detection of metastatic neuroblastoma in bone marrow core biopsies: a proposed immunohistochemical approach. Pediatr Dev Pathol 2016; 19(3):230–6.

22. Parsons LN, Gheorghe G, Yan K, et al. An evidence-based recommendation for a standardized approach to detecting metastatic neuroblastoma in staging bone marrow biopsies. Pediatr Dev Pathol 2017;20(1):38–43.

23. Hata JL, Correa H, Krishnan C, et al. Diagnostic utility of PHOX2B in primary and treated neuroblastoma and in neuroblastoma metastatic to the bone marrow. Arch Pathol Lab Med 2015;139(4): 543–6.

24. Nagai J, Kigasawa H, Tomioka K, et al. Immunocytochemical detection of bone marrow-invasive neuroblastoma cells. Eur J Haematol 1994;53(2):74–7.

25. Peuchmaur M, d'Amore ES, Joshi VV, et al. Revision of the International Neuroblastoma Pathology Classification: confirmation of favorable and unfavorable prognostic subsets in ganglioneuroblastoma, nodular. Cancer 2003;98(10):2274–81.

26. Hassan SF, Mathur S, Magliaro TJ, et al. Needle core vs open biopsy for diagnosis of intermediate- and high-risk neuroblastoma in children. J Pediatr Surg 2012;47(6):1261–6.

27. Deeney S, Stewart C, Treece AL, et al. Diagnostic utility of core needle biopsy versus open wedge biopsy for pediatric intraabdominal solid tumors: results of a prospective clinical study. J Pediatr Surg 2017;52(12):2042–6.

28. Sano H, Bonadio J, Gerbing RB, et al. International neuroblastoma pathology classification adds independent prognostic information beyond the prognostic contribution of age. Eur J Cancer 2006; 42(8):1113–9.

29. Sokol E, Desai AV, Applebaum MA, et al. Age, diagnostic category, tumor grade, and mitosis-karyorrhexis index are independently prognostic in neuroblastoma: an INRG project. J Clin Oncol 2020;38(17):1906–18.

30. Beltran H. The N-myc oncogene: maximizing its targets, regulation, and therapeutic potential. Mol Cancer Res 2014;12(6):815–22.

31. Shiloh Y, Shipley J, Brodeur GM, et al. Differential amplification, assembly, and relocation of multiple DNA sequences in human neuroblastomas and neuroblastoma cell lines. Proc Natl Acad Sci U S A 1985;82(11):3761–5.

32. Tornóczky T, Semjén D, Shimada H, et al. Pathology of peripheral neuroblastic tumors: significance of prominent nucleoli in undifferentiated/poorly differentiated neuroblastoma. Pathol Oncol Res 2007; 13(4):269–75.

33. Campbell K, Shyr D, Bagatell R, et al. Comprehensive evaluation of context dependence of the prognostic impact of MYCN amplification in neuroblastoma: a report from the International Neuroblastoma Risk Group (INRG) project. Pediatr Blood Cancer 2019;66(8):e27819.

34. Suganuma R, Wang LL, Sano H, et al. Peripheral neuroblastic tumors with genotype-phenotype discordance: a report from the Children's Oncology Group and the International Neuroblastoma Pathology Committee. Pediatr Blood Cancer 2013;60(3):363–70.

35. Wang LL, Teshiba R, Ikegaki N, et al. Augmented expression of MYC and/or MYCN protein defines highly aggressive MYC-driven neuroblastoma: a Children's Oncology Group study. Br J Cancer 2015;113(1):57–63.

36. Mossé YP, Laudenslager M, Longo L, et al. Identification of ALK as a major familial neuroblastoma predisposition gene. Nature 2008;455(7215): 930–5.

37. Bresler SC, Weiser DA, Huwe PJ, et al. ALK mutations confer differential oncogenic activation and sensitivity to ALK inhibition therapy in neuroblastoma. Cancer Cell 2014;26(5):682–94.

38. Mossé YP, Lim MS, Voss SD, et al. Safety and activity of crizotinib for paediatric patients with refractory solid tumours or anaplastic large-cell lymphoma: a Children's Oncology Group phase 1 consortium study. Lancet Oncol 2013;14(6): 472–80.

39. Koneru B, Lopez G, Farooqi A, et al. Telomere maintenance mechanisms define clinical outcome in high-risk neuroblastoma. Cancer Res 2020; 80(12):2663–75.

40. Valentijn LJ, Koster J, Zwijnenburg DA, et al. TERT rearrangements are frequent in neuroblastoma and identify aggressive tumors. Nat Genet 2015;47(12): 1411–4.

41. Kurihara S, Hiyama E, Onitake Y, et al. Clinical features of ATRX or DAXX mutated neuroblastoma. J Pediatr Surg 2014;49(12):1835–8.

42. Ambros PF, Ambros IM, Brodeur GM, et al. International consensus for neuroblastoma molecular diagnostics: report from the International Neuroblastoma Risk Group (INRG) Biology Committee. Br J Cancer 2009;100(9):1471–82.

43. Okamatsu C, London WB, Naranjo A, et al. Clinicopathological characteristics of ganglioneuroma and ganglioneuroblastoma: a report from the

CCG and COG. Pediatr Blood Cancer 2009;53(4): 563–9.

44. Brodeur GM, Minturn JE, Ho R, et al. Trk receptor expression and inhibition in neuroblastomas. Clin Cancer Res 2009;15(10):3244–50.

45. Sausen M, Leary RJ, Jones S, et al. Integrated genomic analyses identify ARID1A and ARID1B alterations in the childhood cancer neuroblastoma. Nat Genet 2013;45(1):12–7.

46. Vermeulen J, De Preter K, Naranjo A, et al. Predicting outcomes for children with neuroblastoma using a multigene-expression signature: a retrospective SIOPEN/COG/GPOH study. Lancet Oncol 2009;10(7):663–71.

47. Oberthuer A, Hero B, Berthold F, et al. Prognostic impact of gene expression-based classification for neuroblastoma. J Clin Oncol 2010;28(21):3506–15.

48. Tolbert VP, Matthay KK. Neuroblastoma: clinical and biological approach to risk stratification and treatment. Cell Tissue Res 2018;372(2):195–209.

49. Cohn SL, Pearson AD, London WB, et al. The International Neuroblastoma Risk Group (INRG) classification system: an INRG Task Force report. J Clin Oncol 2009;27(2):289–97.

50. Altekruse SF, Kosary CL, Krapcho M, et al, editors. SEER cancer statistics review, 1975-2007. Bethesda (MD): National Cancer Institute; 2010. Available at: https://seer.cancer.gov/csr/1975_2007/, based on November 2009 SEER data submission, posted to the SEER web site.

51. Hsing AW, Nam JM, Co Chien HT, et al. Risk factors for adrenal cancer: an exploratory study. Int J Cancer 1996;65(4):432–6.

52. Weiss LM. Comparative histologic study of 43 metastasizing and nonmetastasizing adrenocortical tumors. Am J Surg Pathol 1984;8(3):163–9.

53. Wieneke JA, Thompson LD, Heffess CS. Adrenal cortical neoplasms in the pediatric population: a clinicopathologic and immunophenotypic analysis of 83 patients. Am J Surg Pathol 2003;27(7):867–81.

54. Dehner LP, Hill DA. Adrenal cortical neoplasms in children: why so many carcinomas and yet so many survivors? Pediatr Dev Pathol 2009;12(4): 284–91.

55. Hough AJ, Hollifield JW, Page DL, et al. Prognostic factors in adrenal cortical tumors: a mathematical analysis of clinical and morphologic data. Am J Clin Pathol 1979;72:390–9.

56. van Slooten H, Schaberg A, Smeenk D, et al. Morphologic characteristics of benign and malignant adrenocortical tumors. Cancer 1985;55: 766–73.

57. Michalkiewicz E, Sandrini R, Figueiredo B, et al. Clinical and outcome characteristics of children with adrenocortical tumors: a report from the International Pediatric Adrenocortical Tumor Registry. J Clin Oncol 2004;22(5):838–45.

58. Sandrini R, Ribeiro RC, DeLacerda L. Childhood adrenocortical tumors. J Clin Endocrinol Metab 1997;82(7):2027–31.

59. Erickson LA. Challenges in surgical pathology of adrenocortical tumours. Histopathology 2018; 72(1):82–96.

60. Mete O, Asa SL, Giordano TJ, et al. Immunohistochemical biomarkers of adrenal cortical neoplasms. Endocr Pathol 2018;29(2):137–49.

61. Sung TY, Choi YM, Kim WG, et al. Myxoid and sarcomatoid variants of adrenocortical carcinoma: analysis of rare variants in single tertiary care center. J Korean Med Sci 2017;32(5):764–71.

62. Gulack BC, Rialon KL, Englum BR, et al. Factors associated with survival in pediatric adrenocortical carcinoma: an analysis of the National Cancer Data Base (NCDB). J Pediatr Surg 2016;51(1):172–7.

63. Pinto EM, Rodriguez-Galindo C, Pounds SB, et al. Identification of clinical and biologic correlates associated with outcome in children with adrenocortical tumors without germline TP53 mutations: a St Jude Adrenocortical Tumor Registry and Children's Oncology Group study. J Clin Oncol 2017; 35(35):3956–63.

64. Sabbaga CC, Avilla SG, Schulz C, et al. Adrenocortical carcinoma in children: clinical aspects and prognosis. J Pediatr Surg 1993;28(6):841–3.

65. American Joint Committee on Cancer. Adrenal Cortical. In: Amin MB, Greene FL, Edge SB, et al. editors. AJCC cancer staging manual. 8th edition. New York: Springer; 2017. p. 911–8.

66. Tucci S Jr, Martins AC, Suaid HJ, et al. The impact of tumor stage on prognosis in children with adrenocortical carcinoma. J Urol 2005;174(6):2338–42.

67. Bugg MF, Ribeiro RC, Roberson PK, et al. Correlation of pathologic features with clinical outcome in pediatric adrenocortical neoplasia. A study of a Brazilian population. Brazilian Group for Treatment of Childhood Adrenocortical Tumors. Am J Clin Pathol 1994;101(5):625–9.

68. Cagle PT, Hough AJ, Pysher TJ, et al. Comparison of adrenal cortical tumors in children and adults. Cancer 1986;57(11):2235–7.

69. Weiss LM, Medeiros LJ, Vickery ALJ. Pathologic features of prognostic significance in adrenocortical carcinoma. Am J Surg Pathol 1989;13:202–6.

70. Chatterjee G, DasGupta S, Mukherjee G, et al. Usefulness of Wieneke criteria in assessing morphologic characteristics of adrenocortical tumors in children. Pediatr Surg Int 2015;31(6):563-571.

71. Das S, Sengupta M, Islam N, et al. Wieneke criteria, Ki-67 index and p53 status to study pediatric adrenocortical tumors: is there a correlation? J Pediatr Surg 2016;51(11):1795–800.

72. Soon PS, Gill AJ, Benn DE, et al. Microarray gene expression and immunohistochemistry analyses of adrenocortical tumors identify IGF2 and Ki-67 as

useful in differentiating carcinomas from adenomas. Endocr Relat Cancer 2009;16(2):573–83.

73. Duregon E, Fassina A, Volante M, et al. The reticulin algorithm for adrenocortical tumor diagnosis: a multicentric validation study on 245 unpublished cases. Am J Surg Pathol 2013;37(9):1433–40.

74. Volante M, Bollito E, Sperone P, et al. Clinicopathological study of a series of 92 adrenocortical carcinomas: from a proposal of simplified diagnostic algorithm to prognostic stratification. Histopathology 2009;55(5):535–43.

75. Parise IZS, Parise GA, Noronha L, et al. The prognostic role of CD8+ T lymphocytes in childhood adrenocortical carcinomas compared to Ki-67, PD-1, PD-L1, and the weiss score. Cancers (Basel) 2019;11(11):1730.

76. Leite FA, Lira RC, Fedatto PF, et al. Low expression of HLA-DRA, HLA-DPA1, and HLA-DPB1 is associated with poor prognosis in pediatric adrenocortical tumors (ACT). Pediatr Blood Cancer 2014;61(11):1940–8.

77. Magro G, Esposito G, Cecchetto G, et al. Pediatric adrenocortical tumors: morphological diagnostic criteria and immunohistochemical expression of matrix metalloproteinase type 2 and human leucocyte-associated antigen (HLA) class II antigens. Results from the Italian Pediatric Rare Tumor (TREP) Study project. Hum Pathol 2012;43(1):31–9.

78. Achatz MI, Olivier M, Le Calvez F, et al. The TP53 mutation, R337H, is associated with Li-Fraumeni and Li-Fraumeni-like syndromes in Brazilian families. Cancer Lett 2007;245(1–2):96-102.

79. Wasserman JD, Novokmet A, Eichler-Jonsson C, et al. Prevalence and functional consequence of TP53 mutations in pediatric adrenocortical carcinoma: a Children's Oncology Group study. J Clin Oncol 2015;33(6):602–9.

80. Latronico AC, Pinto EM, Domenice S, et al. An inherited mutation outside the highly conserved DNA-binding domain of the p53 tumor suppressor protein in children and adults with sporadic adrenocortical tumors. J Clin Endocrinol Metab 2001; 86(10):4970–3.

81. Ragazzon B, Libé R, Gaujoux S, et al. Transcriptome analysis reveals that p53 and {beta}-catenin alterations occur in a group of aggressive adrenocortical cancers. Cancer Res 2010;70(21):8276–81.

82. Faria AM, Almeida MQ. Differences in the molecular mechanisms of adrenocortical tumorigenesis between children and adults. Mol Cell Endocrinol 2012;351(1):52–7.

83. Pinto EM, Chen X, Easton J, et al. Genomic landscape of paediatric adrenocortical tumours. Nat Commun 2015;6:6302.

84. Ribeiro TC, Latronico AC. Insulin-like growth factor system on adrenocortical tumorigenesis. Mol Cell Endocrinol 2012;351(1):96–100.

85. Wilkin F, Gagné N, Paquette J, et al. Pediatric adrenocortical tumors: molecular events leading to insulin-like growth factor II gene overexpression. J Clin Endocrinol Metab 2000;85(5): 2048–56.

86. West AN, Neale GA, Pounds S, et al. Gene expression profiling of childhood adrenocortical tumors. Cancer Res 2007;67(2):600–8.

87. Peixoto Lira RC, Fedatto PF, Marco Antonio DS, et al. IGF2 and IGF1R in pediatric adrenocortical tumors: roles in metastasis and steroidogenesis. Endocr Relat Cancer 2016;23(6):481–93.

88. Creemers SG, van Koetsveld PM, van Kemenade FJ, et al. Methylation of IGF2 regulatory regions to diagnose adrenocortical carcinomas. Endocr Relat Cancer 2016;23(9):727–37.

89. Gicquel C, Bertagna X, Schneid H, et al. Rearrangements at the 11p15 locus and overexpression of insulin-like growth factor-II gene in sporadic adrenocortical tumors. J Clin Endocrinol Metab 1994;78(6):1444–53.

90. Rosati R, Cerrato F, Doghman M, et al. High frequency of loss of heterozygosity at 11p15 and IGF2 overexpression are not related to clinical outcome in childhood adrenocortical tumors positive for the R337H TP53 mutation. Cancer Genet Cytogenet 2008;186(1):19–24.

91. Almeida MQ, Fragoso MC, Lotfi CF, et al. Expression of insulin-like growth factor-II and its receptor in pediatric and adult adrenocortical tumors. J Clin Endocrinol Metab 2008;93(9):3524–31.

92. Doghman M, El Wakil A, Cardinaud B, et al. Regulation of insulin-like growth factor-mammalian target of rapamycin signaling by microRNA in childhood adrenocortical tumors. Cancer Res 2010;70(11): 4666–75.

93. Figueiredo BC, Stratakis CA, Sandrini R, et al. Comparative genomic hybridization analysis of adrenocortical tumors of childhood. J Clin Endocrinol Metab 1999;84(3):1116–21.

94. James LA, Kelsey AM, Birch JM, et al. Highly consistent genetic alterations in childhood adrenocortical tumours detected by comparative genomic hybridization. Br J Cancer 1999;81(2):300–4.

95. Wong M, Ikeda Y, Luo X, et al. Steroidogenic factor 1 plays multiple roles in endocrine development and function. Recent Prog Horm Res 1997;52: 167–84.

96. Almeida MQ, Soares IC, Ribeiro TC, et al. Steroidogenic factor 1 overexpression and gene amplification are more frequent in adrenocortical tumors from children than from adults. J Clin Endocrinol Metab 2010;95(3):1458–62.

97. Sbiera S, Schmull S, Assie G, et al. High diagnostic and prognostic value of steroidogenic factor-1 expression in adrenal tumors. J Clin Endocrinol Metab 2010;95(10):E161–71.

98. Pianovski MA, Cavalli LR, Figueiredo BC, et al. SF-1 overexpression in childhood adrenocortical tumours. Eur J Cancer 2006;42(8):1040–3.

99. Letouzé E, Rosati R, Komechen H, et al. SNP array profiling of childhood adrenocortical tumors reveals distinct pathways of tumorigenesis and highlights candidate driver genes. J Clin Endocrinol Metab 2012;97(7):E1284–93.

100. Kulshrestha A, Suman S, Ranjan R. Network analysis reveals potential markers for pediatric adrenocortical carcinoma. Onco Targets Ther 2016;9: 4569–81.

101. Zerbini C, Kozakewich HPW, Weinberg DS, et al. Adrenocortical neoplasms in childhood and adolescence: analysis of prognostic factors including DNA content. Endocr Pathol 1992;3(3):116–28.

102. Pilon C, Pistorello M, Moscon A, et al. Inactivation of the p16 tumor suppressor gene in adrenocortical tumors. J Clin Endocrinol Metab 1999;84(8):2776–9.

103. Pinheiro C, Granja S, Longatto-Filho A, et al. GLUT1 expression in pediatric adrenocortical tumors: a promising candidate to predict clinical behavior. Oncotarget 2017;8(38):63835–45.

104. Abduch RH, Carolina Bueno A, Leal LF, et al. Unraveling the expression of the oncogene YAP1, a Wnt/beta-catenin target, in adrenocortical tumors and its association with poor outcome in pediatric patients. Oncotarget 2016;7(51): 84634–44.

105. Tissier F, Cavard C, Groussin L, et al. Mutations of beta-catenin in adrenocortical tumors: activation of the Wnt signaling pathway is a frequent event in both benign and malignant adrenocortical tumors. Cancer Res 2005;65(17):7622–7.

106. Gomes DC, Leal LF, Mermejo LM, et al. Sonic hedgehog signaling is active in human adrenal cortex development and deregulated in adrenocortical tumors. J Clin Endocrinol Metab 2014;99(7): E1209–16.

107. de Sousa GR, Ribeiro TC, Faria AM, et al. Low DICER1 expression is associated with poor clinical outcome in adrenocortical carcinoma. Oncotarget 2015;6(26):22724–33.

108. Caramuta S, Lee L, Ozata DM, et al. Clinical and functional impact of TARBP2 over-expression in adrenocortical carcinoma. Endocr Relat Cancer 2013;20(4):551–64.

109. Schultz KA, Yang J, Doros L, et al. DICER1-pleuropulmonary blastoma familial tumor predisposition syndrome: a unique constellation of neoplastic conditions. Pathol Case Rev 2014; 19(2):90–100.

110. Almeida MQ, Azevedo MF, Xekouki P, et al. Activation of cyclic AMP signaling leads to different pathway alterations in lesions of the adrenal cortex caused by germline PRKAR1A defects versus those due to somatic GNAS mutations. J Clin Endocrinol Metab 2012;97(4):E687–93.

Pediatric Cystic Lung Lesions: Where Are We Now?

Nahir Cortes-Santiago, MD, PhD[a,b], Gail H. Deutsch, MD[c,d],*

KEYWORDS

- Bronchogenic cyst • Bronchial atresia • Pulmonary airway malformation • Sequestration
- Congenital lobar overinflation • Pleuropulmonary blastoma • Birt-Hogg-Dubé syndrome

Key points

- Airway obstruction underlies many congenital cystic lung malformations.
- Revised classifications and nomenclature have been proposed for congenital cystic lung malformations to encompass their pathogenesis and clinical behavior.
- Genetic conditions and neoplasms can present with cystic lung lesions.

ABSTRACT

Pediatric cystic lung lesions have long been a source of confusion for clinicians, radiologists, and pathologists. They encompass a wide spectrum of entities with variable prognostic implications, including congenital lung malformations, pulmonary neoplasms, and hereditary conditions. As our understanding of the developmental and genetic origins of these conditions has evolved, revised nomenclature and classifications have emerged in an attempt to bring clarity to the origin of these lesions and guide clinical management. This review discusses cystic lung lesions and the current understanding of their etiopathogenesis.

pulmonary neoplasms, and hereditary conditions. As the understanding of the developmental and genetic origins of these conditions has evolved, revised nomenclature and classifications have emerged in an attempt to bring clarity to the origin of these lesions and guide clinical management. This review discusses cystic lung lesions and the current understanding of their etiopathogenesis.

OVERVIEW

Pediatric cystic lung lesions have long been a source of confusion for clinicians, radiologists, and pathologists. They encompass a wide spectrum of entities with variable prognostic implications, including congenital lung malformations,

CONGENITAL CYSTIC LUNG MALFORMATIONS

OVERVIEW

Congenital cystic lung malformations are commonly encountered lesions in children, especially with the widespread use of antenatal ultrasound. Although many of these malformations were initially presumed to be distinct entities, they frequently share common etiologic mechanisms and histopathologic features. For example, bronchogenic cysts and extralobar sequestrations (ELS) reflect abnormal budding of the foregut during development, whereas congenital pulmonary airway malformations, intralobar sequestrations

[a] Department of Pathology and Immunology, Baylor College of Medicine, BCM 315, One Baylor Plaza, Houston, TX 77030, USA; [b] Department of Pathology, Texas Children's Hospital, 6621 Fannin Street Suite AB1195, Houston, TX 77030, USA; [c] Department of Pathology, University of Washington School of Medicine, Seattle, WA, USA; [d] Department of Laboratories, Seattle Children's Hospital, OC.8.720, 4800 Sand Point Way Northeast, Seattle, WA 98105, USA
* Corresponding author. Department of Laboratories, Seattle Children's Hospital, OC.8.720, 4800 Sand Point Way Northeast, Seattle, WA 98105.
E-mail address: gail.deutsch@seattlechildrens.org

Surgical Pathology 13 (2020) 643–655
https://doi.org/10.1016/j.path.2020.07.002
1875-9181/20/© 2020 Elsevier Inc. All rights reserved.

(ILSs), pulmonary hyperplasia, and congenital lobar overinflation often arise in the context of airway obstruction during development (**Fig. 1**).[1–3] Although the Stocker classification is still widely used, new radiology- and pathology-based classifications have been proposed to reflect the current understanding of the pathogenesis of these lesions and to guide care (**Box 1**).[4–6]

FOREGUT DUPLICATION/BRONCHOGENIC CYSTS

Introduction

Foregut duplication and bronchogenic cysts arise from anomalous budding of the foregut endoderm from which the respiratory tract and upper gastrointestinal tract develop, as well as other organ systems. Bronchogenic cysts most commonly are found within the mediastinum around the tracheal bifurcation, although intraparenchymal and supra- and subdiaphragmatic locations are well recognized.[7] They do not communicate with the normal tracheobronchial tree unless secondarily infected, which commonly occurs in intraparenchymal cysts.

Gross Features

Foregut duplication and bronchogenic cysts are unilocular lesions without septations or papillary excrescences (**Fig. 2**A). Mucinous viscous fluid generally fills the cystic cavity; the contents may be purulent or bloody in the presence of superimposed infection or hemorrhage, respectively.

Microscopic Features

Most of the foregut duplication cysts are lined by ciliated respiratory epithelium. However, other types of epithelia are well described, including intestinal, gastric, and squamous lining. The term "bronchogenic cyst" is used when respiratory epithelium overlies a wall resembling a bronchus, including smooth muscle and hyaline cartilage plates; bronchial type glands are often present (**Fig. 2**B). In the absence of cartilage in the wall, the more general term "foregut duplication cyst" can be applied.

Differential Diagnosis

When inflamed and intraparenchymal, bronchogenic cysts should be distinguished from an abscess or large cyst congenital pulmonary airway malformation. In contrast to a bronchogenic cyst, both of these entities have multiple lumens.

Diagnosis

Patients with foregut duplication/bronchogenic cysts generally come to medical attention due to symptoms related to compression of adjacent structures, superimposed infection, or incidental detection on imaging performed for unrelated reasons. Diagnosis is ultimately achieved on pathologic examination.

CONGENITAL PULMONARY AIRWAY MALFORMATION

Introduction

Congenital pulmonary airway malformations (CPAMs), formerly congenital cystic

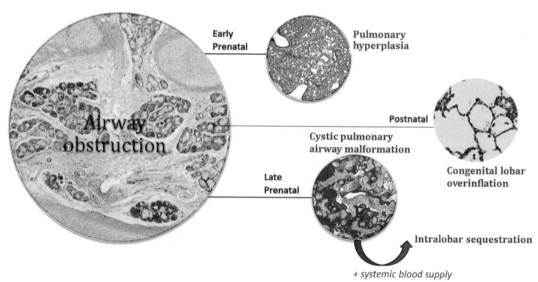

Fig. 1. Proposed pathogenesis of congenital cystic lung malformations. Airway obstruction is a common pathogenetic mechanism underlying many cystic lesions. The timing of insult during development is thought to drive their variable histologic appearance.

Box 1
Langston classification of congenital lung malformations

- Bronchopulmonary malformations
  - Bronchogenic cyst/bronchopulmonary foregut malformation
  - Extralobar sequestration
    - Isolated
    - With cystic pulmonary airway malformation, small cyst type (hybrid lesion)
  - Cystic pulmonary airway malformation, large cyst type (Stocker type 1)
    - Isolated
    - With systemic arterial/venous connection (hybrid lesion/intralobar sequestration)
  - Cystic pulmonary airway malformation, small cyst type (Stocker type 2)
    - Isolated
    - Associated with bronchial atresia (bronchial obstruction sequence)
    - With systemic arterial/venous connection (hybrid lesion/intralobar sequestration)
- Pulmonary hyperplasia and related lesions
  - Congenital high airway obstruction syndrome
  - Solid congenital pulmonary airway malformation (Stocker type 3)
  - Polyalveolar lobe
- Congenital lobar overinflation
- Other cystic lesions
  - Enteric cysts/foregut cysts
  - Type I/Ir pleuropulmonary blastoma
  - Lymphatic/lymphangiomatous cysts
  - Mesothelial cysts
  - Simple parenchymal cysts

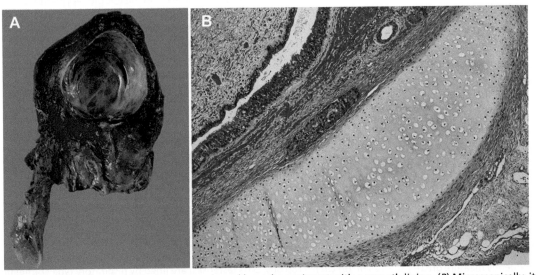

Fig. 2. Bronchogenic cyst. (*A*) An intraparenchymal bronchogenic cyst with a smooth lining. (*B*) Microscopically, it resembles a normal bronchus, lined by respiratory epithelium and containing submucosal glands and cartilage in the wall.

adenomatoid malformations, are the most common malformation of the lower respiratory tract.[8] In a recent study on the distribution of congenital cystic lung malformations, type 2 CPAM was the most frequent lesion followed by ILS.[9] Historically, cystic lung lesions have been divided into subtypes according to the Stocker classification, based on cyst size and their histologic resemblance to segments of the respiratory tree, from trachea and large bronchi to peripheral acini.[5,10] Although this classification proved useful at the time of its inception, our current understanding of the pathogenesis and clinical behavior of these lesions has brought into question its continued utility.[4] Stocker type 0 CPAM is now recognized to be acinar dysplasia, a rare developmental lung disorder associated with mutations in the T-box transcription factor 4 and the fibroblast growth factor signaling pathway.[11–13] Stocker type 3 CPAM is prenatal pulmonary hyperplasia, and Stocker type 4 CPAM represents the cystic variant of pleuropulmonary blastoma (see later discussion). Because of the frequent occurrence of "hybrid lesions" (CPAM in pulmonary sequestrations), Langston divided the most common CPAMs into 2 types: a large cyst type (equivalent to Stocker type 1) and a small cyst type (equivalent to Stocker type 2), with subclassification based on the presence or absence of systemic blood supply.[4] This terminology has been in part adopted in the radiographic literature to guide clinical management.[6,14] The term "bronchial obstruction sequence" also reflects the common pathogenesis and shared histologic features seen in a significant proportion of small cyst CPAM, ILS and ELS.[2,3]

LARGE CYST CONGENITAL PULMONARY AIRWAY MALFORMATION (STOCKER TYPE 1)

Gross Features

Large cyst CPAMs are typically composed of cysts greater than or equal to 2 cm in size, which may be multiloculated (**Fig. 3**A). In a recent large study of congenital cystic lung lesions, features of airway obstruction were seen in 18% of CPAM type 1, and none were associated with a systemic arterial supply.[9]

Microscopic Features

Large cyst CPAMs are lined by columnar respiratory epithelium, with the majority containing clusters of mucinous cells (**Fig. 3**B). The cysts resemble bronchioles with walls generally devoid of cartilage or glands. Papillary infolding of the cyst's respiratory epithelium is commonly seen, as well as abrupt transition from the cyst's columnar epithelium to alveolar parenchyma (**Fig. 3**C).[9]

Differential Diagnosis

The differential includes other large cystic lesions of the lung including bronchogenic cyst, pneumatocele, pulmonary interstitial emphysema, and cystic variant of pleuropulmonary blastoma (PPB). A bronchogenic cyst is a single, self-contained cyst without connection to adjacent lung. Pneumatoceles and pulmonary interstitial emphysema, sequela to pneumonia or positive pressure ventilation, respectively, are air-filled cysts and are not lined by respiratory epithelium. The cysts in the cystic variant of PPB are alveolar versus respiratory in histologic appearance and have nests of primitive spindle cells in the wall and frequent nodules of cartilage.

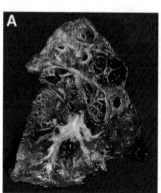 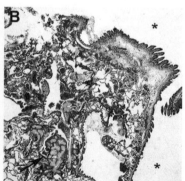 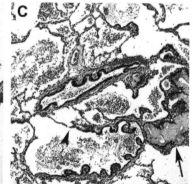

Fig. 3. Congenital pulmonary airway malformation, large cyst type. (*A*) The lesion contains multiple cysts, which frequently measure greater than 2 cm. (*B*) On microscopy, cysts (*asterisks*) are lined by respiratory type epithelium with papillary epithelial infoldings and have smooth muscle in their wall. Mucogenic epithelium (*arrows*, in B and C) is identified in variable proportion. (*C*) Cysts are seen in direct continuity with alveolar spaces (*arrowhead*).

Diagnosis

Because of their size, large cyst CPAMs are commonly recognized via prenatal ultrasound. Most lesions decrease in size with gestational age and are asymptomatic at birth. Persistent large lesions may present with fetal hydrops or neonatal respiratory distress. Postnatal symptom onset may occur with cyst expansion from air influx and compression of adjacent lung. In instances where the lesions are not detected until later childhood, symptoms related to infection may predominate. Imaging findings vary depending on the time of detection, cyst size, and persistence of amniotic fluid in the lesion.[14]

SMALL CYST CONGENITAL PULMONARY AIRWAY MALFORMATION (STOCKER TYPE 2)

Gross Features

Small cyst CPAMs (Stocker type 2) are composed of multiple small cysts that are relatively uniform in size and generally less than 2 cm in diameter. When carefully dissected, an atretic or stenotic bronchus at the lobar, segmental, or subsegmental level may be identified, with or without a mucocele (**Fig. 4**A). Some of these lesions may have a systemic arterial supply, which is termed ILS or hybrid lesion. In other instances, there is isolated bronchial atresia with a single cyst filled with mucus (mucocele) and minimal associated parenchyma.

Microscopic Features

Microscopically, small cyst CPAMs are composed of numerous dilated bronchiole-like structures (microcystic maldevelopment) lined by cuboidal to ciliated respiratory epithelium that have variable amounts of intervening alveolar parenchyma (**Fig. 4**B). These cysts are not accompanied by arteries. Features of airway obstruction, including mucostasis and foamy macrophages, are commonly seen and support the notion that this lesion represents a manifestation of airway obstruction during development. There may be foci of skeletal muscle (rhabdomyomatous differentiation) around the cysts and these should not be construed as evidence of pleuropulmonary blastoma.

Diagnosis

Although small cyst CPAMs were initially thought to carry a poor prognosis due to their association with other anomalies, including renal and cardiac, increased prenatal detection of this malformation has confirmed that they are largely isolated and asymptomatic.[5] Depending on the size, they may present in the neonatal period with respiratory distress. Imaging typically shows a heterogeneous mass with small cystic spaces.[14]

Differential Diagnosis

The main differential diagnosis is an ILS/hybrid lesion, which would require identification of systemic arterial blood supply.

BRONCHOPULMONARY SEQUESTRATION

Introduction

Sequestrations are cystic lung lesions that lack connection to the tracheobronchial tree and have systemic arterial perfusion. Arterial supply is usually derived from the abdominal or thoracic aorta, but other sources have been described, including the celiac and splenic arteries.[15] Venous drainage may occur through either pulmonary or systemic veins. ELS form a separate mass of lung with its own pleural lining, whereas ILS are nonfunctioning lung segments embedded within the pleura of the lung lobe in which they arise. As stated earlier, ILS commonly have small cyst CPAM features and

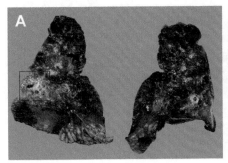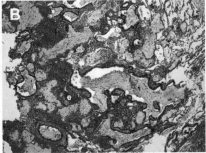

Fig. 4. Congenital pulmonary airway malformation, small cyst type. (*A*) In this bisected lung, a small cluster of small cystic spaces (*rectangle*) is seen in the region of a proximally dilated bronchus (*arrow*). (*B*) Microscopically, the lesion is composed of an increased number of bronchiole-like structures (microcystic maldevelopment), often with prominent mucostasis, which indicates bronchial obstruction.

bronchial obstruction, bringing to question the need for disparate nomenclature.[4] The term "hybrid lesion" is frequently used in this setting. Although ELS arise from abnormal supernumerary budding of the foregut, they also frequently exhibit microcystic maldevelopment due to proximal bronchial atresia.[4,15]

Gross Features

ELS lies outside the visceral pleura of the lung, similar to an accessory lobe, invested by its own pleural lining with or without connection to the gastrointestinal tract. More commonly, they arise within the thoracic cavity, but infradiaphragmatic locations are not uncommon. They contain a vascular pedicle with a systemic artery and draining vein (**Fig. 5A**).

ILS may resemble a small cyst CPAM, including dilated airways filled with mucus and an atretic bronchus at the proximal aspect of the lesion. On cut section, ILS is usually well defined from the adjacent normal lung. It may be altered by prolonged infection and inflammation. Thick-walled feeding systemic arteries may be visible, distinct from the normal vascular structures at the hilum (**Fig. 5B**).

Microscopic Features

Microscopically, ELS have absent or reduced numbers of cartilaginous bronchi and variably mature alveolar spaces. The vessels are large and thick walled, reflecting systemic vascular supply. Features of small cyst CPAM/bronchial atresia sequence with mucus accumulation and a proliferation of bronchiole-like structures are present in a large proportion of cases (**Fig. 5C**). The remainder resemble near-normal lung with enlarged and poorly subdivided airspaces or have features of pulmonary hyperplasia (see later discussion).

Microscopic features of ILS largely depend on when the lesion is detected and excised. In antenatally and incidentally discovered lesions, the microscopic features will overlap with those of ELS and small cyst CPAM. In lesions diagnosed later in life the histologic features may be obscured by the presence of fibrosis and chronic inflammation due to recurring infections.

Differential Diagnosis

Differentiating ILS from small cyst CPAM relies on identification of systemic arterial blood supply. When infected, ILS may be confused with a chronic pneumonia, although the latter has a normal bronchial connection with the involved lung.

Diagnosis

ELS is more commonly seen in association with other congenital abnormalities, including diaphragmatic hernia, cardiovascular anomalies, and other foregut cysts.[16] Imaging in ELS typically shows an echogenic mass, usually in the left lower thoracic region. ILS on the other hand will be an

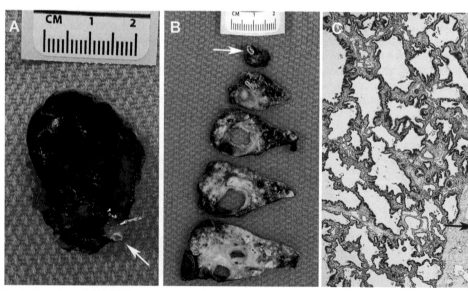

Fig. 5. Bronchopulmonary sequestrations. (*A*) Extralobar sequestration is invested in its own pleura, whereas intralobar sequestration (*B*) is an intraparenchymal lesion. They both have systemic blood supply (*arrows*). (*C*) Microscopically, sequestrations resected early in life will show similar features, with large elastic arteries (*arrow*) and frequent microcystic maldevelopment, identical to small cyst CPAM.

intraparenchymal lesion with a variable imaging appearance that may include a soft tissue mass, focal emphysema, or cystic lesion.[14] Identification of anomalous systemic blood supply radiographically and surgically is a defining feature for both entities.

PULMONARY HYPERPLASIA AND CONGENITAL LOBAR OVERINFLATION

Introduction

Pulmonary hyperplasia (polyalveolar lobe) is characterized by an excessive growth of pulmonary parenchyma. It is the result of airway obstruction early in prenatal life, which blocks the outflow of fetal fluid in the lung, leading to an increase in alveoli.[17] Similarly, congenital high airway obstruction (eg, laryngeal atresia, tracheal stenosis) leads to diffuse, bilateral pulmonary hyperplasia.[18]

Congenital lobar overinflation (CLO) is progressive air trapping of a pulmonary lobe. CLO may be caused by intrinsic (abnormal bronchial cartilage, mucous plugging) or extrinsic (mass lesions) compression of an airway, leading to a one-way valve effect in which air passes to the distal lung but cannot exit. In many cases no identifiable cause is uncovered.[19,20] CLO can be seen in isolation, or complicating cases of pulmonary hyperplasia, in which there has been time for air trapping to occur after birth.

Gross Features

In both pulmonary hyperplasia and CLO, the involved lung lobes are enlarged, bulky, and often pale (**Fig. 6**A, C). CLO commonly affects the left upper lobe. No grossly identifiable cysts are seen.

Microscopic Features

Pulmonary hyperplasia is characterized by a marked increase in radial alveolar count, with normal or near-normal number of bronchial generations.[21] Although increased in number, alveoli are often enlarged and simplified (**Fig. 6**B). Small cyst CPAM changes may be present. In CLO there is marked alveolar distension, similar to pulmonary emphysema[22] (**Fig. 6**D). The histology of CLO may be seen in isolation or in combination with pulmonary hyperplasia. Hybrid lesions containing features of CLO and small cyst CPAM also occur, which underscores airway obstruction as a common cause of cystic lung malformations.

Differential Diagnosis

Pulmonary hyperplasia is differentiated from CLO in that the parenchymal enlargement is due to absolute increase in number of alveoli versus alveolar distension. Radial alveolar count (RAC) is helpful in distinguishing these entities. In a term infant, RAC should average 5 alveolar spaces, which increases to approximately 8 to 10 by 1 year of age. Although CLO is often referred as congenital lobar emphysema, the term "emphysema" is incorrect, as alveolar wall destruction does not accompany alveolar distension.

Diagnosis

Pulmonary hyperplasia can present in utero with polyhydramnios or fetal hydrops, the latter from compression of venous return. Marked expansion of the involved lobe in CLO may lead to mediastinal shift with compression of adjacent lung and tension pneumothorax. In both entities, patients typically present with respiratory distress, which often necessitates surgical intervention and resection.[17,19,23] Chest radiographs show diffuse hazy opacities when there is retained fetal lung liquid in pulmonary hyperplasia, or progressive hyperinflation or hyperlucency of the affected lobe in CLO. Infants may have associated anomalies, including cardiovascular, diaphragmatic, and omphalocele, among others.[20]

General Prognosis of Congenital Cystic Lung Malformations

Overall, the prognosis of congenital lung malformations is favorable after complete surgical resection. Patients with large CPAMs and sequestrations may have pulmonary hypoplasia and/or hypertension due to compression of normal lung and adjacent structures.[4] Mucogenic epithelium in type 1 CPAM is thought to harbor the potential for progression to neoplasia, given the reported occurrence of adenocarcinoma, predominantly bronchioloalveolar type, arising in these lesions and detection of genetic alterations akin to those seen in de novo bronchioloalveolar carcinoma.[24,25]

Clinical Care Points

- Congenital lung malformations carry a good prognosis in the absence of associated anomalies, pulmonary hypoplasia, or hypertension.
- Although most lung malformations are diagnosed by prenatal ultrasound or in the neonatal period, they may be asymptomatic for years or present with episodes of recurrent pneumonia.
- Complete resection of congenital lung malformations is frequently recommended to prevent compression of adjacent structures, superimposed infection, and the rare risk of malignant transformation.

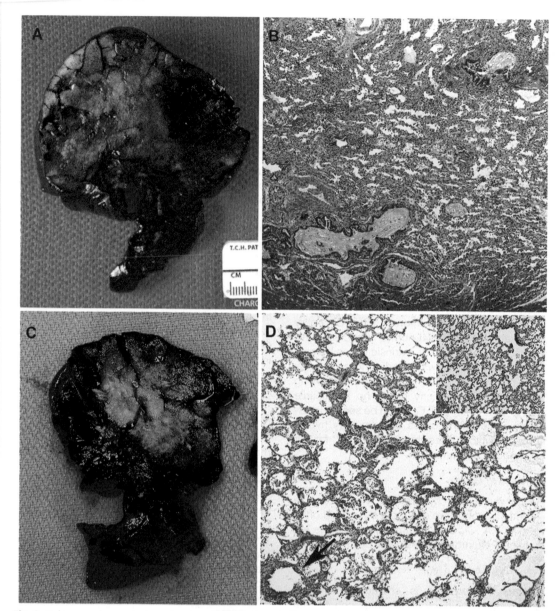

Fig. 6. Pulmonary hyperplasia and congenital lobar overinflation. In both pulmonary hyperplasia (A) and congenital lobar overinflation (C) the involved lung is enlarged, bulky, and pale compared with the adjacent normal lung. (B). Pulmonary hyperplasia shows an increased number of alveoli, which are immature in appearance; features of airway obstruction may be present. (D) Histologically congenital lobar overinflation shows markedly dilated airspaces, relative to an airway (arrow), and normal term lung (insert).

GENETIC CONDITIONS AND NEOPLASMS

PLEUROPULMONARY BLASTOMA

Introduction

Pleuropulmonary blastoma (PPB) is the most common primary parenchymal lung malignancy in the pediatric population.[26] Three types are recognized delineating a spectrum of malignant transformation from type I PPB, which is purely cystic, type II with cystic and solid components, to type III, which is predominantly a solid sarcomatous tumor. Consistent with malignant progression of the 3 types, differences in age of presentation exist.[27] Type I PPB typically presents within the first year of life and may be detected prenatally, type III predominates in patients older than 2 years, and type II presents in between these 2 age extremes.[27,28] Similarly, prognosis is affected by age, with older children faring worse with more aggressive tumors than younger patients.[27] PPB should not be confused with the adult biphasic pulmonary blastoma, an entirely different entity both histologically and pathogenetically.

It is now widely recognized that PPB is largely a genetically driven tumor caused by mutations in the *DICER1* gene.[28,29] DICER1 is a small RNA-processing enzyme with critical functions in the processing and activation of microRNAs, which are themselves critical for regulation of gene expression.[30] Although initially thought that 25% to 30% of PPBs were associated with *DICER1* mutations, newer data suggest that up to 70% of patients with PPB may carry an inherited or de novo germline inactivating *DICER1* mutation, whereas most of the remaining 30% have *DICER1* mutations in a mosaic or tumor-specific manner.[31] Autosomal dominant inherited mutations in *DICER1* form the basis of the *DICER1* tumor predisposition syndrome. Importantly, *DICER1* is considered a tumor suppressor gene, and it conforms to the Knudson two-hit hypothesis in which a second hit (ie, inactivation of the second allele) is required for tumorigenesis. However, the existence of a regressed type Ir PPB suggests that additional genetic or environmental hits are required for progression of disease. In this regard, loss of p53 and activating NRAS mutations have been identified in a subset of patients.[32]

Gross Features

Types I and Ir PPB usually present as peripheral, multiloculated cysts, with thin walls containing no solid components, although they may be hemorrhagic (**Fig. 7**A).[28] Type II PPB is a mixed cystic and solid mass with plaque-like thickening of the cyst walls, solid nodules, or polypoid projections toward the cyst lumen. Type III PPB is almost an entirely solid tumor with frank malignant features commonly seen (**Fig. 7**E). These include regions of hemorrhage, necrosis, and degenerative features. The interface with adjacent parenchyma is variable and may range from sharply delineated to diffusely infiltrative.[33]

Microscopic Features

Type I PPB generally shows thin cyst walls lined by flattened to cuboidal epithelium with varying degrees of primitive mesenchymal cells condensing beneath the epithelial lining, resulting in a cambium layer (**Fig. 7**B). Although most of the cases show a well-formed cambium layer, this can be focal and requires extensive sampling to identify. Skeletal muscle differentiation may be seen within the septa as well as mature cartilage. In a minority of cases there are blastema-like components. Occasionally, nodules of spindle cells resembling mature fibroblasts may be the only component distinguishing a PPB versus a benign lung cyst. By immunohistochemistry, scattered tumor cells are positive for markers of skeletal muscle differentiation (desmin, myogenin, and MyoD1) similar to that seen in embryonal rhabdomyosarcoma; however, lack of expression of these markers does not exclude the diagnosis of PPB.[28,33]

Type Ir PPB is distinguished from type I PPB by the absence of neoplastic cells in conjunction with features of tumor regression, including coagulative necrosis of the septae, hemorrhage, dystrophic calcification, and stromal fibrosis.[28] (**Fig. 7**C).

Type II and type III PPB both contain frankly malignant features composed of sarcomatous and blastematous elements, although type II retains a partial cystic architecture.[33] Sarcomatous elements generally display a fascicular pattern of growth resembling that of fibrosarcoma, although multiple mesenchymal components may be present including rhabdomyoblastic, cartilaginous, and lipoblastic differentiation (**Fig. 7**D, F). Blastematous elements are composed of immature cells with hyperchromatic nuclei, high nuclear to cytoplasmic ratio, and often increased mitotic activity. Anaplasia usually accompanies malignant progression and is characterized by bizarre, giant, and pleomorphic cells. Solid, tumefactive growths tend to have varying degrees of necrosis, which may be grossly visible.

Differential Diagnosis

The differential diagnosis varies with the type of PPB, with the most challenging being distinguishing type I PPB from a CPAM. Although a solitary type 1 PPB may resemble a large cyst CPAM on imaging and gross appearance, cystic PPBs are lined by alveolar type airspaces with a well-circumscribed border from adjacent lung parenchyma, whereas large cyst CPAMs are lined by bronchiolar type epithelium and transition to adjacent lung parenchyma. Rhabdomyomatous differentiation in a CPAM may occur but is not accompanied by small primitive cells within the septa as in type I PPB. As mentioned earlier, there is strong evidence to support that CPAM type 4, composed of alveolar type airspaces, is the cystic variant (type I) of PPB.[34,35] The solid components in types II and III PPB may resemble other sarcomas, such as embryonal rhabdomyosarcoma, but PPBs are typically heterogeneous with varying morphology and cell differentiation.

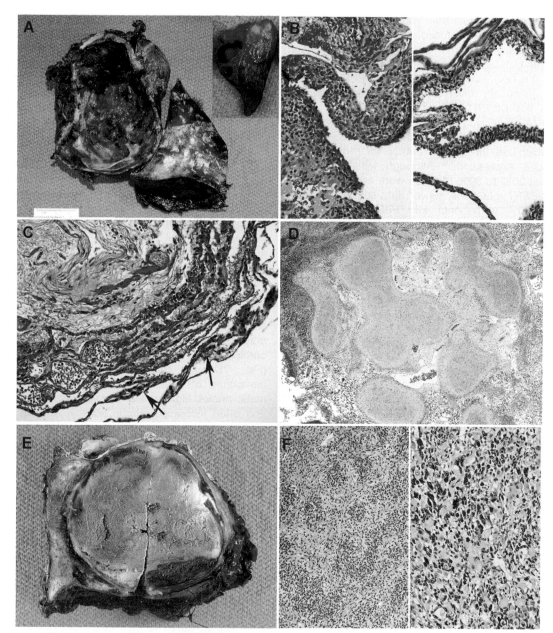

Fig. 7. Pleuropulmonary blastoma. (*A*) Type I pleuropulmonary blastoma (PPB) as a peripheral cystic lesion with extensive hemorrhage. Insert demonstrates a type Ir PPB composed of simple cysts. (*B*) Histologically type I PPB is composed of alveolar type septa with a condensation of primitive mesenchymal cells in the cyst wall, which may be subtle (right panel). (*C*) Type Ir PPB is composed of a thin cyst wall with features of regression including fibrosis and hemosiderin-laden macrophages (*arrows*) (*D*). Nodules of cartilage may be present in all types of PPB. (*E*). Type III PPB is a solid tumor with necrosis. (*F*) Histologically type III PPB is composed of blastematous and sarcomatous elements, which often include anaplasia and mesenchymal differentiation (*right panel*, note rhabdomyoblasts).

Diagnosis

Patients generally present with respiratory distress and may have failure to thrive, fever, irritability, and lethargy. Pneumothorax is a common presentation in type I and type Ir PPB. An abdominal mass may be present in patients with DICER1 predisposition syndrome, related to the presence of cystic nephroma in the kidneys. This may be the initial presentation in a subset of patients, with lung cysts found incidentally on further workup. Diagnosis is generally achieved by imaging, the findings of which will vary depending on the type of lesion present. Type I PPB and type Ir PPB will present as a multiloculated cystic lesion, whereas a mixed cystic and solid lesion or a completely solid mass will be seen in cases of type II and type III PPB, respectively. A subset of patients may be diagnosed on prenatal ultrasound and depending on the extent of the lesion may present with hydrops. In several cases lesions may be multiple and bilateral.[27,28]

Prognosis

Prognosis is intimately associated with age at diagnosis and histopathology, which themselves are tightly related. In a large study from the International Pleuropulmonary Blastoma Registry, overall survival was 91%, 71%, and 53% for type I/Ir, type II, and type III PPB, respectively.[27] Mortality in the type I PPB group was associated with progression of disease to type II and type III PPB, which occurs in approximately 10% of patients.[27]

OTHER CONDITIONS PRESENTING WITH CYSTIC LUNG LESIONS

Other much less common entities in which the primary presentation may be cystic lung lesions in a child, includes Langerhan cell histiocytosis (LCH), Birt-Hogg-Dubé syndrome (folliculin gene-associated syndrome), and lymphangioleiomyomatosis. Connective tissue disorders including Ehler-Danlos syndrome and Marfan syndrome often present with spontaneous pneumothorax but rarely with lung cysts.

LCH is a predominantly adult disease but although rare, can occur in pediatric patients either as a manifestation of systemic disease (more common) or as isolated pulmonary LCH. Patients are either asymptomatic or may present with malaise, dyspnea, and cough. Although nodular and reticulonodular infiltrates are the main early imaging findings, cystic lung lesions predominate in advanced disease.[36] Histopathologically, the lesions are composed of aggregates of histiocytic cells with indented nuclei and diffuse and strong positivity for CD1a and S100. An accompanying eosinophilic infiltrate is common.

Birt-Hogg-Dubé syndrome is an autosomal dominant genodermatosis caused by mutations in the FLCN gene (folliculin protein) that can manifest with skin lesions, kidney tumors, and lung cysts.[37] On imaging the lung cysts vary in number and size, tend to be basal and subpleural in distribution, and elliptical or lentiform in shape. Patients with lung cysts often present with spontaneous pneumothorax. Although on microscopy these cysts may resemble common blebs or bullae,

they are lined by epithelial cells, sometimes with type II pneumocyte-like cells.[38] They occasionally have internal septa consisting of alveolar walls, giving an "alveoli within an alveolus" pattern.

Lymphangioleiomyomatosis (LAM) is a progressive lung disorder that primarily affects women of reproductive age but has also been described in men and pediatric patients.[39] LAM can be sporadic or occur in patients with tuberous sclerosis, an autosomal dominant neurocutaneous syndrome caused by mutations in TSC1 (hamartin) or TSC2 (tuberin) genes. Pneumothorax is the most common presenting sign of LAM.[40] On imaging the cysts are typically thin walled, round, and multiple; other findings such as infiltrates and pleural effusions may be present. On microscopy, there is a disorderly proliferation of spindle cells within the interstitium and alveolar septa that surrounds small air-filled cysts. The cells are positive for smooth muscle markers and a subset coexpress HMB-45 by immunohistochemistry.

GENETIC CONDITIONS AND NEOPLASMS

SUMMARY

Although lung cysts in children are commonly benign and congenital in origin, genetic and neoplastic conditions should be considered, especially when cysts are multifocal and present in older children and adolescents. Manifestations of disease in other organ systems and in family members is frequent in this setting.

CLINICAL CARE POINTS

- Types I and Ir PPB should be in the differential when evaluating a cystic lung lesion in a child and may require extensive sampling to demonstrate the key histologic features.
- Testing for a DICER1 mutation is indicated in a patient with a PPB, which may be the first manifestation of familial DICER1 predisposition syndrome.
- Proliferative lesions can rarely present in older children with lung cysts by imaging.
- Lung cysts in Birt-Hogg-Dubé syndrome may resemble common blebs or bullae.

DISCLOSURE

The authors have nothing to disclose.

REFERENCES

1. Imai Y, Mark EJ. Cystic adenomatoid change is common to various forms of cystic lung diseases of children: a clinicopathologic analysis of 10 cases with

emphasis on tracing the bronchial tree. Arch Pathol Lab Med 2002;126(8):934–40.

2. Kunisaki SM, Fauza DO, Nemes LP, et al. Bronchial atresia: the hidden pathology within a spectrum of prenatally diagnosed lung masses. J Pediatr Surg 2006;41(1):61–5, [discussion: 61–5].

3. Riedlinger WF, Vargas SO, Jennings RW, et al. Bronchial atresia is common to extralobar sequestration, intralobar sequestration, congenital cystic adenomatoid malformation, and lobar emphysema. Pediatr Dev Pathol 2006;9(5):361–73.

4. Langston C. New concepts in the pathology of congenital lung malformations. Semin Pediatr Surg 2003;12(1):17–37.

5. Stocker JT, Madewell JE, Drake RM. Congenital cystic adenomatoid malformation of the lung. Classification and morphologic spectrum. Hum Pathol 1977;8(2):155–71.

6. Adzick NS, Harrison MR, Glick PL, et al. Fetal cystic adenomatoid malformation: prenatal diagnosis and natural history. J Pediatr Surg 1985;20(5):483–8.

7. Nobuhara KK, Gorski YC, La Quaglia MP, et al. Bronchogenic cysts and esophageal duplications: common origins and treatment. J Pediatr Surg 1997; 32(10):1408–13.

8. Sfakianaki AK, Copel JA. Congenital cystic lesions of the lung: congenital cystic adenomatoid malformation and bronchopulmonary sequestration. Rev Obstet Gynecol 2012;5(2):85–93.

9. Pogoriler J, Swarr D, Kreiger P, et al. Congenital cystic lung lesions: redefining the natural distribution of subtypes and assessing the risk of malignancy. Am J Surg Pathol 2019;43(1):47–55.

10. Stocker JT. Congenital pulmonary airway malformation: A new name and an expanded classification of congenital cystic adenomatoid malformation of the lung. Histopathology 2002;41:424–31.

11. Barnett CP, Nataren NJ, Klingler-Hoffmann M, et al. Ectrodactyly and lethal pulmonary acinar dysplasia associated with homozygous FGFR2 mutations identified by exome sequencing. Hum Mutat 2016; 37(9):955–63.

12. Szafranski P, Coban-Akdemir ZH, Rupps R, et al. Phenotypic expansion of TBX4 mutations to include acinar dysplasia of the lungs. Am J Med Genet A 2016;170(9):2440–4.

13. Karolak JA, Vincent M, Deutsch G, et al. Complex compound inheritance of lethal lung developmental disorders due to disruption of the TBX-FGF pathway. Am J Hum Genet 2019;104(2):213–28.

14. Biyyam DR, Chapman T, Ferguson MR, et al. Congenital lung abnormalities: embryologic features, prenatal diagnosis, and postnatal radiologic-pathologic correlation. Radiographics 2010;30(6):1721–38.

15. Newman B. Congenital bronchopulmonary foregut malformations: concepts and controversies. Pediatr Radiol 2006;36(8):773–91.

16. Corbett HJ, Humphrey GM. Pulmonary sequestration. Paediatr Respir Rev 2004;5(1):59–68.

17. Cleveland RH, Weber B. Retained fetal lung liquid in congenital lobar emphysema: a possible predictor of polyalveolar lobe. Pediatr Radiol 1993;23(4):291–5.

18. Silver MM, Thurston WA, Patrick JE. Perinatal pulmonary hyperplasia due to laryngeal atresia. Hum Pathol 1988;19(1):110–3.

19. Hardy Hendren W. Lobar emphysema of infancy. J Pediatr Surg 1966;1(1):24–39.

20. Ozcelik U, Gocmen A, Kiper N, et al. Congenital lobar emphysema: evaluation and long-term follow-up of thirty cases at a single center. Pediatr Pulmonol 2003;35(5):384–91.

21. Tapper D, Schuster S, McBride J, et al. Polyalveolar lobe: anatomic and physiologic parameters and their relationship to congenital lobar emphysema. J Pediatr Surg 1980;15(6):931–7.

22. Tander B, Yalcin M, Yilmaz B, et al. Congenital lobar emphysema: a clinicopathologic evaluation of 14 cases. Eur J Pediatr Surg 2003;13(2):108–11.

23. Kunisaki SM, Saito JM, Fallat ME, et al. Current operative management of congenital lobar emphysema in children: A report from the Midwest Pediatric Surgery Consortium. J Pediatr Surg 2019;54(6): 1138–42.

24. Ioachimescu OC, Mehta AC. From cystic pulmonary airway malformation, to bronchioloalveolar carcinoma and adenocarcinoma of the lung. Eur Respir J 2005;26(6):1181–7.

25. Lantuejoul S, Nicholson AG, Sartori G, et al. Mucinous cells in type 1 pulmonary congenital cystic adenomatoid malformation as mucinous bronchioloalveolar carcinoma precursors. Am J Surg Pathol 2007;31(6):961–9.

26. Dishop MK, Kuruvilla S. Primary and metastatic lung tumors in the pediatric population: a review and 25-year experience at a large children's hospital. Arch Pathol Lab Med 2008;132(7):1079–103.

27. Messinger YH, Stewart DR, Priest JR, et al. Pleuropulmonary blastoma: a report on 350 central pathology-confirmed pleuropulmonary blastoma cases by the International Pleuropulmonary Blastoma Registry. Cancer 2015;121(2):276–85.

28. Hill DA, Jarzembowski JA, Priest JR, et al. Type I pleuropulmonary blastoma: pathology and biology study of 51 cases from the international pleuropulmonary blastoma registry. Am J Surg Pathol 2008; 32(2):282–95.

29. Hill DA, Ivanovich J, Priest JR, et al. DICER1 mutations in familial pleuropulmonary blastoma. Science 2009;325(5943):965.

30. Foulkes WD, Priest JR, Duchaine TF. DICER1: mutations, microRNAs and mechanisms. Nat Rev Cancer 2014;14(10):662–72.

31. Dehner LP, Messinger YH, Schultz KA, et al. Pleuropulmonary blastoma: evolution of an entity as an

entry into a familial tumor predisposition syndrome. Pediatr Dev Pathol 2015;18(6):504–11.

32. Pugh TJ, Yu W, Yang J, et al. Exome sequencing of pleuropulmonary blastoma reveals frequent biallelic loss of TP53 and two hits in DICER1 resulting in retention of 5p-derived miRNA hairpin loop sequences. Oncogene 2014;33(45):5295–302.

33. Priest JR, McDermott MB, Bhatia S, et al. Pleuropulmonary blastoma: a clinicopathologic study of 50 cases. Cancer 1997;80(1):147–61.

34. Hill DA, Dehner LP. A cautionary note about congenital cystic adenomatoid malformation (CCAM) type 4. Am J Surg Pathol 2004;28(4):554–5, [author reply: 555].

35. Priest JR, Williams GM, Hill DA, et al. Pulmonary cysts in early childhood and the risk of malignancy. Pediatr Pulmonol 2009;44(1):14–30.

36. Bano S, Chaudhary V, Narula MK, et al. Pulmonary Langerhans cell histiocytosis in children: a spectrum of radiologic findings. Eur J Radiol 2014;83(1): 47–56.

37. Toro JR, Pautler SE, Stewart L, et al. Lung cysts, spontaneous pneumothorax, and genetic associations in 89 families with Birt-Hogg-Dube syndrome. Am J Respir Crit Care Med 2007;175(10): 1044–53.

38. Furuya M, Tanaka R, Koga S, et al. Pulmonary cysts of Birt-Hogg-Dube syndrome: a clinicopathologic and immunohistochemical study of 9 families. Am J Surg Pathol 2012;36(4):589–600.

39. von Ranke FM, Zanetti G, e Silva JL, et al. Tuberous sclerosis complex: state-of-the-art review with a focus on pulmonary involvement. Lung 2015; 193(5):619–27.

40. Ryu JH, Moss J, Beck GJ, et al. The NHLBI lymphangioleiomyomatosis registry: characteristics of 230 patients at enrollment. Am J Respir Crit Care Med 2006;173(1):105–11.

Strategies for the Neonatal Lung Biopsy
Histology to Genetics

Jill Lipsett, BMBS, PhD, FRCPA, FISQua[a],
Megan K. Dishop, MD[b],*

KEYWORDS

- Neonate • Lung biopsy • Hypoplasia • Prematurity • Surfactant • Alveolar capillary dysplasia
- Genetic disorders

Key points

- Neonatal lung biopsies are infrequently performed and require planning with a multidisciplinary team to allow optimal tissue handling for special studies.
- Neonatal lung biopsies require careful microscopic assessment of alveolar architecture and vascular architecture to aid in identifying genetic and acquired disorders of lung development.
- Biopsy findings should be correlated with clinical findings, chest computed tomography abnormalities, and molecular studies for optimal interpretation.
- If a definitive diagnosis is not reached, the lung biopsy may narrow the differential diagnosis for the neonatologist, may exclude specific diseases of interest to guide continued medical therapy, and may assist in selection of additional diagnostic tests, such as genetic testing or cardiac imaging.

ABSTRACT

Neonatal lung biopsy guides important medical decisions when the diagnosis is not clear from prior clinical assessment, imaging, or genetic testing. Common scenarios that lead to biopsy include severe acute respiratory distress in a term neonate, pulmonary hypertension disproportionate to that expected for gestational age or known cardiac anomalies, and assessment of suspected genetic disorder based on clinical features or genetic variant of unknown significance. The differential diagnosis includes genetic developmental disorders, genetic surfactant disorders, vascular disorders, acquired infection, and meconium aspiration. This article describes pathologic patterns in the neonatal lung and correlation with molecular abnormalities, where appropriate.

OVERVIEW

Lung biopsy in the neonatal period is clinically indicated when either preterm or term infants have unusually severe diffuse lung disease of uncertain nature where more definitive diagnosis will help guide management decisions, including in some cases, transition to palliative care. Biopsy is not undertaken lightly and the diagnostic yield is optimized by considered planning before biopsy to ensure appropriate samples are triaged. Family and pregnancy history, neonatal clinical course, and imaging studies all provide valuable context for assessment of the biopsy. Identification of possible underlying genetic conditions has implications for both the index case and family members, including siblings yet born. Developmental abnormalities may be secondary to other comorbidities such as congenital heart disease or

---

[a] Department of Anatomical Pathology, S.A. Pathology, Women's and Children's Hospital, King William Street, North Adelaide, South Australia 5006, Australia; [b] Department of Pathology and Laboratory Medicine, Phoenix Children's Hospital, 1919 East Thomas Road, Phoenix, AZ 85016, USA
* Corresponding author.
E-mail address: mdishop@phoenixchildrens.com

Surgical Pathology 13 (2020) 657–682
https://doi.org/10.1016/j.path.2020.08.011
1875-9181/20/© 2020 Elsevier Inc. All rights reserved.

surgpath.theclinics.com

skeletal dysplasia that may have impacted during in utero development, and often secondary iatrogenic effects from intensive care will complicate the biopsy appearances with features dependent on the duration and developmental maturity of the lung when impacted. Acute and congenital infections contribute to the differential and may occur secondarily, whereas noninfectious inflammatory conditions exist but are rare. This article reviews procedures optimizing diagnostic yield of the neonatal lung biopsy with sections highlighting diagnostic features, ancillary studies, the state of genetic knowledge and prognostic features for this complex group of diseases (**Table 1**).

PREPARATION FOR NEONATAL LUNG BIOPSY

To maximize the diagnostic yield from neonatal lung biopsies, it is important to work closely within a multidisciplinary team so that the pathologist understands the differential diagnosis and the need for special studies. The neonatologist and/or pulmonologist should provide obstetric history, family history, clinical progress to date, differential diagnosis, and specific questions to be answered. The radiologist is helpful in describing imaging characteristics, change over time, and imaging differential diagnosis. Communication between the surgeon and pathologist is helpful in guiding where to biopsy and number of biopsies. It is advisable to avoid the right middle lobe and left lingula in most cases due to the risk of over estimating severity of disease at these sites, compared with other lobes. The size of the biopsy should be at least 1 cm deep to include bronchioles and muscular pulmonary arteries for evaluation. Using thoracoscopic technique, if a wedge biopsy is obtained at this minimum depth, then the width of the biopsy should be approximately 2 cm, allowing adequate tissue for both histologic examination and special studies. The tissue should be submitted fresh to the laboratory immediately after biopsy, and the pathologist should be notified to allow for special handling. Guidelines for handling of the pediatric lung biopsies have been published previously[1] and are summarized here (**Tables 2 and 3**). It is particularly important in neonatal lung biopsies to reserve tissue for electron microscopy, given its important in evaluating genetic disorders of surfactant metabolism. In addition, it is critical to gently inflate the lung biopsy before sectioning, so that the airspaces are distended. Inflation allows assessment of the size and shape of alveoli, as well as the thickness of the alveolar walls, character of the interstitial cells, and the capillary architecture. The importance of these microscopic

Table 1 Differential diagnosis in neonatal lung biopsy	
Abnormal parenchymal development	Pulmonary hypoplasia, primary (Acinar dysplasia, TBX4 abnormality, TTF1/ NKX2.1 abnormality) Pulmonary hypoplasia, secondary, due to in utero lung restriction Chronic neonatal lung disease due to prematurity Abnormal alveolarization associated with chromosomal disorders (Down syndrome, other) Abnormal alveolarization associated with congenital heart disease
Vascular disease	Alveolar capillary dysplasia Pulmonary arteriopathy associated with congenital heart disease Pulmonary venous disease associated with congenital heart disease Lymphangiectasia, primary and secondary
Genetic disorders of surfactant metabolism	ABCA3 deficiency Surfactant protein B deficiency Surfactant protein C deficiency TTF1/NKX2.1 deficiency
Congenital infection	Congenital bacterial pneumonia secondary to amniotic fluid infection syndrome Herpes simplex virus Cytomegalovirus
Airway disease	Meconium aspiration Neuroendocrine cell hyperplasia of infancy
Systemic disease	Metabolic storage disorders Langerhans cell histiocytosis Congenital leukemia Primary immunodeficiency

Table 2
Guidelines for triaging neonatal lung biopsy tissue

Microbiology	Obtain piece sterilely for bacterial, viral, fungal and acid fast cultures, as appropriate.
Electron microscopy	Obtain small pieces of tissue in glutaraldehyde for possible ultrastructural examination.
Frozen tissue	Obtain piece in cryovial for possible molecular studies (microbiology or genetic disease).
Frozen tissue in CryoMatrix	Obtain piece inflated and embedded in CryoMatrix for possible immunofluorescence study.
Histology	Inflate remaining wedge with formalin. Fix for 20 minutes or more. Section perpendicular to the cut edge to create wedge-shaped sections, and submit entirely for processing and routine hematoxylin-eosin staining.

findings will be evident in the description of the following diseases of the neonate and infant.

HYALINE MEMBRANE DISEASE AND ACUTE LUNG INJURY

Neonatal respiratory distress syndrome is most often associated with prematurity, but may also occur in term infants due to lung hypoplasia or other acute lung injury in the perinatal period.

MICROSCOPIC FEATURES

Hyaline membrane disease is the pathologic correlate of neonatal respiratory distress syndrome, and is characterized by formation of linear fibrinoproteinaceous membranes lining the alveolar walls. These membranes are composed of proteins from fluid associated with vascular endothelial injury, as well as admixed necrotic debris from sloughed epithelial cells (**Fig. 1A**). The alveoli are stiff and noncompliant due to increased surface tension due to the deficiency of normal surfactant in the premature lung. One complication of high ventilatory pressures required in some babies with hyaline membrane disease is the production of pulmonary interstitial emphysema (PIE). PIE is caused by rupture of alveoli with air leak into the interstitium and tracking along interlobular septa to the pleura, sometimes associated with pneumothorax. Microscopically, PIE is characterized by fusiform air-filled cystic spaces in these locations (**Fig. 1B**).

Ancillary stains
- Special Stains: periodic acid–Schiff (PAS) stain is negative in the hyaline membranes.
- Immunohistochemistry: Cytokeratin may demonstrate associated epithelial loss or regeneration, such as type II pneumocyte hyperplasia.

Prognosis: Dependent on severity of prematurity, and associated comorbidities.
Associated Genetic Changes/Alterations: None.

> **Key Features: Hyaline Membrane Disease**
>
> *Diagnostic features:* Hyaline membranes and karyorrhectic debris lining alveolar walls and some bronchioles.

Table 3
Selected single gene disorders affecting the neonatal lung

TBX4	T-Box Transcription Factor 4	Acinar Dysgenesis and Congenital Alveolar Dysplasia
FOXF1	Forkhead box F1	Alveolar capillary dysplasia
TTF1/NKX2.1	Thyroid transcription factor 1/NK2 homeobox 1	Abnormal alveolar development Genetic disorder of surfactant regulation
SFTPB	Surfactant protein B	Genetic disorder of surfactant metabolism
SFTPC	Surfactant protein C	Genetic disorder of surfactant metabolism
ABCA3	ATPase binding cassette transporter subfamily A3	Genetic disorder of surfactant metabolism

Clues: Clinical history of prematurity or other perinatal acute lung injury. Peak formation of hyaline membranes between 12 and 24 hours.

Pitfalls: Organizing hyaline membranes form round aggregates that may mimic alveolar proteinosis.

Differential Diagnosis: Pulmonary edema, pulmonary alveolar proteinosis.

CHRONIC NEONATAL LUNG DISEASE DUE TO PREMATURITY

Chronic neonatal lung disease is clinically defined as persistent oxygen requirement after 30 days of age. From a pathologic perspective, chronic neonatal lung disease due to prematurity equates with abnormal alveolar growth and development, signified by enlarged airspaces with deficient septation. If mild, this alveolar simplification may be difficult to recognize, especially for those who are

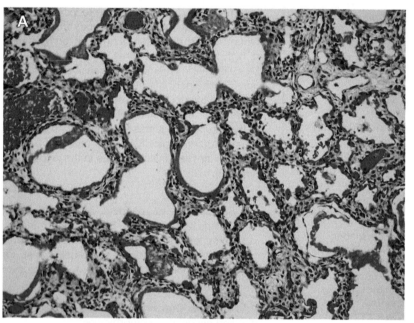

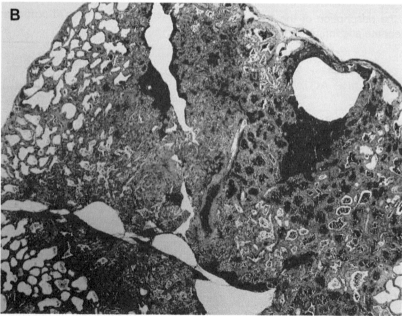

Fig. 1. Neonatal respiratory distress syndrome. (*A*) Hyaline membranes form during acute lung injury from a combination of epithelial necrotic debris and transudate of proteins due to vascular endothelial injury, and peak during the first 24 hours after premature delivery. (*B*) Acute pulmonary interstitial emphysema is a complication of ventilation of stiff lungs, and results from rupture of alveoli with leak of air into the interstitium and interlobular septa. Cystic spaces in the septa can mimic developmental abnormalities of lymphatics, such as primary lymphangiectasia.

unfamiliar with the microscopic architecture of normal preterm and term neonatal lungs. This form of alveolar simplification is sometimes referred to as "new" bronchopulmonary dysplasia, because it is morphology seen in the era of artificial surfactant therapy. Before widespread use of artificial surfactant, premature neonate typically developed a pattern of classical bronchopulmonary dysplasia, characterized by alternating areas of atelectasis and hyperinflation, associated with airway injury and some degree of pulmonary fibrosis, resulting in distortion of the pleural contours and abnormal pseudofissures, due to retraction from underlying interlobular septal fibrosis. With current therapies, bronchopulmonary dysplasia is unusual, but still occurs in extremely premature neonates and in neonates with multifactorial disease (for example, prematurity and pulmonary hypoplasia).

MICROSCOPIC FEATURES

Normal alveolar development in a full-term neonate (Fig. 2A) is compared with abnormal alveolarization in a former premature infant (Fig. 2B). Pulmonary arterial hypertension is often reflected by medial hypertrophy of pulmonary arteries and muscularization of the intra-acinar arterioles (Fig. 2C).

Ancillary stains
- Special Stains: Trichrome or Movat pentachrome stain may highlight collagen deposition in the most severe forms (bronchopulmonary dysplasia). The stains are also helpful in highlighting any associated pulmonary arteriopathy.
- Immunohistochemistry: Cytokeratin stain may be helpful in demonstrating alveolar architecture in poorly inflated lung biopsies.

Prognosis: Dependent on severity of prematurity, and severity of comorbidities.
Associated Genetic Changes/Alterations: None.

 y Features: Chronic Neonatal Lung Disease due to Prematurity

Diagnostic features: Alveolar enlargement and simplification of varying degree.

Clues: Variation in size and shape of alveoli. Round or ovoid alveolar shapes due to insufficient alveolar septation. Presence of primary septa, but lack of secondary septa.

Pitfalls: May mimic or coincide with alveolar hyperinflation due to air trapping.

Differential Diagnosis: Emphysema, air trapping.

CHRONIC NEONATAL LUNG DISEASE DUE TO SECONDARY PULMONARY HYPOPLASIA

Pulmonary hypoplasia is diagnosed when there is a reduction in lung volume, reflected by simplification of the lobular parenchyma, defined as "primary" when there is no related underlying disorder and "secondary" when it is associated with conditions that restrict intrauterine lung excursion. Genetic abnormalities are increasingly being recognized and defined as the cause of primary forms of pulmonary hypoplasia (see later in this article). Secondary pulmonary hypoplasia is more common, and causes include congenital diaphragmatic hernia, fetal hydrops, oligohydramnios, skeletal dysplasia and akinesia syndromes, thoracic mass or cyst, intrauterine growth restriction, and renal agenesis. Imaging studies can suggest pulmonary hypoplasia with reduction of lung fields and high diaphragms and clinically it is suspected with respiratory distress and need for high ventilation pressures, unresponsive to surfactant therapy. A diagnosis of pulmonary hypoplasia can be suggested at biopsy when there is a reduction in the radial alveolar count, the method developed by Emery and Mithal,[2] obtained by dropping a perpendicular from the junction of conducting and respiratory epithelia to the nearest connective tissue septum/pleura and counting the number of alveoli this line transects, normally increasing from around 2 at 26 weeks to 5-6 by term to 9 alveoli by 10 years of age.

MICROSCOPIC FEATURES

The microscopic appearances of pulmonary hypoplasia alone can vary from normal to near normal appearance with only a reduction in the number of alveoli in the terminal acinar unit through varying degrees of architectural distortion including enlargement of respiratory and alveolar ducts and alveoli present. This can be overlooked and the comparison with age matched control tissue, expanded to a similar degree, can assist in identification of subtle changes. Often, effects of mechanical ventilation, other treatment effects and superimposed infection can add to the picture and separating out the different components can be difficult. Greater irregularity of architectural distortion will suggest secondary pathology.

Ancillary stains
- Special Stains: Movat pentachrome stain will help highlight different elements for assessment. PAS stain will assist identification and

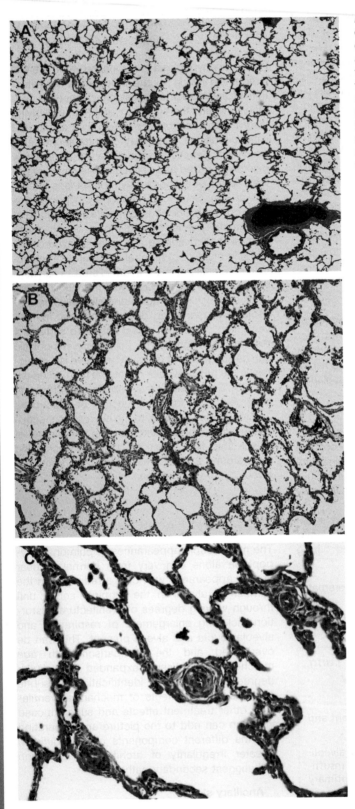

Fig. 2. Chronic neonatal lung disease due to prematurity. (*A*) Normal alveolar development at full term. (*B*) Abnormal alveolarization in an 8-month-old former premature infant with architectural remodeling following hyaline membrane disease. (*C*) Pulmonary arteriopathy occurs secondary to the simplified capillary bed associated with alveolar simplification, in this case showing significant muscularization of the intra-acinar arterioles.

degree of secondary pulmonary interstitial glycogenosis

- Immunohistochemistry: Pan-cytokeratin AE1/3, CD31 and CD34 to assist assessment of capillary and alveolar relationships.

Prognosis: The prognosis depends on the degree of hypoplasia. Many of these children can be supported while lung growth continues, whereas severe pulmonary hypoplasia for example, secondary to congenital diaphragmatic hernia or prolonged oligohydramnios are often lethal.

ASSOCIATED GENETIC CHANGES/ ALTERATIONS

Some reports of primary pulmonary hypoplasia, including some familial cases have now been identified to have genetic changes affecting the TBX4-FGF10-FGFR2 epithelial-mesenchymal signaling (see later in this article).[3]

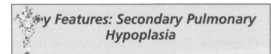

Key Features: Secondary Pulmonary Hypoplasia

Diagnostic features: Reduction in the acinar complexity and number of alveoli with or without a degree of architectural change and simplification.

Clues: Impression of conducting airways extending closer to lobular septa or pleura. Use of control tissue helps demonstrate growth abnormality and lobular volume reduction.

Pitfalls: Features can be subtle, identification aided by comparison to age-matched control sections. Superimposed changes from prolonged respiratory support or infections can produce lobular remodeling.

Differential Diagnosis: Chronic neonatal lung disease, Primary forms of pulmonary hypoplasia.

PULMONARY ARTERIAL HYPERTENSION AND CHANGES ASSOCIATED WITH CONGENITAL HEART DISEASE

Pulmonary arterial hypertension may be reflected in neonatal lung biopsy by the presence of medial hypertrophy or intimal proliferation within the muscular pulmonary artery branches, as well as muscularization of the intra-acinar arterioles. The cause of pulmonary arteriopathy is often related

to lung parenchymal disorders, such as chronic neonatal lung disease due to prematurity or pulmonary hypoplasia, however may also reflect abnormal pulmonary hemodynamics related to underlying congenital heart disease. Neonatal lung biopsies may be performed in fact to discriminate between the relative contribution of congenital heart disease and parenchymal lung disease in the pathogenesis of respiratory insufficiency in this age group (**Box 1**). Other diagnostic considerations include exclusion of pulmonary venous hypertension as a cause of severe pulmonary arterial hypertension. In pulmonary vein stenosis or obstructive physiology due to total anomalous pulmonary venous return, the pulmonary veins in the lung biopsy appear thickened and/or arterialized. The constellation of findings in pulmonary venous hypertension includes diffuse congestion, acute hemorrhage, abundance of hemosiderin laden macrophages, lymphatic dilation and muscularization, and pulmonary arteriopathy. This pattern is sometimes referred to as "chronic congestive vasculopathy."

Key Features: Pulmonary arteriopathy

Diagnostic features: Medial hypertrophy and/or intimal proliferation of muscular pulmonary artery branches. Muscularization of intra-acinar arterioles is indicated by presence of a smooth muscle cuff associated with the smallest arterial branches within the interstitium near periphery.

Clues: Movat pentachrome, trichrome, or SMA stains helps to highlight the vascular architecture.

Pitfalls: Presence of pulmonary arteriopathy does not always correlate with clinical evidence of pulmonary hypertension. When evaluating the pulmonary arteries, always remember to evaluate the pulmonary veins, as some of the most severe forms of pulmonary arterial hypertension are secondary to pulmonary venous obstruction.

Differential Diagnosis: The cause of pulmonary arteriopathy is often multifactorial. The clinical differential diagnosis includes abnormal lung growth and development, pulmonary overcirculation due to cardiovascular shunt, pulmonary venous hypertension due to pulmonary vein stenosis or obstruction, and chronic hypoxia.

> **Box 1**
> **Diagnostic considerations for neonates with known congenital heart disease**
>
> - Alveolar simplification: associated with chromosomal disorders and/or congenital heart disease
> - Diffuse alveolar damage: acute lung injury in the setting of pulmonary hypoperfusion or cardiogenic shock
> - Pulmonary arteriopathy: cardiac left to right shunt lesions with pulmonary overcirculation, associated with pulmonary venous hypertension, associated with alveolar simplification
> - Pulmonary venous disease: pulmonary vein stenosis, obstructive physiology in total anomalous pulmonary venous connection
> - Alveolar capillary dysplasia: may be associated with hypoplastic left heart syndrome and other cardiovascular anomalies
> - Primary lymphangiectasia: Down syndrome, Turner syndrome, isolated
> - Secondary lymphangiectasia: associated with pulmonary edema or pulmonary venous hypertension

MICROSCOPIC FEATURES

The muscular pulmonary artery branches accompanying the terminal and respiratory bronchioles may be thickened due to medial hypertrophy. Intimal proliferation or concentric intimal fibrosis may develop. In long-standing pulmonary arterial hypertension due to unrecognized or unrepaired congenital heart disease, other changes such as necrotizing arteritis, plexiform lesions, and dilation lesions, may evolve, so-called Eisenmenger syndrome. The severity of pulmonary arterial hypertension in the setting of congenital heart disease may be characterized by modified Heath-Edwards grading or Rabinovich classification.

Ancillary stains
- Special Stains: Movat pentachrome, trichrome, elastic stain
- Immunohistochemistry: Smooth muscle actin (SMA).

Prognosis: Dependent on underlying parenchymal lung disease, and ability to repair the congenital heart defect.
Associated Genetic Changes/Alterations: None.

LYMPHANGIECTASIA

Lymphangiectasia occurs in primary and secondary forms. Primary lymphangiectasia is a developmental disorder of lymphatics resulting in severe diffuse lymphatic dilation, often associated with intrauterine and congenital chylothoraces, variable extrapulmonary lymphangiectasia, and anasarca. Secondary lymphangiectasia is more common, and refers to lymphatic dilation due to pulmonary edema or pulmonary venous hypertension.

MICROSCOPIC FEATURES

Both primary and secondary lymphangiectasia shows dilated lymphatic channels in the pleura, interlobular septa, and bronchovascular bundles. Primary lymphangiectasia is typically more severe and obvious at low power (**Fig. 3**), whereas secondary lymphangiectasia may be more variable in distribution and mild to moderate in severity. Definitive diagnosis however relies on clinical correlation.

Ancillary stains
- Special Stains: None.
- Immunohistochemistry: D2-40 (podoplanin)

Prognosis: Primary lymphangiectasia is not amenable to medical therapy, and may be fatal. Secondary lymphangiectasia response to correction of pulmonary hemodynamics.
Associated Genetic Changes/Alterations: None.

> *Key Features: Primary Lymphangiectasia*
>
> *Diagnostic features:* Moderate to severe diffuse dilation of lymphatic channels within pleura, intralobular septa, and bronchovascular bundles. May show cystic dilation.
>
> *Clues:* Fusiform clear cystic spaces. Muscularization of lymphatics.
>
> *Pitfalls:* May mimic secondary lymphangiectasia due to hemodynamic factors (pulmonary edema, pulmonary venous hypertension). The distinction requires clinical correlation. Primary lymphangiectasia is typically more severe and diffuse than secondary lymphangiectasia.
>
> *Differential Diagnosis:* Secondary lymphangiectasia, acute pulmonary interstitial emphysema, technical artifact of biopsy inflation using a fine-needle.

Fig. 3. Lymphangiectasia. The pleural lymphatics are markedly dilated in this lung biopsy from a neonate with primary lymphangiectasia.

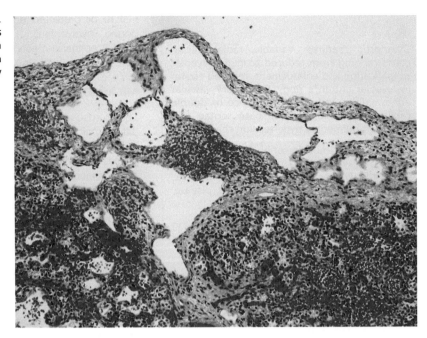

PULMONARY DISEASE IN NEONATES WITH DOWN SYNDROME

Down syndrome (DS) is the most common chromosomal anomaly encountered. Biopsies of neonates with DS may be performed either in the knowledge of the presence of Trisomy 21 or perhaps before diagnosis. These neonates may present with respiratory failure requiring support. Primary lung pathology varies, with pulmonary hypoplasia seen in most, while associated anomalies can impact secondarily on the lungs, particularly congenital heart disease. DS patients are particularly at risk of pulmonary hypertension, in part intrinsically related to an underlying primary lung hypoplasia with associated hypoplastic pulmonary vasculature growth and compounded by any right to left shunts associated with congenital heart disease, aspiration, and increased susceptibility to infections. Down syndrome, regardless of other associated congenital abnormalities has been shown to have an increased incidence of neonatal persistent pulmonary hypertension (PPHT) at 1.2% consistent with an intrinsic predisposition.[4]

MICROSCOPIC FEATURES

Features seen in DS in the neonatal lung biopsy are variable. Although most subjects will have pulmonary hypoplasia the radial:alveolar count may not reflect this and may even be increased to adult levels. Acini can show simplification of alveolar development with enlargement of alveolar ducts and alveoli. Reduced elastic tissue can be seen in the entrance rings of alveoli. Vascular changes include pulmonary hypertensive changes involving arteries and immaturity of the capillary plexus, retaining a double layer in the inter-airspace septae.

Ancillary stains:
- Movat pentachrome stain or Verhoeff–Van Gieson (VVG) can be used to highlight vascular changes and elastin within the alveolar entrance rings.
- Immunohistochemistry: Cytokeratin stains and vascular stains (CD31 and CD34) can be used to highlight the airspace contours and capillary plexus within the septa.

PROGNOSIS

The prognosis of DS overall has improved with survival now to a mean age of 60 years. Pulmonary disease has been identified as the most common cause of morbidity and mortality for this group. As well as the underlying pulmonary abnormality, congenital heart disease and other co-morbidities, particularly obstructive sleep apnea, aspiration and recurrent infections all may contribute.[5]

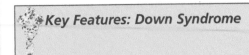

Key Features: Down Syndrome

Diagnostic features: Variable radial:alveolar count ranging from reduced to high. Alveolar simplification and enlargement, reduced elastin in alveolar entrance rings. Pulmonary vascular abnormalities, including persistence of double capillary plexus in inter-airspace septae and persistent pulmonary hypertension changes

Clues: Look for multifactorial disease. Patients with DS may have superimposed changes of impaired alveolar growth and development, vasculopathy from congenital heart disease, and susceptibility to aspiration.

Differential Diagnosis: Chronic neonatal lung disease of prematurity, congenital alveolar dysplasia

PRIMARY PULMONARY HYPOPLASIA: ACINAR DYSGENESIS AND CONGENITAL ALVEOLAR DYSPLASIA

Acinar dysgenesis (AD) is a rare developmental lung abnormality with immediate respiratory failure at delivery and death shortly after, such is the severity, there is typically no time for neonatal biopsy with diagnosis made if an autopsy is performed. The lungs are severely hypoplastic, globally small, with marked decrease in lobular and acinar development such that conceptually the appearances have been likened to an arrest of development in the pseudoglandular phase.

Congenital alveolar dysplasia (CAD) is a rarer condition still, presenting usually as a term neonate with early respiratory failure and near 100% mortality. Unlike AD, the lungs are not obviously hypoplastic and can be of normal or increased weight reflecting some congestion. These lungs are characterized by a diffuse immature appearance more resembling saccular stage of lung development, and while the acinar maldevelopment can resemble that seen in ACDMPV, vein misalignment is not observed, nor the prominent hypertensive arterial changes characterizing the latter.

The molecular etiology of these conditions is largely unknown, however TBX4 mutations have been reported associated with AD[6] and deletions in TBX4 identified in an infant with CAD.[7] Another infant with AD and ectrodactyly was described with a homozygous missense FGFR2 mutation.[8] Some case pedigrees with consanguinity and recurrences of AD have been suggestive of autosomal-recessive inheritance.[8,9] A recent study of 26 cases including AD, CAD and other lethal lung hypoplasias found various deletions and mutations involving TBX4 or

FGF10 or predicted enhancer regions that supported involvement of disrupted TBX4-FGF10-FGFR2 epithelial-mesenchymal signaling in these rare developmental lung abnormalities.[3]

MICROSCOPIC FEATURES

The microscopic features of acinar dysplasia are of a diffuse maldevelopment with larger conducting airways including islands of cartilage, and some bronchioles without cartilage lying in loose mesenchyme. There is increased stromal tissue in between small and irregular islands of maldeveloped acinar elements comprising few airspace structures that if present are immature and alveolar development is absent. The vascular bed is deficient and air:blood membranes are not formed (**Fig. 4**A).

CAD microscopically features more advanced acinar development with distal airspaces readily identified though appearing relatively immature and simplified with increased septae between them. Alveolar development is not seen. The acinar appearance more resembles saccular phase of development while the capillary bed present is not obviously deficient and retains its sub-epithelial position with air:blood membranes evident (**Fig. 4**B).

ANCILLARY STAINS

- Special Stains: Movat pentachrome stain can highlight vascular elements.
- Immunohistochemistry: Pankeratin AE1/AE3 can be used to outline the airspace component, whereas CD31 or CD34 can identify the vessels, including the capillary bed.

Prognosis: The prognosis of both AD and CAD is uniformly poor. Newborns with AD typically die within hours of delivery.

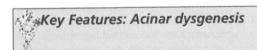

Key Features: Acinar dysgenesis

Diagnostic features: Relative prominence of larger airway structures with severe reduction in acinar tissue with few airspaces evident. Increased mesenchyme and septal tissue.

Clues: AD is not likely to be biopsied in the neonatal period due to severity and death within the first day of life. The lung architecture is composed almost entirely of conducting airways, leading to presence of cartilage near the periphery or even within the pleura.

Pitfalls: Acinar dysgenesis is distinctive due to the very primitive lobular development.

Differential Diagnosis:

- CAD. Like AD, CAD can be considered a primary form of pulmonary hypoplasia, but it is less severe than AD, resembling saccular stage of development. CAD should not be diagnosed in a premature neonate, due to overlapping features with immature lung.

- Alveolar capillary dysplasia (ACD). Like AD, ACD may be associated with simplified lobules, but there is typically a greater degree of alveolar development in ACD as compared with after dysgenesis. Dilated shunt vessels and deficient capillary density also help to distinguish ACD from acinar dysgenesis.

ALVEOLAR CAPILLARY DYSPLASIA

ACD is a severe lung developmental abnormality that presents in the neonatal period usually within hours but up to a couple of weeks of birth with respiratory failure and accelerating pulmonary hypertension resulting in death within a few months. Vascular maldevelopment manifests in a deficient pulmonary capillary bed and blood:gas interface and small to medium-sized pulmonary veins are identified abnormally positioned accompanying arterioles. Refractory, accelerated pulmonary

Fig. 4. Primary pulmonary hypoplasia. (*A*) Acinar dysgenesis is characterized by a severe developmental arrest of acinar development, resulting in conducting airways surrounded by markedly simplified lobules. (*B*) Congenital alveolar dysplasia is a primary form of maldevelopment in which the lung architecture of a term neonate resembles saccular stage of development, including a widened interstitium and incomplete alveolar septation.

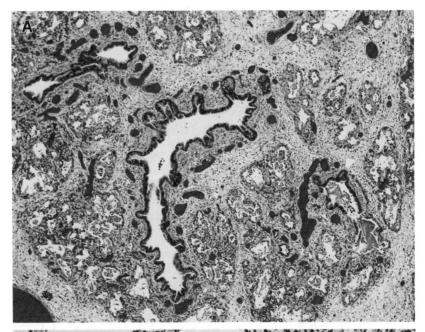

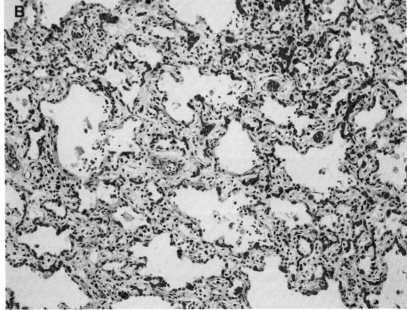

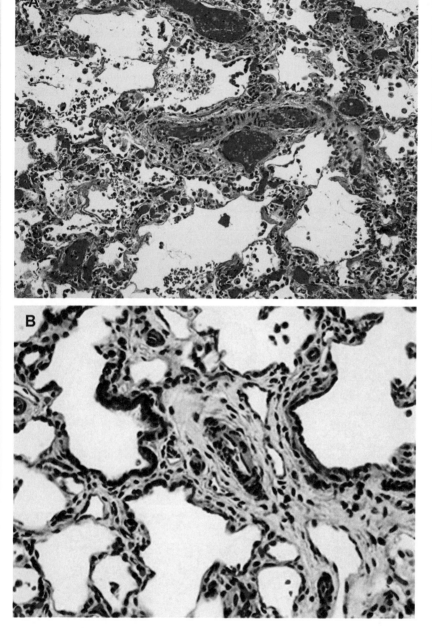

Fig. 5. Alveolar capillary dysplasia. (*A*) Abnormal dilated shunt vessels accompany hypertrophied muscular pulmonary arteries. (*B*) Alveolar walls contain deficient numbers of capillaries centrally positioned in the interstitium, without normal juxtaposition to the alveolar epithelial interface.

arterial hypertension develops. Most infants (80%) have additional congenital abnormalities involving the heart, and gastrointestinal, genitourinary, and other systems.[10–13]

MICROSCOPIC FEATURES

Lobular architecture is abnormal with airspaces appearing variably more immature and widening of the inter-airspace septae where capillaries are reduced in number and positioned more centrally in the interstitium (**Fig. 5**). Congestion and engorgement of the misaligned lobular venules aids their identification as they can be identified abnormally located adjacent to intralobular arterioles and arterioles that travel with terminal and smaller bronchioles. Pulmonary hypertensive changes including muscularization of intralobular arterioles and marked medial hyperplasia of the muscular pulmonary artery branches are also evident. A degree of lymphangiectasia is seen in approximately one-third of cases.

Ancillary stains are not always necessary but may help identify the changes present.

- Special Stains:
  - VVG or Movat stain to highlight arterial generations.
- Immunohistochemistry:
  - Cytokeratins demonstrate the airspace linings
  - CD31 or CD34 vascular makers to identify capillary profiles within the airspace septa
  - D240 to identify lymphatic vascular channels and differentiate from veins
  - SMA to demonstrate muscularization of vessel walls
  - Perls stain to highlight iron when considering the differentials

The differential diagnosis includes other causes of pulmonary arteriopathy in the neonate, including chronic neonatal lung disease due to prematurity and/or congenital heart disease. These disorders have normal capillary density in the alveolar walls, with normal positioning of capillaries adjacent to alveolar epithelium, forming blood air membranes. The differential diagnosis of severe pulmonary arterial hypertension in a neonate also includes pulmonary venous hypertension due to pulmonary vein stenosis, obstructive physiology of anomalous pulmonary venous return, or cardiomyopathy with elevated left-sided pressures. Pulmonary venous hypertension can mimic alveolar capillary dysplasia due to vascular congestion, lymphatic dilation, and severe pulmonary arterial disease, but is distinguished by pulmonary venous arterialization and presence of abundant hemosiderin laden macrophages. Lymphangiectasia can be a prominent feature in some patients with ACD. Primary lymphangiectasia may be associated with intrauterine pleural effusions, secondary pulmonary hypoplasia, and therefore abnormal alveolarization with pulmonary arterial disease. The key difference is that ACD shows deficient capillaries, centrally placed within alveolar walls.

PROGNOSIS

The prognosis of ACD is uniformly poor, refractory to medical interventions and surgery with heart-lung transplant only really a theoretic possibility at this time. Affected infants usually die within a few weeks with exceptional cases surviving months.[14–16] Infants with severe PHT may undergo lung biopsy to determine continuation or withdrawal of active management based on the pathologist's diagnosis of ACD.

Key Features

Diagnostic features: Deficient capillary bed displaced away from the alveolar epithelium. Misaligned pulmonary veins and venules. Pulmonary arterial medial hypertrophy (often severe).

Clues: Severe pulmonary arterial medial hypertrophy. Associated congestion and engorgement of the intra-acinar veins, visible at low-power. Lymphangiectasia (one-third of cases). Simplified acinar alveolar architecture, enlarged airspaces, widened septae.

Pitfalls: Prominence of the pulmonary arteriopathy can dominate and lead to misdiagnosis without focused attention on the other features. Misalignment of veins is more reliably detected in lobules where they are seen adjacent to small muscularized arterioles. Larger veins in ACD may be found normally positioned in interlobular septa.

Differential Diagnosis: Pulmonary arteriopathy secondary to chronic lung disease, cardiac disease, or pulmonary venous disease. Pulmonary hypoplasia. Primary and secondary lymphangiectasia.

ASSOCIATED GENETIC ABNORMALITIES

Long suspected, a genetic basis for ACD was first identified in 2009[17] and since then the vast majority of patients with ACD have demonstrated heterozygous point mutations in FOXF1 and genomic copy number variants (CNVs) at 16q24.1 involving FOXF1 and its upstream regulatory region. FOXF1 (Forkhead box F1) encodes a transcription factor, regulated by the sonic hedgehog signaling pathway, active during lung development. A large study in 2016 of 141 families worldwide identified 86 pathogenic variants of the FOXF1 locus (38 deletion CNVs, a complex rearrangement and 47 point mutations). When parental origin was identified, the vast majority have identified maternal inherited chromosome 16 with the implication being maternal imprinting of the FOXF1 locus in human lungs. Cases associated with severe cardiac defects were associated with deletion CNVs involving FOXF1 and its upstream enhancer. These investigators suggested long-range regulation of FOXF1 expression may be responsible for key phenotypic differences. They reported one family with de novo missense variant in ESRP1, potentially implicating FGF signaling in the etiology of ACD.[13] The story is not yet over, as new phenotypic linked genetic variants, variations in inheritance and epigenetic influences as well as replication/repair errors are being recognized.[18]

SURFACTANT DYSFUNCTION DISORDERS

Respiratory function and adaptation to air-breathing at birth requires adequate surfactant activity to allow alveolar inflation and stabilization with surfactant deficiency now recognized as the cause of an estimated 10% to 15% of respiratory failure in the term neonate.[19] Following the identification of Surfactant Protein B (SFTPB) deficiency in the early 1990s, approximately a decade later, Surfactant Protein C (SFTPC) deficiency was recognized with an expanded spectrum of disease from neonates through to adults. Mutations in the ATPase binding cassette transporter subfamily A3 (ABCA3) gene were next identified and emerged the most common genetic defect associated with impaired surfactant metabolism, with a spectrum of pathology overlapping both SFTPB and SFTPC and presenting in all ages. Mutations and deletions in TTF1/NKX2.1 gene on chromosome 14q13 that can also affect development of the thyroid and the brain impact also on production of surfactant proteins and phenotypes affect the lung variably including neonatal respiratory distress, interstitial lung disease in childhood and presenting in adulthood. Abnormal pulmonary development and increased susceptibility to infections is seen. An isolated respiratory phenotype has been reported in 25%, with the respiratory effects often accounting for the morbidity.[19] Somewhat separated from these deficiency states, is pulmonary alveolar proteinosis (PAP) thought associated with macrophage dysfunction and includes mutations in the granulocyte-macrophage colony-stimulating factor (GM-CSF) receptor genes coding both alpha and beta subunits, showing X-linked and autosomal recessive inheritance respectively. Pulmonary alveolar proteinosis with hypogammaglobulinemia (PAPHG) with which mutations in the OAS1 gene have been identified, as an example of immunodeficiency associated disease.[20–22] While GM-CSF receptor mutations are reported only in older children to date, PAPHG presents within a few months of birth, often triggered by a viral infection. The histopathology for PAPHG has not been reported from biopsy but BAL confirms PAP material. The pathology described with GM-CSF receptor mutations (CSF2RA, CSF2RB) is similar to classic adult PAP due to antibodies to GM-CSF. PAS lipoproteinaceous surfactant material accumulates in airspaces with a lack of type II cell reactive hyperplasia and no features of chronic lung disease.

MICROSCOPIC FEATURES

The inherited surfactant deficiency disorders, SFTPB, SFTPC, ABCA3, and TTF1/NKX2.1 can all present with similar clinical and pathologic features in the neonate with some features that may favor specific genotypes over others in some cases. At any age, the presence of PAS-D positive proteinaceous exudate (PAP) in airspaces, even focally, should raise the possibility of one of the surfactant disorders. Early on the exudate is finely granular, with time it can become coarse and admixed with globular and dense bodies and areas with cholesterol clefts associated with multinucleated giant cells. In surfactant dysfunction disorders in neonates, PAP is typically accompanied by type II cell alveolar epithelial hyperplasia. With time, the acinar architecture undergoes remodeling, with larger disordered alveolar spaces, interstitial widening due to smooth muscle, fibrosis and variable inflammation.

The morphology of surfactant disorders due to ABCA3 (Fig. 6) is contrasted with other types of surfactant disorders due to SFTPB (Fig. 7A), SFTPC (Fig. 7B), and TTF1 deficiency (Fig. 7C).

- ABCA3 mutations may present early and more resemble SFTPB mutations, or in older children and adolescents with features more akin to SFTPC deficiency. Electron microscopy shows small "fried egg" lamellar bodies.
- SFTPB mutations are the most likely to present in the neonatal period, radiologically resembling preterm infants with hyaline membrane disease. The clues on histology are the PAP material and prominent type II cell reactive hyperplastic changes.
- SFTPC mutations typically present in older infants, through childhood or even in adults. The pattern of chronic pneumonitis of infancy should raise consideration of SFTPC mutation. PAP material and type II cell reactive hyperplasia are less pronounced than SFTPB deficiency. There is evolving lobular remodeling, with interstitial widening comprising some inflammatory cells, muscle and/or fibrosis. The intra-airspace material includes foamy macrophages and cholesterol clefts. Patterns seen in older children and adults include nonspecific interstitial pneumonia (NSIP) and usual interstitial pneumonia (UIP).
- TTF1/NKX2.1 mutations show a very heterogeneous phenotype with 25% showing only

Fig. 6. Genetic disorder of surfactant metabolism due to ABCA3 deficiency. (*A*) The genetic disorders of surfactant metabolism result in pulmonary alveolar proteinosis associated with alveolar epithelial hyperplasia. Alveolar remodeling begins within the first few weeks of life. (*B*) The pulmonary alveolar proteinosis may be variable in distribution and is typically accompanied by macrophages and cell debris.

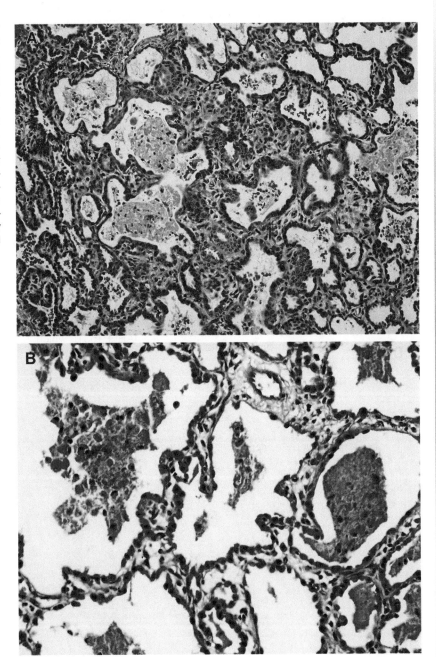

lung pathology and 56% with brain-lung-thyroid syndrome. Lack of brain or thyroid pathology should not exclude it from the differential diagnosis.[23,24] Biopsies may show lung pathology including focal PAP material with increased alveolar macrophages, a degree of type II cell hyperplasia as well as abnormal airway and alveolar development and altered expression of surfactant proteins.

It can present with neonatal respiratory distress syndrome and increased susceptibility to infections, particularly viral infections.[23] NKX2.1 mutations should be considered even in the child without associated brain or thyroid pathology.

- PAP caused by mutations in CSF2RA and CSF2RB has only been reported in older children. PAPHG is reported in the first months of

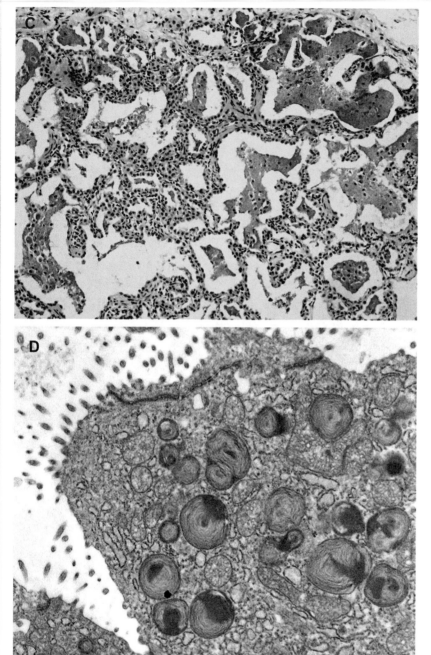

Fig. 6. (continued). (C) PAS stain highlights the proteinosis material, allowing distinction from edema fluid or fibrin. (D) Electron microscopy in ABCA3 deficiency shows small lamellar bodies with increased round or wedge-shaped densities.

life, and is associated with hypogammaglobulinemia. Pathology features include copious PAP material without destructive or inflammatory or reactive type II cell change.

The differential diagnosis of the surfactant disorders includes necrotizing viral pneumonitis and chronic aspiration. Intra-airspace granular sloughed material and debris associated with viral pneumonitis can mimic PAP material, and aspiration pneumonia can show foamy macrophages and cholesterol clefts. Both are differentiated by PAS negativity. Positive viral PCR, culture or immunohistochemistry, and presence of necrosis

Fig. 7. Genetic disorders of surfactant metabolism. (*A*) Surfactant protein B deficiency is typically diagnosed in the first days to weeks of life due to abundant proteinosis filling the airspaces. (*B*) Surfactant protein C deficiency may present in the first weeks to months of life, and is typically associated with more abundant foamy macrophages, cholesterol clefts, and less conspicuous proteinosis. (*C*) TTF1/NKX2.1 deficiency may result in dysregulation of surfactant and pathologic features resembling chronic pneumonitis of infancy. In this case, foamy macrophages and cholesterol clefts are accompanied by occasional dense globules of proteinosis material.

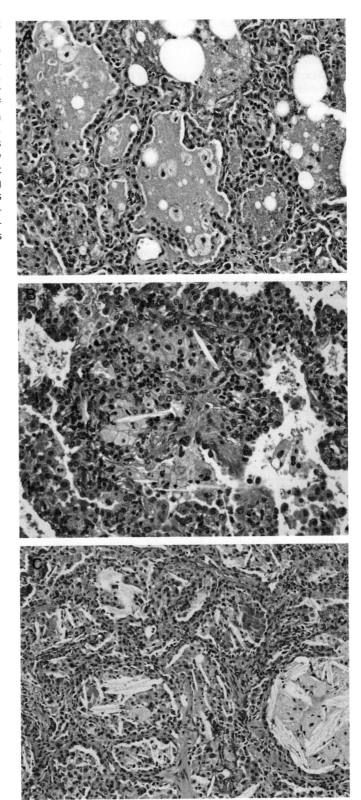

and viral cytopathic changes aid in the diagnosis of necrotizing viral infections in the neonate.

Ancillary stains:
- Special Stains: PAS stains positively PAP material, whereas it is negative with hyaline membranes or edema fluid. Masson trichrome can be used to highlight fibrous tissue in the pulmonary interstitium.
- Immunohistochemistry: Stains are available for SFPTB and SFTPC, though histology is generally sufficient to raise the suspicion and initiate genetic testing.

PROGNOSIS

The prognosis of genetic surfactant disorders that present with respiratory failure in the neonatal period is poor with diagnosis of one of these conditions useful in management considerations by the clinician and the family. Genetic screening for surfactant related mutations may identify variants of unknown significance which, particularly in infants with comorbidities, may require lung biopsy for confirmation of diagnosis.

Key Features: Surfactant Dysfunction Disorders

Diagnostic features: Variable degree of pulmonary alveolar proteinosis. Reactive alveolar epithelial hyperplasia. Variable chronic lobular remodeling depending on postnatal age. Lamellar body abnormalities, especially in SFTPB disease (multivesiculation and multilamellation) and ABCA3 disease (small lamellar bodies with round densities).

Clues: Pulmonary alveolar proteinosis may be granular or globular, and is highlighted by PAS stain. After a period of weeks to months, there is lobular remodeling, signaled by increased interstitial smooth muscle, interstitial widening, and change in shape and size of airspaces. Older infants and children tend to have less conspicuous proteinosis, and more conspicuous foamy macrophages and cholesterol clefts. SFTPB and ABCA3 mutations are most likely to be diagnosed in the neonatal period due to respiratory insufficiency, whereas SFTPC, NKX2.1, CSF2RA, and CSF2RB mutations are more likely to cause chronic disease in older infants and children.

Pitfalls:
- PAS stain also highlights mucus, which accumulates in the setting of airway obstruction.

- Electron microscopy of lamellar bodies can be normal in the surfactant disorders. Some reactive conditions also cause eccentric wedge-shaped electron densities, which should not be overinterpreted as the "fried egg" densities of ABCA3 deficiency.

Differential Diagnosis:
- Alveolar epithelial necrosis, as in the setting of necrotizing viral pneumonitis, can be confused for pulmonary alveolar proteinosis material.

- *Pneumocystis jiroveci* infection is characterized by a frothy airspace exudate similar to PAP, but organisms are easily highlighted on Gomori methenamine silver (GMS) stain.

PULMONARY INTERSTITIAL GLYCOGENOSIS

Pulmonary interstitial glycogenosis with, previously called infantile cellular interstitial pneumonia, is characterized by increased mesenchymal cells expanding the interstitium of alveolar walls of neonates and young infants, typically less than 6 months of age. Initially described in 2002 as a new form of interstitial lung disease,[25] it has now been recognized in association with a variety of neonatal lung diseases, especially chronic neonatal lung disease due to prematurity, and in the setting of pulmonary arterial hypertension. Although the pathogenesis is not well understood, it is thought to be a secondary reactive phenomenon in light of its many associated diseases. It is also thought to be self-limited, resolving spontaneously over time, but has some anecdotal clinical response to steroid therapy in some patients.

MICROSCOPIC FEATURES

Alveolar walls are expanded by interstitial cells with ovoid nuclei and indistinct clear to eosinophilic cytoplasm , which is PAS positive and diastase labile (**Fig. 8**). The interstitial cells are not lymphocytic or histiocytic, but rather show vimentin positivity and ultrastructural features suggesting mesenchymal cells similar to fibroblasts. The cytoplasm of these cells is glycogen rich, which may be demonstrated by PAS positivity or by electron microscopy. It may be seen diffusely within a lung biopsy, but more often is focal or patchy in distribution. The cells of pulmonary interstitial glycogenosis should not be confused with fibroblasts, as in bronchopulmonary dysplasia, as fibroblasts are more spindled in shape with tapered cytoplasm. The morphologic differential diagnosis includes Langerhans cell histiocytosis

Fig. 8. Pulmonary interstitial glycogenosis. (*A*) The interstitium is expanded by increased mesenchymal cells with ovoid nuclei and ill-defined vacuolated cytoplasm. In contrast to fibroblasts, these cells do not have spindled nuclei. (*B*) PAS stain highlights the cytoplasm within the interstitial glycogenosis cells.

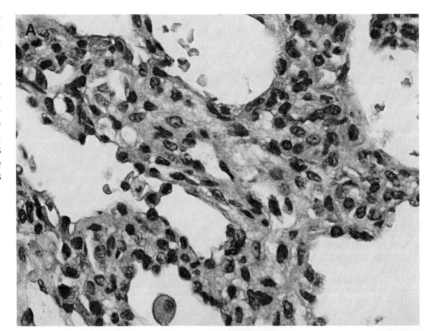

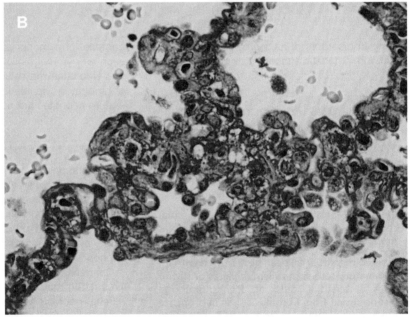

(Fig. 9), leukemia, lymphoma, other histiocytic processes, and metabolic storage disease with interstitial foamy histiocytes, such as glycogen-storage disease or lysosomal storage disease.

Ancillary stains
- Special Stains: PAS positive.
- Immunohistochemistry: Vimentin positive. Negative for lymphocyte markers (CD45) or histiocyte markers (S100, CD68, CD1a).

Prognosis: Very good. Pulmonary interstitial glycogenosis will resolve over time without therapy, but may also respond to steroid therapy. Long-term prognosis is determined by the presence and severity of underlying chronic neonatal lung disease.

Associated Genetic Changes/Alterations: There are no known primary genetic abnormalities causing pulmonary interstitial glycogenosis. This finding may however be seen as a secondary

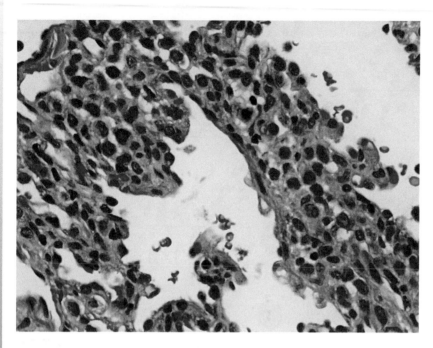

Fig. 9. Langerhans cell histiocytosis. Disseminated Langerhans cells in the infantile form of LCH may infiltrate the alveolar walls, resembling pulmonary interstitial glycogenosis focally. The indented nuclei, lack of foamy cytoplasm, and presence of CD1a or CD207 expression allows recognition of LCH cells.

finding in disorders of lung growth and development and in genetic surfactant disorders.

Key Features: Pulmonary Interstitial Glycogenosis

Diagnostic features: Interstitial widening with increased mesenchymal cells containing ovoid nuclei and indistinct bubbly cytoplasm.

Clues: PAS-positive cytoplasm of interstitial cells. PIG is often associated with alveolar simplification and/or pulmonary arteriopathy.

Pitfalls: Interstitial cells can be confused with inflammatory cells such as lymphocytes or histiocytes. Interstitial cells of PIG should be distinguished from fibroblasts seen in bronchopulmonary dysplasia, as fibroblasts have a more spindled shape and may be associated with collagen deposition.

Differential Diagnosis: Viral pneumonitis or other inflammatory disease. Langerhans cell histiocytosis, leukemia, or other neoplastic interstitial infiltrate.

CONGENITAL AND NEONATAL INFECTIONS

The differential diagnosis of congenital and neonatal lung infection includes congenital bacterial pneumonia and systemic viral infection such as cytomegalovirus and herpes simplex virus. Neonates may also be exposed to a variety of respiratory viruses in the community, and premature neonates are particularly susceptible.

MICROSCOPIC FEATURES

Congenital pneumonia refers to the accumulation of neutrophils within air spaces, sometimes associated with squames and/or bacterial organisms. These foci of pneumonia are associated with inhalation of infected amniotic fluid, and correlation with placental findings may reveal acute chorioamnionitis.

Congenital viral infection due to herpes simplex virus (HSV) may cause fulminant liver failure and adrenal necrosis with cutaneous lesions and, in some neonates, presence of viral pneumonitis. HSV causes patchy zones of necrosis and hemorrhage, associated with occasional cells containing intranuclear inclusions (**Fig. 10**). These Cowdry inclusions may be difficult to identify amidst the cell necrosis, but are easily highlighted on HSV immunohistochemistry.

Respiratory syncytial virus in a neonate with a normal immune system specifically results in lymphocytic bronchiolitis and interstitial pneumonitis. However, when respiratory syncytial virus (RSV) presents fulminantly in an immunosuppressed neonate or a neonate with primary immunodeficiency, RSV will cause a necrotizing giant cell

Fig. 10. Herpes simplex virus infection can be acquired in utero or during delivery, and results in a necrotizing pneumonia with occasional viral cytopathic effect. Due to fulminant presentation, this is most often recognized on postmortem examination rather than on lung biopsy.

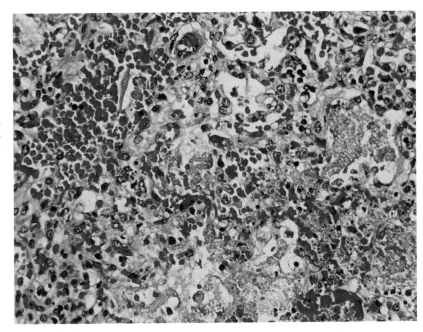

pneumonitis, not dissimilar from HSV pneumonitis. There are typically numerous large multinucleate syncytial type giant cells, some of which contain intracytoplasmic small eosinophilic viral inclusions. The extensive epithelial necrosis results in granular debris within airspaces. Presence of syncytial giant cells should trigger consideration for acquired or primary immunodeficiency in a neonate, and also warrants search for other associated infections, such as pneumocystis (Fig. 11).

Ancillary stains
- Special Stains: Gram stain for bacteria. GMS for disseminated yeast, fungal infection, and Pneumocystis.
- Immunohistochemistry: HSV, RSV, varicella zoster virus, measles.

Prognosis: Dependent on severity of infection.
Associated Genetic Changes/Alterations: None.

Fig. 11. Respiratory syncytial virus infection in a neonate with severe combined immunodeficiency results in a pattern of giant cell pneumonitis. The syncytial-type giant cells with cytoplasmic globules indicate overwhelming viral load in an immunosuppressed or immunocompromised state. The necrotic epithelial debris within airspaces can mimic the alveolar proteinosis seen in genetic disorders of surfactant metabolism.

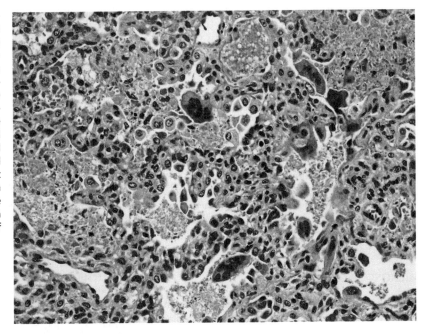

MECONIUM ASPIRATION

Meconium aspiration is a common complication in newborns following prolonged delivery or stress in utero. It may be recognized clinically by the presence of brown-stained mucoid fluid aspirated from the nose and mouth at the time of delivery. However, it may be unrecognized or the severity may be underestimated in some neonates.

MICROSCOPIC FEATURES

Meconium aspiration may be recognized in postmortem lung examination of neonates to survive hours to days, but may also be recognized in neonatal lung biopsy occasionally. If there is no prior history of meconium aspiration, then the persistent tachypnea and ground glass opacities may lead to neonatal lung biopsy to investigate other causes of interstitial and alveolar lung disease. Microscopically, meconium resembles airway and alveolar mucus, but is typically associated with admixed aggregates of anucleated squames and a few yellow to brown pigmented macrophages (**Fig. 12**).

Ancillary stains
- Special Stains: Movat pentachrome stain highlights both mucus and meconium.
- Immunohistochemistry: Cytokeratin stain may help to confirm the anucleated squames within the meconium.

Prognosis: Depending on extent of meconium aspiration and airway obstruction. Small amounts of meconium will typically resolve over time, but may persist for weeks to months after delivery.

Associated Genetic Changes/Alterations: None.

NEUROENDOCRINE CELL HYPERPLASIA OF INFANCY

Neuroendocrine cell hyperplasia of infancy (NEHI) was described in 2005 as a histologic correlate for persistent tachypnea of infancy.[26] It is typically diagnosed in older infants and toddlers, but also could present in the neonatal period. These children have an oxygen requirement, with tachypnea and chronic hypoxia, but no wheezing. Chest computed tomography (CT) is characterized by patchy ground glass opacities, most often hilar in distribution. The severity of symptoms is often greater than expected based on lung biopsy findings.

MICROSCOPIC FEATURES

The lung biopsy in NEHI is normal or near normal at low power. Subtle findings may include alveolar distention or alveolar duct distention, focal alveolar edema fluid, mild bronchiolar respiratory epithelial hyperplasia, or mild prominence of airway lymphoid tissue. Hyperplasia of neuroendocrine cells can only be recognized by immunohistochemistry, defined as neuroendocrine cells representing 10% or more of total respiratory epithelial cells in peak airways (**Fig. 13**). Large neuroepithelial bodies at the interface between the respiratory bronchiole and alveolar duct are also typical. It is important to note that there are a number of other neonatal and pediatric lung diseases associated with secondary neuroendocrine cell hyperplasia, most importantly chronic neonatal lung disease of prematurity/bronchopulmonary dysplasia. NEHI is therefore diagnosis of exclusion, and any evidence of significant alveolar simplification, airway fibrosis, or pulmonary vascular disease would exclude NEHI, which implies an idiopathic form of NEH.

Ancillary stains
- Special Stains: Trichrome or Movat pentachrome, to exclude airway fibrosis and to assess pulmonary arteries.
- Immunohistochemistry: Bombesin (preferred), chromogranin, synaptophysin

Prognosis: Good. Neuroendocrine cell hyperplasia of infancy typically improves slowly over time, with decreasing oxygen dependence over a period of months to years. Conservative management includes optimization of nutrition and oxygen supplementation, but discontinuation of steroids or other inflammatory modulators. There is no mortality associated with NEHI.

Associated Genetic Changes/Alterations: There is a report of TTF1/NKX2.1 mutation in association with familial NEHI, but most patients have no known genetic abnormality.[27]

Key Features: Neuroendocrine Cell Hyperplasia of Infancy

Diagnostic features: Increased numbers of neuroendocrine cells in the airways (>10%) and large neuroepithelial bodies, demonstrated on Bombesin stain.

Clues: Near-normal lung biopsy in a child with history of hypoxia, tachypnea, and patchy ground glass opacities on chest CT. Lung biopsy may show subtle alveolar duct dilation, mild bronchiolar respiratory epithelial hyperplasia, mild prominence of bronchiolar-associated lymphoid tissue, and/or scant alveolar edema fluid.

Pitfalls: Any degree of alveolar simplification, chronic lung disease, or pulmonary arteriopathy excludes the diagnosis of NEHI. Neuroendocrine cell hyperplasia is a secondary finding in these diseases. Other neuroendocrine markers such as chromogranin or synaptophysin may not meet diagnostic criteria, and bombesin stain is preferred as the most sensitive diagnostic marker for airway neuroendocrine cells.

Differential Diagnosis: Constrictive/obliterative bronchiolitis may also show a near-normal lung biopsy with subtle hyperinflation. Trichrome or Movat pentachrome stain highlight the airway fibrosis, and bombesin stain excludes NEHI.

SUMMARY

Neonatal lung biopsy remains a diagnostically challenging area of pediatric pathology, due to the infrequency of biopsy in this age group, and the rarity of certain developmental and genetic disorders in this population. Assessment of alveolar growth and development is of paramount importance in recognizing chronic neonatal lung disease of prematurity, pulmonary hypoplasia, and rare disorders such as acinar dysgenesis, congenital alveolar dysplasia, and alveolar capillary

Fig. 12. Meconium aspiration. (*A*) Aspirated meconium material resembles mucus, and is admixed with anucleate squames and yellow-brown pigmented macrophages. (*B*) The mucoid nature of meconium is highlighted in blue on Movat pentachrome stain.

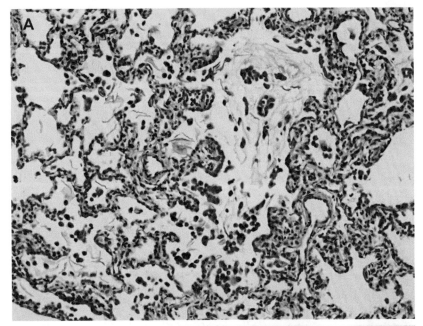

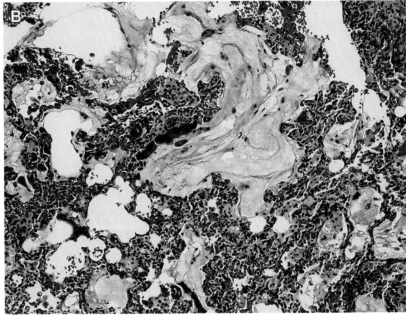

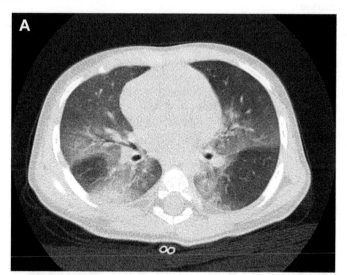

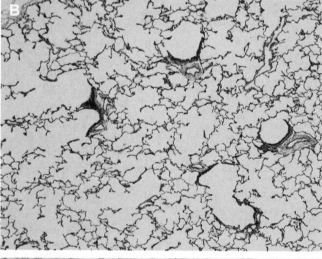

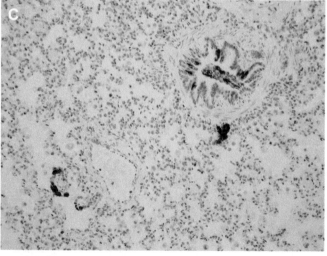

Fig. 13. Neuroendocrine cell hyperplasia of infancy. (*A*) CT scan demonstrates patchy zones of ground-glass opacities bilaterally. (*B*) At low power, the lung architecture is normal except for slight dilation of alveolar ducts, consistent with parenchymal hyperinflation. (*C*) Bombesin stain highlights the increased number of airway neuroendocrine cells and the large neuroepithelial bodies at the interface of alveolar ducts and alveoli.

dysplasia. Abnormal alveolarization (alveolar simplification) may be particularly difficult to recognize for pathologists who more often interpret the emphysematous lungs of adults. Although molecular diagnosis of the genetic disorders of surfactant metabolism may preclude the need for invasive procedures such as lung biopsy, it is nevertheless important for pathologists to recognize the distinctive pathologic features on biopsy to allow correlation with existing molecular results, or further recommendation for genetic testing if not already performed. Neonatal lung biopsy still has an important role in guiding medical therapy for babies in neonatal intensive care, and in some cases allows early recognition of fatal disease which would allow early referral for lung transplantation for palliative care. The diagnostic yield of neonatal lung biopsy is optimized when the pathologist works in close coordination with radiologists and the clinical care team, both before and after the biopsy, to understand the differential diagnosis and to determine potential therapy.

CLINICAL CARE POINTS

- Optimal interpretation of neonatal lung biopsy requires coordination and communication with a multidisciplinary care team to plan the biopsy, to understand the differential diagnosis, and to obtain special studies.
- Microscopic examination of neonatal lung biopsy should focus on assessment of lung growth and development, associated findings such as pulmonary interstitial glycogenosis and pulmonary arteriopathy, vasculopathy associated with congenital heart disease, genetic disorders of surfactant metabolism, perinatal infection, and complications of delivery such as meconium aspiration.
- Special stains such as Movat pentachrome (or Trichrome and Elastic stains) aid in the assessment of the pulmonary vasculature and early fibrosis. PAS stain is used to distinguish pulmonary alveolar proteinosis from hyaline membranes or edema, and can also be used to recognize pulmonary interstitial glycogenosis.
- Lung biopsy findings should be correlated with germline molecular testing, including consideration of the genetic disorders of surfactant metabolism (SFTPB, SFTPC, ABCA3, NKX2.1) and genetic disorders of lung growth and development (FOXF1, TBX4, NKX2.1). Lung biopsy may help to clarify the pathogenicity of genetic variants of unknown significance.

DISCLOSURE

Dr M.K. Dishop is a consultant for Boehringer-Ingelheim pharmaceuticals. Dr J. Lipsett has no commercial or financial conflicts of interests or funding sources to disclose.

REFERENCES

1. Langston C, Patterson K, Dishop MK, chILD Pathology Cooperative Group. A protocol for the handling of tissue obtained by operative lung biopsy: recommendations of the child pathology cooperative group. Pediatr Dev Pathol 2006;9:173–80.
2. Emery JL, Mithal A. The number of alveoli in the terminal respiratory unit of man during late intrauterine life and childhood. Arch Dis Child 1960;35:544–57.
3. Karolak JA, Vincent M, Deutsch G, et al. Complex compound inheritance of lethal lung developmental disorders due to disruption of TBX-FGF pathway. Am J Hum Genet 2019;104:213–28.
4. Cua CL, Blankenship A, North AL, et al. Increased incidence of idiopathic persistent pulmonary hypertension in Down syndrome neonates. Pediatr Cardiol 2007;28:250–4.
5. McDowell KM, Craven DI. Pulmonary complications of Down syndrome during childhood. J Pediatr 2011;158:319–25.
6. Szafranski P, Coban-Akdemir ZH, Rupps R, et al. Phenotypic expansion of TBX_4 mutations to include acinar dysplasia of the lungs. Am J Med Genet 2016;170:2440–4.
7. Suhrie K, Pajor NM, Ahlfeld SK, et al. Neonatal lung disease associated with TBX4 mutations. J Pediatr 2018. https://doi.org/10.1016/j.jpeds.2018.10.018.
8. Barnett CP, Nataren NJ, Klingler-Hoffmann M, et al. Ectrodactyly and lethal pulmonary acinar dysplasia associated with homozygous FGFR2 mutations identified by exome sequencing. Hum Mutat 2016;37:955–63.
9. Chow CW, Massie J, Ng J, et al. Acinar dysplasia of the lungs: variation in the extent of involvement and clinical features. Pathology 2013;45:38–43.
10. Garola RE, Thibeault DW. Alveolar capillary dysplasia, with and without misalignment of pulmonary veins: an association of congenital anomalies. Am J Perinatol 1998;15:103–7.
11. Sen P, Thakur N, Stockton DW, et al. Expanding the phenotype of alveolar capillary dysplasia (ACD). J Pediatr 2004;145:646–51.
12. Eulmesekian P, Curtz E, Parvez B, et al. Alveolar capillary dysplasia: a six-year single center experience. J Pernat Med 2005;33:347–52.
13. Szafranski P, Gambin T, Dharmadhikari AV, et al. Pathogenetics of Alveolar Capillary Dysplasia with Misalignment of Pulmonary Veins. Hum Genet 2016;135:569–86.

14. Abdallah HI, Karmazin N, Marks LA. Late presentation of misalignment of lung vessels with alveolar capillary dysplasia. Crit Care Med 1993;21: 628–30.

15. Al-Hathlol K, Phillips S, Seshia MK, et al. Alveolar capillary dysplasia. Report of a case of prolonged life without extracorporal membrane oxygenation (ECMO) and review of the literature. Early Hum Dev 2000;57:85–94.

16. Licht C, Schickendantz S, Sreeram N, et al. Prolonged survival in alveolar capillary dysplasia syndrome. Eur J Pediatr 2004;163:181–2.

17. Stankiewicz P, Sen P, Bhatt SS, et al. Genomic and genic deletions of the FOX gene cluster on 16q24.1 and inactivating mutations of FOXF1 cause alveolar alveolar capillary dysplasia and other malformations. Am J Hum Genet 2009;84:780–91.

18. Karolak J, Bacolla A, Liu Q, et al. A recurrent 8bp frameshifting indel in FOXF1 defines a novel mutation hotspot associated with alveolar capillary dysplasia with misalignment of pulmonary veins. Am J Med Genet 2019;179:2272–6.

19. Whitsett J, Wert S, Weaver T. Diseases of pulmonary surfactant homeostasis. Ann Rev Pathol 2015;10: 371–93.

20. Suzuki T, Sakagami T, Rubin BK, et al. Familial pulmonary alveolar proteinosis caused by mutations in CSF2Ra. J Exp Med 2008;205:2703–10.

21. Martinez-Moczygemba M, Doan ML, Elidemir O, et al. Pulmonary alveolar proteinosis caused by deletion of the GM-CSFR2a gene in the X chromosome pseudoautosomal region 1. J Exp Med 2008; 205:2711–6.

22. Suzuki T, Maranda B, Sakagami T, et al. Hereditary pulmonary alveolar proteinosis caused by recessive CSF2RB mutations, [Letter]. Eur Respir J 2011;37: 201–17.

23. Nattes E, Lejeune S, Carsin A, et al. Heterogeneity of lung disease associated with NK2 homeobox 1 mutations. Respir Med 2017;129:16–23.

24. Hamvas A, Deterding R, Wert S, et al. Heterogenous pulmonary phenotypes associated with mutations in the thyroid transcription factor gene NKX2.1. Chest 2013;144:794–804.

25. Canakis AM, Cutz E, Manson D, et al. Pulmonary interstitial glycogenosis: a new variant of neonatal interstitial lung disease. Am J Respir Crit Care Med 2002;165:1557–65.

26. Deterding RR, Pye C, Fan LL, et al. Persistent tachypnea of infancy is associated with neuroendocrine cell hyperplasia. Pediatr Pulmonol 2005;40: 157–65.

27. Young LR, Deutsch GH, Bokulic RE, et al. A mutation in TTF1/NKX2.1 is associated with familial neuroendocrine cell hyperplasia of infancy. Chest 2013; 144(4):1199–206.

Wilms Tumor
Challenges and Newcomers in Prognosis

Lauren N. Parsons, MD[a,b,*]

KEYWORDS

- Wilms tumor • Children's oncology group • International Society of Pediatric Oncology
- Biomarkers

Key points

- Wilms tumor is a morphologically and biologically heterogeneous tumor.
- Challenges in the pathologic assessment of Wilms tumor include difficulties with gross examination, easily overlooked or misinterpreted histologic elements of staging, and failure to detect anaplasia.
- Biomarkers of prognostic significance have been evaluated/validated in Wilms tumor; new methodologies continue to identify new potential therapeutic targets and prognostic indicators.

ABSTRACT

Wilms tumor is the most common renal tumor of childhood. It is a biologically and morphologically diverse entity, with ongoing studies contributing to our understanding of the pathobiology of various subgroups of patients with Wilms tumor. The interplay of histologic examination and molecular interrogation is integral in prognostication and direction of therapy. This review provides an overview of some of the challenging aspects and pitfalls in pathologic assessment of Wilms tumor, along with discussion of current and up-and-coming markers of biological behavior with prognostic significance.

modern therapeutic interventions, long-term survival in patients with WT, when considered as a group, approaches 85% to 90%.[3] As such, current objectives for WT therapy are primarily (1) reducing the risk of long-term therapy–related sequelae in low-risk WT and (2) identifying and improving outcomes for WT patient subsets who currently have less favorable outcomes. Risk stratification of patients with WT incorporates a variety of components, including gross pathologic findings, histologic classification, and molecular alterations. This review focuses on common challenges and pitfalls encountered by pathologists in the examination of WT specimens, as well as, current and up-and-coming factors associated with prognosis in patients with WT.

OVERVIEW

Wilms tumor (WT) is the most common malignant renal tumor of childhood. It accounts for approximately 80% to 90% of renal tumors in the pediatric population and has an incidence of approximately 8.2 cases per one million children.[1,2] As a result of

DIAGNOSTIC OVERVIEW

WT is an embryonal malignancy of childhood derived from nephrogenic blastemal cells. It often shows various features of the developing kidney, along with other patterns of differentiation. The classic appearance of WT is triphasic, with

---

[a] Medical College of Wisconsin, Milwaukee, WI, USA; [b] Children's Hospital of Wisconsin, Milwaukee, WI, USA
* 9000 West Wisconsin Avenue, MS#701, Milwaukee, WI 53226.
E-mail address: lparsons@mcw.edu

Surgical Pathology 13 (2020) 683–693
https://doi.org/10.1016/j.path.2020.08.007

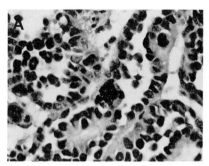
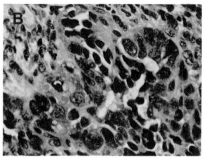

Fig. 1. Features of nuclear anaplasia in WT include enlarged, multipolar mitotic figures (A, H&E, 40x) and enlarged, hyperchromatic nuclei that are greater than 3 times the size of surrounding nonanaplastic nuclei (B, H&E, 40x). H&E, hematoxylin and eosin.

undifferentiated blastemal cells along with stromal cells and epithelial cells, the latter 2 of which may show varying degrees of differentiation. For example, it is not uncommon for the epithelial component of WT to form primitive tubules and glomeruloid structures, whereas the stromal component may display heterologous elements such as skeletal muscle and cartilage.[4] These cell types may be present in varying proportions; when one component represents greater than 66% of the tumor, that component is considered to be "predominant"; for example, blastema predominant WTs are tumors in which greater than two-thirds of the tumor are composed of blastema.[5]

WTs are divided into tumors with favorable histology and those with unfavorable histology. Unfavorable histology tumors are those that demonstrate diffuse anaplasia. The designation of anaplasia requires the presence of 2 features. First, the tumor must contain cells with hyperchromatic, markedly enlarged nuclei that are greater than 3 times the size of nearby nonanaplastic nuclei. In addition, abnormal multipolar/polyploid mitotic figures must be present (Fig. 1).[4,5] Anaplasia is further characterized as diffuse or focal. The designation of focal anaplasia is reserved for WTs in which anaplasia is confined to the kidney parenchyma (not within vascular spaces or metastatic lesions) and is present only in one or a few sharply circumscribed areas. Anaplasia discovered in a small biopsy specimen is considered evidence of diffuse anaplasia and is managed as such. Some tumors may show areas of nuclear hyperchromasia/marked enlargement in the absence of abnormal mitoses, therefore falling short of the anaplasia designation; such tumors are said to display "nuclear unrest," a feature with similar outcomes to favorable histology/nonanaplastic WT.[4] However, in an otherwise focally anaplastic tumor, the remainder may not show areas of nuclear unrest. If nuclear unrest is present in these situations, the tumor must be classified as diffuse anaplasia and unfavorable histology. Anaplasia in WT correlates with a lack of response to therapy and is associated with a poorer prognosis in the context of higher stage tumors.[4]

DIFFERING APPROACHES: CHILDRENS ONCOLOGY GROUP AND SOCIÉTÉ INTERNATIONALE dOncologie PÉDIATRIQUE

Most North American patients with WT are managed according to Children's Oncology Group (COG) protocols, in which up-front nephrectomy is followed by evaluation of untreated tumor. Staging according to this system is summarized here: (https://documents.cap.org/protocols/cp-pediatric-wilms-resection-19-4000.pdf).[6] Subsequent chemotherapy for these patients is dictated by a variety of clinical, pathologic, and biological factors, many of which are discussed later in this review. Stage 3 tumors—in which there has been tumor spillage/disruption, positive margins, or spread to lymph nodes—receive abdominal radiation therapy, whereas lower stage tumors generally do not unless anaplasia is identified.[7] Notably, tumor biopsy before resection/nephrectomy automatically corresponds with a local stage 3 in the COG system and is therefore discouraged if the tumor/kidney is safely resectable with negative margins.[6]

In contrast, in Europe the Société Internationale d'Oncologie Pédiatrique (SIOP; also known as International Society of Pediatric Oncology) protocols—in which neoadjuvant chemotherapy precedes nephrectomy—are the standard of care. On resection, posttherapy tumors are evaluated for degree of necrosis/treatment effect and, in the case of viable tumor, the proportion of blastema present (See table 1 here: https://www.nature.com/articles/s41585-018-0100-3).[8] Tumors that are entirely necrotic are considered low risk, whereas those showing blastema predominance in the viable tumor component are designated as high risk. The remaining subtypes are considered intermediate risk. SIOP staging of posttherapy WT is summarized in box 2 here: https://www.na-ture.com/articles/s41585-018-0100-3. It should be noted that stage 2 tumors are the same in both staging systems, in that the tumor in the renal sinus or capsule of a pretreated tumor must be viable to qualify as stage 2. There is a notable change to stage 3 tumors in the 2016 SIOP UM-BRELLA protocol. Previously, a tumor would be designated stage 3 if there were either viable tumor or necrotic tumor present at the resection margin. In the upcoming protocols, only viable tumor at the resection margin is considered stage 3. However, necrotic tumor is still sufficient for stage 3 designation if it is present in a lymph node or as a tumor thrombus in the renal vein, ureter, or vena cava.[8,9]

Despite differences in initial management, there are many similarities between the COG and SIOP approaches. Staging is a crucial component of each system, highlighting the importance of careful pathologic examination. The presence of anaplasia is of great significance in both pre- and posttherapy tumors, as anaplasia cannot be induced by therapy and carries similar implications in both systems (discussed later). Interestingly, patient outcomes are comparable between the SIOP and COG systems despite their inherent ideological differences.[7] However, the significance and utility of some biomarkers may differ between the 2 systems; as such, biomarkers will be discussed in the context of each of the therapeutic methodologies.

CHALLENGES

In the context of WT, there are several important factors for the pathologist to recognize that will directly influence therapy and prognosis. The significance of the gross examination in WT cannot be overstated, as careful and proper sampling is of paramount importance for proper staging. The variable histomorphology of WT can present diagnostic challenges as well as difficulties in designation of risk due to the presence of anaplasia and the effect of chemotherapy in posttherapy nephrectomies. Some of these challenges are discussed later, along with strategies to avoid diagnostic pitfalls.

CHALLENGES RELATED TO GROSS EXAMINATION AND TECHNIQUE

Careful gross examination and dissection is essential for accurate staging of WT. One commonly encountered dilemma in the gross dissection of WT nephrectomies is the friable nature of the tumor itself. Fragments of tumor (or so-called floaters) can complicate histologic interpretation of staging when they are discovered in problematic places, such as artifactually embedded tumor fragments in vessels of the renal sinus or capsule, or minute pieces of tumor that seem to be outside the capsule. Adequate formalin fixation of the nephrectomy before gross examination can reduce the potential for artificial tumor spread. The presence of ink on tumor fragments seen in vessels signals artifact rather than true lymphovascular invasion. In questionable cases of spread outside the kidney versus artifactual tumor contamination, correlation with the operative report or gross appearance can be helpful in making a determination.[6] Another issue that may be encountered when grossing WT nephrectomy specimens is assessment of the renal vein margin for tumor thrombus. In this scenario, retraction of the renal vein following resection (either due to formalin fixation or due to the intrinsic properties of the vessel) can give the false impression of tumor present at the renal vein margin. Examination of this margin while the specimen is fresh and discussion with the surgeon in questionable cases can mitigate this issue.[6]

HISTOLOGIC CHALLENGES: IS IT ACTUALLY A WILMS TUMOR?

Often, the diagnosis of WT is straightforward. However, a variety of circumstances may prompt diagnostic confusion. Some histologic subtypes of WT can show a striking similarity to other tumors of the kidney, other primitive tumors of childhood, or soft tissue tumors. Distinguishing between large hyperplastic nephrogenic rests and WT may also be problematic. Careful attention to certain histomorphologic features is generally the most effective way to confirm the diagnosis of WT. Ancillary studies may be helpful in a handful of situations or to eliminate other entities in the differential diagnosis.

Nephrogenic rests are persistent foci of embryonal cells within otherwise mature kidneys and are considered to be the precursor lesions of WT. They may be classified as intralobar nephrogenic rests (ILNR) or perilobar nephrogenic rests (PLNR). ILNRs often contain stromal elements and are usually located intermingled within the normal renal parenchyma, whereas PLNRs generally contain blastema and epithelial components, are well circumscribed, and are located at the edge of the renal lobule.[4,10] Despite their differences, both types of nephrogenic rests can be difficult to distinguish from WT. Both lesions can be quite large, and they may be almost indistinguishable cytologically from WT. One of the most helpful features for differentiating rests from WT is the presence of a fibrous pseudocapsule separating WT from the surrounding renal parenchyma.[4,10] As stated, INLRs are often found blending with the surrounding normal kidney, which is not typically a feature of WT. Although PLNRs are generally well circumscribed, they should not be encased by a pseudocapsule. Another helpful feature specifically for differentiating between ILNRs and WT is the components of the lesion itself. ILNRs often have a prominent stromal component and frequently display adipocytic differentiation. In contrast, skeletal muscle and cartilage are more often seen in WT; note that this is not entirely specific but in conjunction with other features can be helpful to support the diagnosis of WT over ILNR.[4,10]

Depending on the histologic features of the tumor, other entities may enter the differential diagnosis. Epithelial-predominant WT—in this case composed exclusively of well-differentiated tubules and epithelial elements—may be difficult to distinguish from the benign metanephric adenoma (MA). As discussed earlier, the presence of a fibrous pseudocapsule favors WT over MA. Similarly, elevated mitotic activity has traditionally been associated with WT rather than MA. There is overlap between the immunohistochemical profiles of WT and MA, as both are frequently positive for WT1 and negative for markers of renal cell carcinoma (RCC). CD57 positivity favors MA, as several studies have shown high rates of positivity in MA.[11] BRAFV600E mutations are frequent in MA (up to 90% in some studies) and are not seen in WT.[12] Recent studies suggest that BRAF immunohistochemistry may be useful in detecting this mutation, although approximately 15% to 25% of mutation-positive cases were negative or showed unconvincing staining.[13] Unfortunately, there are challenging cases that show overlapping features of WT and MA; expert consultation may be helpful in such situations, although in some cases the distinction remains elusive.[14,15]

WT may mimic a variety of other pediatric renal malignancies. Variants of RCC may at times be difficult to distinguish from epithelial-predominant WT, particularly in older children where the clinical scenario would favor a diagnosis of RCC. Immunohistochemistry may be useful in these situations. For example, solid variant of papillary RCC should be positive for CK7 and AMACR but negative for WT1, whereas WT should show the inverse staining pattern.[11] Xp11 translocation–associated RCC may also enter the differential, as it is the most common RCC of childhood.[16] Demonstration of TFE3 or TFEB nuclear staining or evidence of translocation of TFE3 or TFEB by fluorescence in-situ hybridization will readily assist in the proper diagnosis.[17] WTs showing prominent stromal or blastemal differentiation may be mistaken for congenital mesoblastic nephroma (CMN—particularly the cellular variant) or clear cell sarcoma of kidney (CCSK). As in the case of MA, recognition of a fibrous pseudocapsule will support a diagnosis of WT, whereas both CMN and CCSK should show an infiltrative border at least focally.[4] Cyclin D1 positivity is generally strong and diffuse in CCSK and is negative in the blastemal component of WT.[18,19] Molecular studies in particular may be helpful in this scenario. The cellular variant of CMN will most often display the characteristic t(12;15) translocation, and a significant proportion of CCSK may show evidence of BCOR internal tandem duplications.[20,21]

Primitive small round blue cell tumors of childhood may be nearly morphologically indistinguishable from blastema-predominant WT. Neuroblastoma and Ewing sarcoma may occur near the kidney (and rarely may occur within the kidney), thus presenting a diagnostic dilemma. PAX-8 immunohistochemistry should be positive in WT and can be a helpful clue to the diagnosis.[16] Immunohistochemical stains for the other entities being considered, such as PHOX2b for neuroblastoma and CD99 for Ewing sarcoma, in conjunction with PAX-8 should delineate these entities from one another.[16]

HISTOLOGIC CHALLENGES: ANAPLASIA

Detection of anaplasia, whether focal or diffuse, may be challenging and has been identified as one of the most frequent reasons for discrepancy between institutional pathologic interpretation and central pathology review. In a study of the first 3000 patients enrolled on COG AREN03B2, approximately 35% of cases of WT with diffuse anaplasia that were identified on central review were not detected by the institutional pathologist.[22] One feature that can be helpful when assessing a WT for anaplasia is the fact that areas of anaplasia can look morphologically distinct from nonanaplastic areas even from low to intermediate power; this is thought to be due at least in part to the idea that areas of anaplasia represent clones that are different from the surrounding WT. Most anaplastic cells can be detected from 10x power, so it may be useful to scan at 10x power to screen for anaplasia in all submitted slides. Special attention must be paid to intravascular, extracapsular, or metastatic WT for detection of anaplasia, as its presence in these locations can be easily over-looked but alone qualifies as diffuse anaplasia.

HISTOLOGIC CHALLENGES: STAGING

For both the pretherapy COG system and the post-therapy SIOP system, WT staging is based on de-gree of extension outside the kidney and presence of tumor left behind in the body following resection (SIOP staging and its associated chal-lenges are discussed later in further detail). COG protocols designate fully resected intact WTs with negative surgical margins and no involved lymph nodes as stage 1. Stage 2 tumors have extension of tumor beyond the renal capsule or invasion of the soft tissue or vasculature of the renal sinus but are still completely resected. Stage 3 tumors are those with positive surgical margins, prior or intraoperative tumor rupture, piecemeal removal or prior biopsy, or lymph nodes containing tumor.[6]

Staging of WT cases also can be challenging due to a variety of factors, including artifact (as discussed earlier in the gross examination section). In addition, invasion of renal sinus vasculature and soft tissue can be overlooked. In fact, failure to appreciate renal sinus involvement is the most common reason for discrepancy between institutional pathology review and central pathology review in WT.[23] It should be noted that although much of the renal sinus is located at the hilum, the renal sinus extends deep into the renal parenchyma in parts of the kidney.[4] Involvement of vasculature or soft tissue in these areas still constitutes renal sinus involvement and corresponds with a stage 2 tumor. Recognition of intrarenal extension of the renal sinus, histologically characterized by vascular structures surrounded by fat and mesenchymal tissue, can help in avoiding this pitfall.[4,6] Determination of the presence of rupture may also present difficulty. Careful review of the operative report and/or discussion with the surgeon may be useful in such situations.[6] If a region is seen grossly that is suspicious for tumor rupture, it may be helpful to overlay that focus in a second color of ink to help identify the area more readily histolog-ically. However, there are instances when rupture is neither suspected/documented by the surgeon nor identified grossly, but there is suspicion of rupture at the time of microscopic examination. Histologic clues to rupture include a fibroblastic reaction and hemorrhage/fibrin overlying or intermixed with tumor at the surface of the kidney (**Fig. 2**).

HISTOLOGIC CHALLENGES: POSTTHERAPY SPECIMENS

Accurate histologic interpretation of posttherapy changes is essential to risk assignment in

posttherapy WT. Posttherapy tumors are assessed for degree of tumor viability and pre-dominant histologic component in the case of viable tumor. An entirely necrotic WT following therapy is classified as low risk; although this designation is generally straightforward, some findings can complicate interpretation. It may be difficult to distinguish paucicellular stromal ele-ments from benign stroma with chemotherapy-induced changes. The presence of foamy histio-cytes favors chemotherapy effect and can be a useful finding.[9] Distinguishing between a true blastema-predominant tumor and a mixed type with a prominent blastemal component has signif-icant prognostic importance, as posttherapy blas-tema predominant tumors are considered high risk. In such cases, some investigators recom-mend estimating the percent of viable tumor that is composed by blastema for each individual slide and averaging these for a total overall percentage.[9]

It is important to recall the key differences be-tween staging of posttherapy WT versus staging of primarily resected tumors, namely due to the incorporation of chemotherapy-induced necrosis into staging evaluation. If viable tumor is present in the soft tissue or vessels of the renal sinus, or is penetrating through the capsule, the tumor re-ceives a designation of stage 2. However, if the tu-mor in these locations is nonviable and the tumor is completely resected, the tumor is assigned a stage of 1. Stage 3 tumors may have either viable *or* necrotic tumor transected at the vascular margin, within a lymph node, in tumor implants in the abdominal cavity or in areas of peritoneal invasion.[8]

PROGNOSTIC INDICATORS

For many years, prognostic information for pa-tients with WT was derived from pathologic and surgical/clinical findings. Before the institution of standard WT therapy regimens, some of these fac-tors—blastemal predominance, for example—were linked to worse outcomes than other favor-able histology tumors. However, with the introduc-tion of dactinomycin and vincristine as standard therapy for patients with WT, many of the differ-ences observed between tumors of differing histo-logic type (epithelial vs blastemal vs stromal) became insignificant.[5] However, there are some important morphologic findings that retain clinical and prognostic significance. In addition, with the advent of new molecular techniques, many bio-markers—both established and forthcoming—have been identified that carry important implica-tions for outcome.

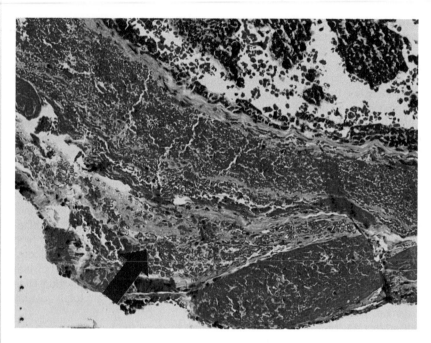

Fig. 2. A section from a stage 3 WT in which rupture was identified intraoperatively. Note the blood and layered fibrin (*arrow*) adjacent to/admixed with tumor, a histologic finding that supports tumor rupture (H&E, 10x). H&E, hematoxylin and eosin.

ANAPLASIA, TP53 ALTERATIONS, AND ASSOCIATION WITH OUTCOMES

Perhaps the most significant pathologic prognostic indicator in WT is anaplasia/unfavorable histology, which continues to show tremendous value with respect to directing therapy and determining outcomes in WT. Tumors with diffuse anaplasia require more aggressive chemotherapy regimens, and despite the more intensive therapy these patients receive, outcomes remain inferior to those observed in favorable histology WT.[7] TP53 alterations have been demonstrated in a significant proportion of diffusely anaplastic WT. A cooperative study between SIOP and COG revealed that half of the tumors showed TP53 mutation and/or loss of 17p and also demonstrated inferior event-free and overall survival in patients with anaplastic WT with TP53 mutation.[24] Additional studies evaluating anaplastic WT samples from patients enrolled in the National Wilms Tumor Study (NWTS)-5 showed a similar percentage of TP53 mutations in the tumors analyzed. Notably, stage 3 and 4 patients with diffuse anaplasia and TP53 alterations displayed a significantly inferior disease-free and overall survival, suggesting that TP53 status may be an important prognostic factor within this subgroup of WT.[25] Further studies assessing the relationship between TP53 status, volume of anaplasia, and outcome are forthcoming.

EPITHELIAL-PREDOMINANT HISTOLOGY AS A MARKER OF BIOLOGICAL BEHAVIOR

Another morphologic finding that has recently been linked to outcome is epithelial-predominant histology, characterized by tumor composed of greater than 66% epithelial differentiation within a WT. These components may show a spectrum of morphology from primitive tubules to immature-appearing glomeruloid forms and (as discussed earlier) at times can be difficult to distinguish from benign metanephric adenomas (**Fig. 3**). For many years, it was evident that a subset of WT characterized by epithelial predominant well-differentiated tubular morphology, low stage, and very young patient age was associated with excellent outcomes.[5] Tumors within this group were found to show a distinct gene expression pattern similar to that of the late postinduction epithelial phase of kidney development.[26] Further investigation has shown that a significant proportion of these tumors demonstrated mutations in TRIM28.[27] A recent study by COG evaluated all stage 1 epithelial predominant WT enrolled on AREN03B2 and found that 4-year overall survival for these patients was 100%, with a very low frequency of recurrence/metastasis regardless of age, tumor size, or therapy status.[28] These findings taken together suggest that these tumors may be a biologically distinct favorable subset within WT and that epithelial predominance in the appropriate context may serve as a marker of this biological behavior.

CHROMOSOMAL ALTERATIONS AS BIOMARKERS

1p and 16q loss of heterozygosity

In the early 1990s, Grundy and colleagues[29] identified the relationship between loss of heterozygosity (LOH) for 1p, 11p, and 16q among a subset of WT in NWTS-3&4 and decreased relapse-free and overall survival. Given the need for improved prognostication and risk stratification within the broad group of favorable histology WT, the association between outcome and LOH for these chromosomes was further examined prospectively in the NWTS-5 cohort. This study showed that within favorable histology WT, LOH for either 1p or 16q was associated with an increased risk of relapse; when taken together, concomitant LOH of 1p and 16q exerted an even more significant impact on patient outcomes.[30] As a result of these findings, LOH of 1p and 16q were incorporated in to the risk stratification schema for subsequent studies. A study examining the impact of LOH of 1p/16q on prognosis in patients with stage 3 WT revealed that, in conjunction with positive lymph nodes, 1p/16q LOH was a negative prognostic factor. Improved outcomes for patients with LOH 1p and 16q have been observed with augmented therapy, reinforcing the value of this biomarker as a prognostic indicator in the setting of up-front nephrectomy.[31] Studies from SIOP have displayed variable results regarding the prognostic significance of LOH 1p and 16q in posttherapy favorable histology WT specimens.[32] The UMBRELLA SIOP-RTSG 2016 protocol, in which biomarker analysis is one of the primary aims, will further investigate 1p/16q LOH among posttherapy tumors to determine its relationship (if any) with outcome.[8] Regardless, combined LOH of 1p and 16q occurs in a small minority of favorable histology WT (overall fewer than 5%), highlighting the need for additional markers of biological behavior in these tumors.[3]

1q gain

Gain of chromosome 1q has been associated with poorer outcomes in a variety of tumors, making it an attractive candidate biomarker to investigate in WT.[33,34] Early studies identified as association between 1q gain and relapse in a cohort of favorable histology WT.[35] An analysis of patients registered on NWTS-4 revealed that 1q gain was associated with shorter event-free survival.[36] This finding was further validated in the NWTS-5 cohort, where the effect of 1q gain on event-free and overall survival was particularly pronounced in stage 1 and stage 4 patients.[37] Given that approximately 30% of favorable histology WT display gain of 1q, this biomarker holds promise as a risk stratifier for a significant subset of patients with WT undergoing upfront nephrectomy.[3] As such, ongoing and upcoming COG protocols are including 1q gain as a biological marker to assess risk and inform therapeutic decisions. Studies from SIOP have demonstrated a similar

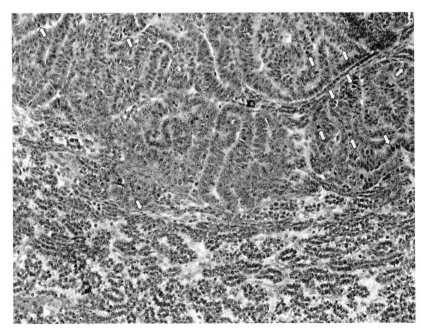

Fig. 3. An epithelial-predominant WT (H&E, 10x), which may be mistaken for metanephric adenoma. Clues to WT as the appropriate diagnosis include presence of a pseudocapsule (not shown) and frequent mitotic figures (*arrows* denote several). H&E, hematoxylin and eosin.

proportion of favorable histology WT displaying 1q gain and thus far have shown association between 1q gain and worse event-free survival; however, the effect on overall survival does not seem to be as significant in posttherapy tumors.[32] As with 1p/16q LOH, the UMBRELLA protocol may provide further insight into the utility of 1q gain as a biomarker in posttherapy favorable histology WT.[8]

11p15 methylation status

11p15 is the site of the WT2 region, within which the *IGF2* gene is located. *IGF2* is highly expressed in primitive metanephric mesenchyme, with reduced expression in renal epithelial cells. Studies have demonstrated abnormalities of 11p15 in nearly 70% of WT.[38] Examination of this region for LOH revealed that a significant proportion of favorable histology WT—approximately 30% to 35%—show LOH for 11p15.[39,40] Gene expression analysis of favorable histology WTs from NWTS-5 demonstrated that among tumors that would typically be considered low risk based on clinicopathologic factors, many of those that relapsed showed LOH for 11p15.[26] This finding was further confirmed in a cohort of very low-risk WT, in which 11p15 methylation was associated with relapse in patients who underwent nephrectomy only.[41] This suggests that 11p15 methylation status may be valuable in risk-stratifying patients within this subset of WT and allow for expansion of patients eligible for nephrectomy only. Additional studies validating the incorporation of 11p15 methylation status for risk stratification are forthcoming.

NEW BIOMARKER CANDIDATES IN WILMS TUMOR

Prohibiton (PHB) is a protein localized to the mitochondria that contributes to multiple cellular processes including apoptosis, cellular proliferation, and gene transcription.[42,43] Alterations in PHB expression levels have been noted in several human cancers, including lymphomas, osteosarcoma, and various carcinomas.[44–46] Recent studies have detected variations in urinary levels of PHB in patients with WT that are associated with increased risk of relapse; in addition, increased expression of PHB by immunohistochemistry was observed in favorable histology WT that ultimately relapsed. Furthermore, renal tumor cell lines (including a WT line) that overexpressed PHB were found to be resistant to conventional WT chemotherapies.[47] Although additional studies to further investigate the role of PHB in WT and its interaction with various cellular components is necessary, PHB may be a

promising prognostic indicator with the advantage of ability to be detected noninvasively.

Hotspot mutations in SIX1 and SIX2 have been identified in a subset of relapsed favorable histology WT. In this study, tumors showing mutations of SIX1/2 concomitant with mutations of the microRNA processing genes DROSHA and DGCR8 were associated with higher rates of both relapse and death.[48] These genetic events occur in combination in a relatively small subgroup of favorable histology WT (approximately 2%) and with a slightly greater frequency in the high-risk WT evaluated (approximately 6.5%).[48] Therefore, although this is an interesting finding that provides further insight into the molecular pathobiology of WT, it is applicable to a fairly small subset of WT. Nonetheless, evaluation of these mutations may offer another tool for predicting clinical behavior and outcomes in WT.

Notably, the studies discussed earlier were performed using pretherapy WT specimens. Molecular biology aims of the SIOP UMBRELLA protocol include provisions for exploration of the above-described molecular alterations (among others) and their implications in the context of posttherapy WT.[8] Examination of drivers in blastema-predominant posttherapy tumors will also be performed, which may provide new insights into targets in these high-risk posttherapy tumors.[8] Biomarker analysis in the SIOP cohort will provide important insights into the significance of these candidate biomarkers in the context of neoadjuvantly treated WT.

SUMMARY

As is evident, WT is a clinically and biologically diverse pediatric tumor. Accurate morphologic assessment remains crucial to diagnosis and prognosis, whereas molecular factors provide important insights into outcomes and guidance of therapy. There are opportunities to fine-tune the histologic classification of WT, including examining the criteria for diffuse anaplasia and exploration of variations in the traditional staging systems. Whole genome/exome sequencing and gene expression analysis have provided new and exciting insights into the molecular events that contribute to the development of WT. As we continue to identify the genes and molecular aberrations implicated in WT, clarification of their roles in tumor development will be key to determining additional prognostic and therapeutic markers. The merging of histopathological observations and molecular biomarkers has—and will continue to—aid pathologists, oncologists, and the entire care team in achieving the best possible outcomes for patients with WT.

CLINICS CARE POINTS

- Wilms tumor therapy and prognosis relies on a variety of histopathologic and molecular factors.
- Common challenges in Wilms tumor diagnosis and pathologic interpretation include staging challenges related to gross examination, histologic detection of renal sinus invasion, identification of anaplasia, and interpretation of post-therapy nephrectomy specimens.
- Important prognostic morphologic findings include anaplasia, epithelial-predominant histology in low stage tumors, and blastema predominant post-therapy tumors.
- Current prognostic indicators of importance include loss of heterozygosity for chromosome 1p and 16q, gain of chromosome 1q, 11p15 methylation status; some of these require validation in post-nephrectomy cohorts.
- Up-and-coming molecular biomarkers have been and continue to be identified via gene expression profiling and genome wide sequencing to better risk-stratify Wilms tumor patients for optimal therapy.

DISCLOSURE

The authors have nothing to disclose.

REFERENCES

1. Davidoff AM. Wilms Tumor. Adv Pediatr 2012;59(1): 247–67.
2. Howlader N, Noone AM, Krapcho M, et al. SEER cancer statistics review (CSR) 1975-2016. Bethesda (MD): National Cancer Institute; 2019.
3. Aldrink JH, Heaton TE, Dasgupta R, et al. Update on Wilms tumor. J Pediatr Surg 2019;54(3):390–7.
4. Kidney tumors in children. In: Murphy WM, Grignon DJ, Perlman EJ, editors. Tumors of the kidney, bladder and related urinary structures. AFIP atlas of tumor pathology 4th series. 2004. Available at: https://www.arppress.org/kidney-bladder-urinary-p/4f01.htm.
5. Beckwith JB, Zuppan CE, Browning NG, et al. Histological Analysis of Aggressiveness and Responsiveness in Wilms Tumor. Med Pediatr Oncol 1996;27: 422–8.
6. Rudzinski E, Perlman E, Kim G, et al. Protocol for the examination of resection specimens from patients with Wilms and other pediatric renal tumors. Wilms tumor resection 4.0.0.0. College of American Pathologists; 2019. https://doi.org/10.14694/EdBook_AM.2014.34.215. PMID: 24857079.
7. Dome JS, Perlman EJ, Graf N. Risk stratification for wilms tumor: current approach and future directions. Am Soc Clin Oncol Educ Book 2014;215–23.
8. Vujanić GM, Gessler M, Ooms AHAG, et al. The UMBRELLA SIOP-RTSG 2016 Wilms tumour pathology and molecular biology protocol. Nat Rev Urol 2018; 15(11):693–701.
9. Vujanić GM, Sandstedt B. The pathology of Wilms' tumour (nephroblastoma): the International Society of Paediatric Oncology approach. J Clin Pathol 2010;63(2):102–9.
10. Perlman E. Nephrogenic Rests and Nephroblastomatosis in SIOP EDUCATION BOOK 2009: International Society of Paediatric Oncology 41st Congress of the International Society of Paediatric Oncology. Sao Paulo, Brazil, October 6–9, 2009. p. 101–5.
11. Kinney S, Eble J, Hes O, et al. Metanephric adenoma: the utility of immunohistochemical and cytogenetic analyses in differential diagnosis, including solid variant papillary renal cell carcinoma and epithelial-predominant nephroblastoma. Mod Pathol 2015;28:1236–48.
12. Caliò A, Eble JN, Hes O, et al. Distinct clinicopathological features in metanephric adenoma harboring BRAF mutation. Oncotarget 2016;8(33):54096–105.
13. Udager AM, Pan J, Magers MJ, et al. Molecular and immunohistochemical characterization reveals novel BRAF mutations in metanephric adenoma. Am J Surg Pathol 2015;39(4):549-557.
14. Goldstein JA, Cajaiba MM, Chi YY, et al. BRAF exon 15 mutations in the evaluation of well-differentiated epithelial nephroblastic neoplasms in children. [abstract] Society for Pediatric Pathology Spring Meeting March 16-18, 2018, Vancouver, BC.
15. Wobker SE, Matoso A, Pratilas CA, et al. Metanephric Adenoma-Epithelial Wilms Tumor Overlap Lesions: An Analysis of BRAF Status. Am J Surg Pathol 2019;43(9):1157–69.
16. Ooms AHAG, Vujanić GM, D'Hooghe E, et al. Renal Tumors of Childhood-A Histopathologic Pattern-Based Diagnostic Approach. Cancers (Basel) 2020;12(3):729.
17. Magers MJ, Udager AM, Mehra R. MiT Family Translocation-Associated Renal Cell Carcinoma: A Contemporary Update With Emphasis on Morphologic, Immunophenotypic, and Molecular Mimics. Arch Pathol Lab Med 2015;139(10):1224–33.
18. Mirkovic J, Calicchio M, Fletcher CD, et al. Diffuse and strong cyclin D1 immunoreactivity in clear cell sarcoma of the kidney. Histopathology 2015;67(3): 306–12.
19. Uddin N, Minhas K, Abdul-Ghafar J, et al. Expression of cyclin D1 in clear cell sarcoma of kidney. Is

it useful in differentiating it from its histological mimics? Diagn Pathol 2019;14(1):13.

20. Gooskens SL, Houwing ME, Vujanic GM, et al. Congenital mesoblastic nephroma 50 years after its recognition: A narrative review. Pediatr Blood Cancer 2017;64(7). https://doi.org/10.1002/pbc.26437.

21. Wong MK, Ng CCY, Kuick CH, et al. Clear cell sarcomas of the kidney are characterised by BCOR gene abnormalities, including exon 15 internal tandem duplications and BCOR-CCNB3 gene fusion. Histopathology 2018;72(2):320–9.

22. Dome JS, Fernandez CV, Mullen EA, et al. Children's Oncology Group's 2013 blueprint for research: renal tumors. Pediatr Blood Cancer 2013;60(6):994–1000.

23. Mullen EA, Geller JI, Gratias EJ, et al. Real-time central review: A report of the first 3,000 patients enrolled on the Children's Oncology Group Renal Tumor Biology and Risk Stratification protocol AREN03B2. J Clin Oncol 2014;32:5s, (suppl; abstr 10000).

24. Maschietto M, Williams RD, Chagtai T, et al. TP53 mutational status is a potential marker for risk stratification in Wilms tumour with diffuse anaplasia. PLoS One 2014;9(10):e109924.

25. Ooms AH, Gadd S, Gerhard DS, et al. Significance of TP53 Mutation in Wilms Tumors with Diffuse Anaplasia: A Report from the Children's Oncology Group. Clin Cancer Res 2016;22(22):5582–91.

26. Gadd S, Huff V, Huang CC, et al. Clinically relevant subsets identified by gene expression patterns support a revised ontogenic model of Wilms tumor: a Children's Oncology Group Study. Neoplasia 2012;14(8):742–56.

27. Armstrong AE, Gadd S, Huff V, et al. A unique subset of low-risk Wilms tumors is characterized by loss of function of TRIM28 (KAP1), a gene critical in early renal development: A Children's Oncology Group study. PLoS One 2018;13(12):e0208936.

28. Parsons LN, Mullen EA, Geller JI, et al. Outcome analysis of stage I epithelial-predominant favorable-histology Wilms tumors: A report from Children's Oncology Group study AREN03B2. Cancer 2020;126(12):2866–71.

29. Grundy PE, Telzerow PE, Breslow N, et al. Loss of heterozygosity for chromosomes 16q and 1p in Wilms' tumors predicts an adverse outcome. Cancer Res 1994;54(9):2331–3.

30. Grundy PE, Breslow NE, Li S, et al. Loss of heterozygosity for chromosomes 1p and 16q is an adverse prognostic factor in favorable-histology Wilms tumor: a report from the National Wilms Tumor Study Group. J Clin Oncol 2005;23(29):7312–21.

31. Dix DB, Fernandez CV, Chi YY, et al. Augmentation of Therapy for Combined Loss of Heterozygosity 1p and 16q in Favorable Histology Wilms Tumor: A Children's Oncology Group AREN0532 and AREN0533 Study Report. J Clin Oncol 2019;37(30):2769–77.

32. Chagtai T, Zill C, Dainese L, et al. Gain of 1q As a Prognostic Biomarker in Wilms Tumors (WTs) Treated With Preoperative Chemotherapy in the International Society of Paediatric Oncology (SIOP) WT 2001 Trial: A SIOP Renal Tumours Biology Consortium Study [published correction appears in J Clin Oncol. 2017 Jun 20;35(18):2100]. J Clin Oncol 2016;34(26):3195–203.

33. Lo KC, Ma C, Bundy BN, et al. Gain of 1q is a potential univariate negative prognostic marker for survival in medulloblastoma. Clin Cancer Res 2007;13:7022–8.

34. Pezzolo A, Rossi E, Gimelli S, et al. Presence of 1q gain and absence of 7p gain are new predictors of local or metastatic relapse in localized resectable neuroblastoma. Neuro Oncol 2009;11:192–200.

35. Hing S, Lu YJ, Summersgill B, et al. Gain of 1q is associated with adverse outcome in favorable histology Wilms' tumors. Am J Pathol 2001;158(2):393–8.

36. Gratias EJ, Jennings LJ, Anderson JR, et al. Gain of 1q is associated with inferior event-free and overall survival in patients with favorable histology Wilms tumor: a report from the Children's Oncology Group. Cancer 2013;119(21):3887–94.

37. Gratias EJ, Dome JS, Jennings LJ, et al. Association of Chromosome 1q Gain With Inferior Survival in Favorable-Histology Wilms Tumor: A Report From the Children's Oncology Group. J Clin Oncol 2016;34(26):3189–94.

38. Scott RH, Murray A, Baskcomb L, et al. Stratification of Wilms tumor by genetic and epigenetic analysis. Oncotarget 2012;3(3):327–35.

39. Satoh Y, Nakadate H, Nakagawachi T, et al. Genetic and epigenetic alterations on the short arm of chromosome 11 are involved in a majority of sporadic Wilms' tumours. Br J Cancer 2006;95(4):541–7.

40. Grundy P, Telzerow P, Moksness J, et al. Clinicopathologic correlates of loss of heterozygosity in Wilm's tumor: a preliminary analysis. Med Pediatr Oncol 1996;27(5):429–33.

41. Perlman EJ, Grundy PE, Anderson JR, et al. WT1 mutation and 11P15 loss of heterozygosity predict relapse in very low-risk wilms tumors treated with surgery alone: a children's oncology group study. J Clin Oncol 2011;29(6):698–703.

42. Theiss AL, Sitaraman SV. The role and therapeutic potential of prohibitin in disease. Biochim Biophys Acta 2011;1813(6):1137–43.

43. Ande SR, Xu YXZ, Mishra S. Prohibitin: a potential therapeutic target in tyrosine kinase signaling. Signal Transduct Target Ther 2017;2:17059.

44. Yang J, Li B, He QY. Significance of prohibitin domain family in tumorigenesis and its implication in cancer diagnosis and treatment. Cell Death Dis 2018;9(6):580.

45. Wang W, Xu L, Yang Y, et al. A novel prognostic marker and immunogenic membrane antigen: prohibitin (PHB) in pancreatic cancer. Clin Transl Gastroenterol 2018;9(9):178.

46. Bentayeb H, Aitamer M, Petit B, et al. Prohibitin (PHB) expression is associated with aggressiveness in DLBCL and flavagline-mediated inhibition of cytoplasmic PHB functions induces anti-tumor effects. J Exp Clin Cancer Res 2019;38(1):450.

47. Ortiz MV, Ahmed S, Burns M, et al. Prohibitin is a prognostic marker and therapeutic target to block chemotherapy resistance in Wilms' tumor. JCI Insight 2019;4(15):e127098.

48. Walz AL, Ooms A, Gadd S, et al. Recurrent DGCR8, DROSHA, and SIX homeodomain mutations in favorable histology Wilms tumors. Cancer Cell 2015; 27(2):286–97.

Pediatric Renal Tumors
Updates in the Molecular Era

Amy L. Treece, MD

KEYWORDS

- Cystic nephroma • Metanephric • Mesoblastic nephroma • Renal cell carcinoma
- Clear cell sarcoma of kidney • Rhabdoid tumor

Key points

- Pediatric cystic nephromas are associated with germline or somatic mutations in *DICER1*; they are distinct from cystic partially differentiated nephroblastoma and adult cystic nephromas.

- Metanephric adenomas, adenofibromas, and stromal tumors are related and carry somatic *BRAF* mutations.

- In addition to NTRK3 fusions, congenital mesoblastic nephromas (CMNs) contain a variety of fusions or alterations in receptor tyrosine kinases or downstream effector molecules.

- Translocation renal cell carcinomas carry fusions of the *TFE3* gene and, less commonly, the *TFEB* gene, with an expanding landscape of fusion partners.

- Alterations in clear cell sarcoma of the kidney include YWHAE-NUTM2B fusions, BCOR internal tandem duplications, and other rare alterations of BCOR, linking them with other BCOR-altered tumors.

- Rhabdoid tumors of the kidney are characterized by alterations in *SMARCB1*, causing loss of INI1 expression and downstream effects on numerous critical cell proliferation pathways.

ABSTRACT

Molecular characterization has led to advances in the understanding of pediatric renal tumors, including the association of pediatric cystic nephromas with DICER1 tumor syndrome, the metanephric family of tumors with somatic BRAF mutations, the characterization of ETV6-NTRK3–negative congenital mesoblastic nephromas, the expanded spectrum of gene fusions in translocation renal cell carcinoma, the relationship of clear cell sarcoma of the kidney with other BCOR-altered tumors, and the pathways affected by SMARCB1 alterations in rhabdoid tumors of the kidney. These advances have implications for diagnosis, classification, and treatment of pediatric renal tumors.

OVERVIEW

Non-Wilms pediatric renal tumors are rare and diverse, affecting different age groups and with different biological origins and clinical behaviors. Widening use of molecular techniques, including cytogenetics and sequencing, has opened the door to insights into the diagnosis, classification, and treatments for these tumors. Many of these advances are very recent, within just the past few years, and may establish the groundwork for even more progress, particularly in the treatment of aggressive tumors.

CYSTIC NEPHROMA

INTRODUCTION

Pediatric cystic nephroma (CN) is a benign neoplasm in children, distinct from adult-type cystic nephromas. Originally thought to be on the most benign end of the spectrum of Wilms tumor and partially differentiated cystic nephroblastoma (CPDN), they have in the past decade been established as primarily *DICER1* mutation–driven tumors, with either germline or somatic *DICER1* mutations (**Box 1**).

Department of Pathology, Children's Hospital Colorado, University of Colorado School of Medicine, 13123 East 16th Avenue, Box 120, Aurora, CO 80045, USA
E-mail address: Amy.treece@childrenscolorado.org

Surgical Pathology 13 (2020) 695–718
https://doi.org/10.1016/j.path.2020.08.003
1875-9181/20/© 2020 Elsevier Inc. All rights reserved.

surgpath.theclinics.com

> **Box 1**
> **Molecular features and their clinical impact in pediatric cystic nephroma**
>
> - Molecular alterations:
>   - Somatic (usually missense) or germline (usually loss of function) *DICER1* mutations
> - Clinicopathologic features:
>   - Molecularly distinct from CPDN and adult cystic nephroma
>   - *DICER1* tumor predisposition syndrome (eg, pleuropulmonary blastoma, ovarian Sertoli-Leydig cell tumors, thoracic or uterine cervical embryonal rhabdomyosarcoma, multinodular goiter)
>   - CN is an indication for germline testing, often paired with tumor
> - Diagnostic molecular testing:
>   - *DICER1* mutations detected by next-generation sequencing (NGS), but exon-based sequencing may miss intronic mutations
>   - Rare larger deletion events or loss of heterozygosity (LOH) may require specific deletion/duplication technologies (microarray or multiplex ligation-dependent probe amplification [MLPA])
>   - Interpretation of germline status complicated by mosaicism

GROSS AND MICROSCOPIC FEATURES

Pediatric CNs are grossly multicystic tumors, identical in appearance to CPDN, with thin septa and lacking solid areas (**Fig. 1**). The cyst linings are smooth, and the cysts may contain clear fluid. Microscopically, the cysts are lined by flattened to cuboidal or hobnailed epithelium. The septa are composed of fibrous tissue and may have a layer of spindle cells (see **Fig. 1**). Mature tubular structures may be present in the septa, but no blastemal or primitive epithelial elements are seen, in contrast with CPDN.[1]

DIFFERENTIAL DIAGNOSIS

Before molecular characterization, CNs were reported in patients with pleuropulmonary blastoma (PPB) or their family members.[2–6] PPB was first linked with germline *DICER1* mutations a decade ago and, in a larger study, 12% of patients with PPB had or had a family member with CN.[7–9] A high proportion of histologically defined pediatric CNs were shown to have *DICER1* mutations, whereas mutations were absent in patients with CPDN, distinguishing CN from the CPDN spectrum.[10]

Pediatric CNs are also distinct from adult CNs, which are now included in the spectrum of mixed epithelial and stromal tumors.[11] On histology, pediatric tumors lack the classic ovarian-type stroma and the ropy collagen of adult tumors. The stroma of the adult type is inhibin positive, but both can show estrogen receptor (ER) positivity.[12] Nearly all adult patients are negative for *DICER1* mutations, and rare exceptions likely represent pediatric patients with CN that were not recognized in childhood.[12,13]

MOLECULAR PATHOLOGY FEATURES AND DIAGNOSIS

DICER1-associated tumors have biallelic mutations in *DICER1*. They may carry an autosomal dominant germline plus a somatic mutation or may be entirely somatic. As more tumors have been studied, a mutational pattern has emerged, with most somatic mutations clustering in hotspots in the ribonuclease (RNase) IIIB domain and germline mutations more commonly spread throughout the gene and resulting in loss of function.[14] In patients who present with a *DICER1*-associated tumor in the absence of a family history, testing of both the tumor and a germline specimen by sequencing and deletion/duplication testing can be helpful in determining whether the tumor is sporadic or whether there is a risk for the family of *DICER1* tumor predisposition syndrome. Pediatric CN is considered a major indication for germline testing in published recommendations.[15] Note that 2 mutations are not always identified in the tumor tissue, possibly because of intronic mutations or deletion/duplication events that may not be detected depending on the sequencing approach used. Interpretation of sequencing results may be further complicated by the possibility of low-level mosaicism in the germline.[15]

Similar to PPB, multiple *DICER1*-associated tumors have now been documented to have a spectrum of histologic and clinical features from benign

Fig. 1. Pediatric CN. (*A, B*) CN in a patient with a concurrent pleuropulmonary blastoma and a germline *DICER1* mutation showing cystic spaces lined by a hobnail epithelium. Septa are fibrous and contain hemorrhage and chronic inflammation and sparse mesenchymal cells.

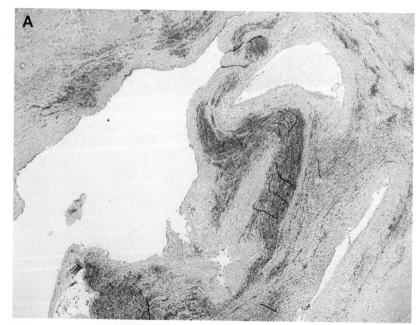

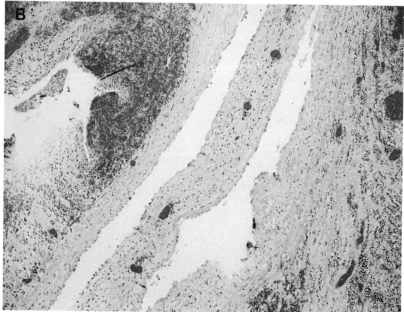

to highly aggressive. Tumors with more aggressive features are characterized by undifferentiated spindled and small round blue cells with marked pleomorphism or anaplasia and heterologous differentiation, including rhabdomyoblastic, chondroblastic, and bone or osteoid formation.[16] Anaplastic sarcoma of the kidney (ASK) has these same features, as well as cystic spaces lined by a hobnail epithelium and separated by thin fibrous septa. ASK also lacks primitive nephrogenic elements, similar to CN.[17] ASKs have the same *DICER1* mutational pattern as CNs, with both sporadic and familial/germline mutations.[18] Although most pediatric CNs are bland and benign, they seem to be on a spectrum with ASK and may progress from CN to these more aggressive lesions. In small reports, ASKs are associated with higher rates of metastasis and local recurrence.[16–20]

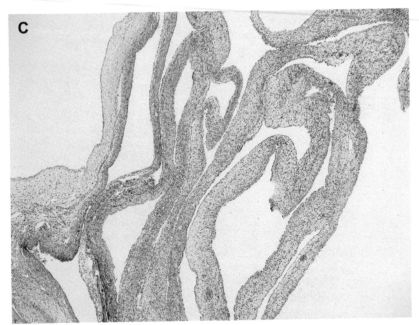

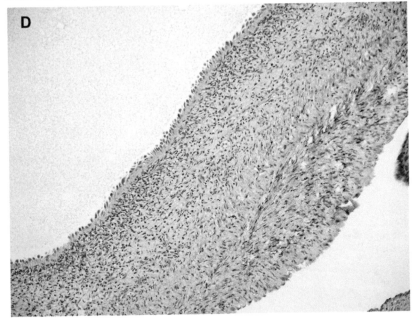

Fig. 1. (continued). (C, D) Sporadic CN in a patient with negative germline testing for DICER1. Septa show the same hobnail epithelium and increased numbers of mesenchymal spindle cells in septa. The histologic differences between these samples are not specific for the presence or absence of germline DICER1 mutations (hematoxylin-eosin, original magnification ×50 [A, C] and ×100 [B, D]).

METANEPHRIC TUMORS

INTRODUCTION

The family of metanephric tumors comprises metanephric adenoma (MA), metanephric adenofibroma (MAF; previously known as nephrogenic adenofibroma), and metanephric stromal tumor (MST). These tumors are related by their overlapping histopathologic spectrum of features and by the presence of a *BRAF* mutation in most cases,

throughout the histologic spectrum. Although MAs are more common in adults, MAFs are seen in children and young adults and MSTs are primarily seen in younger children[21–23] (**Box 2**).

GROSS AND MICROSCOPIC FEATURES

MSTs are a benign renal neoplasm arising from the renal medulla. Grossly, they appear well circumscribed and lobulated and may have cystic areas.[22] Calcification or ossification may be seen

---

Box 2
Molecular features and their clinical impact in metanephric tumors

- Molecular alterations:
  - *BRAF* V600E mutations, and rarely other codon V600 mutations
- Clinicopathologic features:
  - Established molecular link between MA, MAF, and MST, which in most cases distinguishes them from nephroblastic lesions
  - Immunohistochemistry (IHC) for *BRAF* V600E may be helpful in difficult cases and offers a rapid molecular correlation, but will be negative in cases with other *BRAF* mutations
- Diagnostic molecular testing:
  - Testing for *BRAF* codon V600 mutations available by multiple modalities, including real-time polymerase chain reaction (PCR), NGS, and traditional sequencing technologies

---

in the wall.[24] On microscopic examination, they are unencapsulated and can show growth into the surrounding parenchyma, entrapping normal structures and undermining the urothelium of the renal pelvis. The tumor is composed of a spindled to stellate to epithelioid stroma with variable cellularity with areas of brisk mitotic activity. Other characteristic features include collarettes of the stromal cells surrounding entrapped vessels with angiodysplasia and entrapped tubules that may show cystic dilatation. Juxtaglomerular cell hyperplasia and heterologous differentiation, particularly glial or chondroid, may also be present, as are focal hyperplastic embryonal proliferations. The stromal component is generally positive for CD34 and negative for desmin and cytokeratins.[22]

MAFs are also benign and are seen in children and young adults, occasionally presenting with polycythemia. Similar to MSTs, MAFs arise in the medulla, but are more likely to be cystic. The growth pattern and the stroma are identical to that seen in MST and are accompanied by an epithelial component identical to that seen in MA. The epithelial component is characterized by densely packed tubular and papillary structures, sometimes with psammoma bodies. Juxtaglomerular cell hyperplasia is lacking. The immunohistochemical profile of the stroma is identical to that of MST, with CD34 positivity, and the epithelial component shows variable cytokeratin expression and positivity for WT1, consistent with that seen in MA.[23,25–27]

MAs are the most common of the metanephric tumors and represent the epithelial end of the spectrum of metanephric tumors and are generally unencapsulated, but well-circumscribed neoplasms with a sharply demarcated interface with the surrounding parenchyma. They are composed of bland tumor cells that form an acinar pattern of varying density set in an acellular stroma. Tubular or papillary patterns can also be seen. The tumor cells are round to ovoid without prominent nucleoli and with scant cytoplasm[21] (**Fig. 2**). Most MAs completely lack mitoses and a fibrous capsule; however, more recently it has been shown that these may be present, although to a very limited extent. Dystrophic ossification may be seen in long-standing tumors.[21,28] MAs may show variable staining for cytokeratins but are consistently positive for WT1 (see **Fig. 2**) and CD57.[21,29]

MOLECULAR PATHOLOGY FEATURES

Before molecular characterization of these tumors, metanephric tumors were thought to be related to Wilms tumors and intralobar nephrogenic rests.[22,23] Early molecular studies were performed primarily in MAs because of the higher numbers of cases available for study, and numerous studies showed the presence of *BRAF* V600E mutations, by sequencing in most cases, with rare reports of other *BRAF* codon V600 mutations.[27,30–33] These studies were followed by molecular evaluations of MSTs and MAFs that again showed a high proportion of tumors with *BRAF* mutations.[27,34–36] Immunohistochemistry is now available for evaluation of the *BRAF* V600E mutation and has been highly correlated with mutational status in these tumors, although *BRAF* codon V600 mutations other than the V600E, such as the V600D, are not be detected by the antibody.[27,28,31,32,34,37]

Additional molecular studies of MAs have shown chromosomal abnormalities, including complex gains of the long arm of chromosome 17 and amplification of the short arm of chromosome 19, although many cases showed no gains or losses.[38–40] Broader sequencing analysis of MAs showed variable mutations in other neoplasia-associated genes, including *NF1*, *NOTCH1*, and *SPEN*. Rare fusions between *BRAF* and other genes were also identified.[33] The clinical

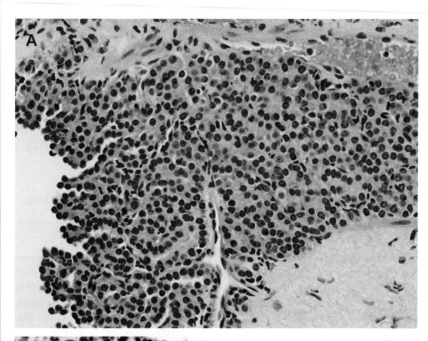

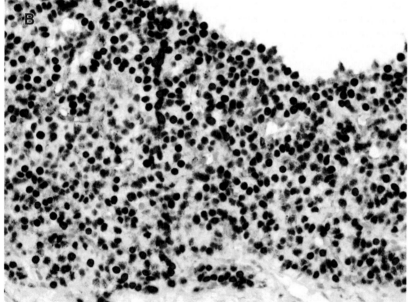

Fig. 2. MA. (A) Monomorphic ovoid cells with indistinct nucleoli in an acinar to tubular pattern (hematoxylin-eosin, original magnification ×400). (B) Nuclei are strongly positive for WT1 (WT1, original magnification ×400).

significance of these alterations and their applicability to the other metanephric tumors have not been determined.

MOLECULAR PATHOLOGY DIAGNOSIS

The identification of *BRAF* mutations in metanephric tumors has been most useful to establish the relatedness of these tumor to each other and their distinct origins from other tumor types. Detection of *BRAF* mutations by sequencing or

by immunohistochemistry may help to different these tumors from others with overlapping histology or in cases where a biopsy is performed before resection.

CONGENITAL MESOBLASTIC NEPHROMA

INTRODUCTION

Congenital mesoblastic nephromas (CMNs) are low-grade tumors of infancy with classic, cellular, and mixed subtypes. Although an *ETV6-NTRK3* translocation has been described for more than 2 decades in the cellular subtype, the molecular underpinnings of cases lacking this fusion, including in the classic subtype, a proportion of the mixed subtype, and rare cellular cases, have been unclear until recently (**Box 3**).

GROSS AND MICROSCOPIC FEATURES

Classic CMNs account for 35% to 50% and cellular for 35% to 45%, with the mixed subtype making up the remaining 15% to 20% of mesoblastic nephromas.[41,42] CMNs of all subtypes are unencapsulated tumors that may show invasion into the parenchyma or perirenal soft tissues, usually at the hilum. The cut surface shows a whorled appearance in the classic subtype, whereas the cellular is more homogeneous and may show areas of hemorrhage, necrosis, or cystic degeneration (**Fig. 3**). The mixed subtype may have features of either.

Microscopically, classic CMNs are composed of sweeping and interlacing fascicles of tumor cells with elongated, ovoid nuclei (see **Fig. 3**). Nucleoli are indistinct and mitoses are generally rare, but in rare cases may be increased. These tumors show an irregular, fingerlike interface with the parenchyma and entrap normal structures. The vasculature is open and thin walled and may have a branching, hemangiopericytomalike pattern. Nodules of cartilage may also be present. The cellular subtype is composed of more densely packed tumor cells arranged in shorter fascicles, but may also have a haphazard architecture. Nuclei are more plump than in the classic type,

and mitotic activity is higher (see **Fig. 3**). Areas of necrosis or hemorrhage may be present. The mixed subtype shows more variable cellularity and may or may not have distinct classic or cellular areas.[43,44] Classic immunohistochemical staining is nonspecific.

CLINICAL FEATURES

CMN is the most common congenital renal tumor, with up to 16% diagnosed prenatally.[41] Most cases are diagnosed in the first year of life, with the classic subtype presenting within days to weeks and the cellular presenting within 3 to 5 months of birth.[41] CMN has an overall survival rate of approximately 95% to 96%.[41,42,45] Local recurrence rate is less than 5%; metastasis is rare. Tumor progression is most common within the first year and in the cellular subtype and those cellular CMNs lacking the *ETV6-NTRK3* fusion.[41,42,46] Overall, approximately half of patients with recurrence or metastasis die of disease.[46] Surgical resection is the preferred treatment, although neoadjuvant chemotherapy may be required for unresectable tumors, and postoperative chemotherapy may be used in high-stage presentations and tumors.[45,46] Of note, treatment strategies are currently in flux and likely will change, given the advent of targeted therapeutic options, particularly the high success rate of targeted therapies for tumors containing *NTRK*-gene fusions.

MOLECULAR PATHOLOGY FEATURES

Early studies of the molecular characteristics of CMN focused on cytogenetics, specifically the

---

Box 3
Molecular features and their clinical impact in congenital mesoblastic nephroma

- Molecular alterations:
  - *ETV6-NTRK3* fusion present in most cellular and a subset of mixed CMNs
  - A subset of cellular and mixed cases have a growing set of alternative fusions or alterations in *NTRK* genes, *RET*, *BRAF*, among others
  - Most classic and fusion-negative cellular and mixed cases have *EGFR* internal tandem duplications
- Clinicopathologic features:
  - Pan-TRK IHC may allow rapid characterization of *NTRK* fusion–positive cases
  - Identification of *NTRK* or other targetable mutations may allow the use of inhibitor therapies in advanced-stage patients
- Diagnostic molecular testing:
  - Fusions can be detected by karyotype, fluorescence in situ hybridization (FISH), reverse-transcriptase PCR (RT-PCR), or RNA-based NGS technologies
  - If negative, consider NGS covering *BRAF* and *EGFR*

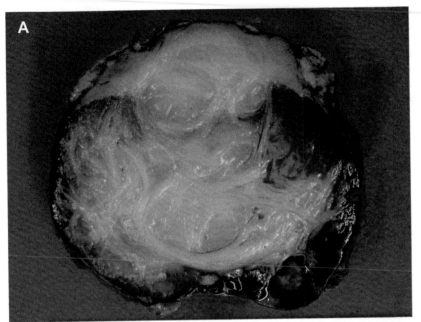

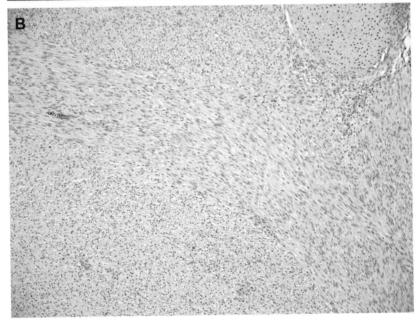

Fig. 3. CMN. (*A*) Gross appearance of classic CMN with a whirled appearance and indistinct borders with the surrounding parenchyma. (*B*) Classic CMN with sweeping fascicles and bland spindle cells. A nodule of cartilage is present in the upper right corner (hematoxylin-eosin, original magnification ×100).

t(12;15)(p13;q25) translocation resulting in the fusion of *ETV6* and *NTRK3*, after it was described in the cellular and mixed subtypes (**Fig. 4**).[47] This finding was confirmed in numerous studies, with most cellular and a variable proportion of the mixed cases showing the fusion.[48–51] Fusion-positive cases that show mixed histology seem to be positive for the fusion in all histologic components.[50] Immunohistochemical antibodies against the TRK family of proteins (panTRK) in small series showed that 2 of 3 fusion-positive CMN cases were positive by immunohistochemical staining, indicating that this may be a useful low-cost tool to identify fusion-positive cases.[52]

The standard molecular work-up for CMNs has long relied on fluorescence in situ hybridization (FISH), most commonly using a break-apart probe for *ETV6*, and, less commonly, FISH for rearrangement of the *NTRK3* gene. Until recently, cases negative for these rearrangements were generally not investigated further. In the last 2 years, and with the rapidly growing application of broad

Fig. 3. (*continued*). (*C*) Homogeneous cut surface of cellular CMN. (*D*) Cellular CMN with shorter, more densely packed fascicles composed of plump spindle cells with scattered thin-walled, dilated vessels (hematoxylin-eosin, original magnification ×100).

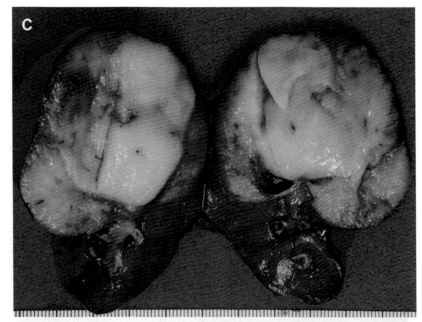

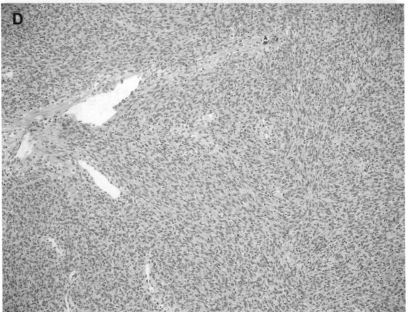

next-generation sequencing (NGS) for DNA and RNA alterations, the understanding of fusion-negative CMN has grown significantly. The spectrum of fusions in CMN has expanded to include variant NTRK fusions (eg, EML4-NTRK3 fusions, fusions involving the NTRK1 gene), RET fusions, and BRAF fusions.[53–57] Cellular and mixed tumors were among the cases with these alternative fusions. Other fusion-negative tumors, including classic, cellular, and mixed subtypes, have been identified with intragenic BRAF compound deletion and duplication events and, more commonly,

EGFR internal tandem duplications.[52,57] Although these studies have been limited, this growing set of additional molecular alterations seem to account for most ETV6-NTRK3–negative cases. It remains to be seen whether these newly identified molecular categories correlate with clinical behavior.

MOLECULAR PATHOLOGY DIAGNOSIS

FISH or targeted reverse-transcriptase polymerase chain reaction to identify the ETV6-NTRK3

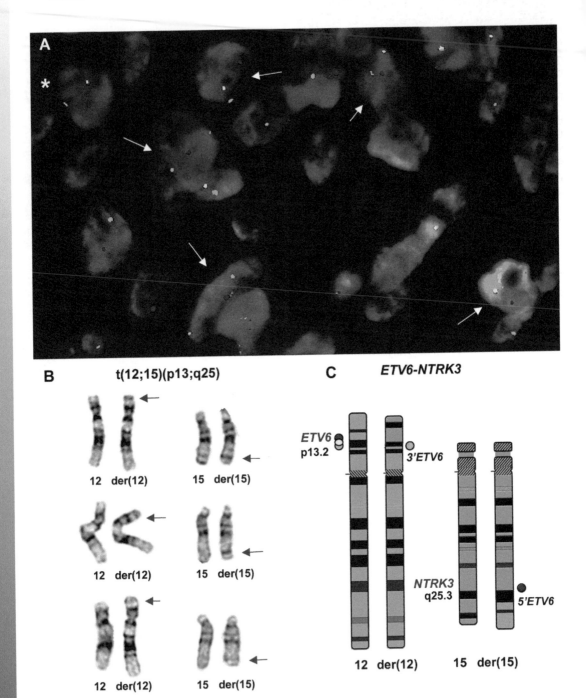

Fig. 4. Cellular CMN showing a positive rearrangement of ETV6 and tumor chromosome culture with a t(12;15)(p13;q25) consistent with an ETV6-NTRK3 fusion. (A) Interphase fluorescence in situ hybridization (FISH) using the dual-color, break-apart assay for ETV6 (12p13). Positive ETV6 rearrangement cells are indicated by the arrows. These cells show a positive pattern with 1 normal fusion signal (*yellow*) and 1 split signal of separated red and green representing a positive rearrangement of the ETV6 probe. An asterisk indicates a normal cell with a normal pattern of 2 fusion signals. (B) Composite of chromosome 12 and 15 homologues from tumor cytogenetic culture. Arrows point to the breakpoints of the rearrangement on the abnormal chromosomes. (C) A colored ideogram representing the t(12;15) and showing the FISH probe signal chromosome locations. (*Courtesy* of the Colorado Genetics Laboratory, University of Colorado Anschutz Medical Campus, Aurora, CO; with permission.)

fusion is commonly used for the diagnostic work-up. If negative, expanded NGS-based testing may be considered. This expanded testing may be particularly useful in high-stage patients that could benefit from TRK or other targeted inhibitor therapies. Although very few cases of CMN treated with TRK inhibitors have been reported in the literature, these and other tumors have shown considerable responses with less chemotherapy-associated morbidity, highlighting the importance of the pathologist's role in identifying these cases.[53,58]

TRANSLOCATION RENAL CELL CARCINOMA

INTRODUCTION

Renal cell carcinomas (RCCs) are uncommon in children, accounting for less than 5% of renal tumors.[59] Most cases are in the World Health Organization–defined category of the microphthalmia-associated transcription factor (MiT) family of translocation RCCs (tRCCs), with an ever-growing spectrum of fusions involving genes in the MiT family of transcription factors[11] (Box 4).

GROSS AND MICROSCOPIC FEATURES

The earliest-described and most common translocations involve the TFE3 gene at the chromosome Xp11 locus and include fusions with ASPSCR1 (previously known as ASPL) on chromosome 17, and with PRCC on chromosome 1.[60–62] The ASPSCR1 fusion is identical to that seen in alveolar soft part sarcoma (ASPS) but is generally balanced in tRCC and unbalanced in ASPS.[61]

Cases with the ASPSCR1-TFE3 fusion are characterized by a pseudopapillary to organoid architecture with delicate fibrovascular septa and psammomatous calcifications. The cells may be discohesive, resulting in an alveolar pattern. Tumor cells have abundant clear to finely granular cytoplasm that may be eosinophilic. Nuclei are irregular with vesicular chromatin and prominent nucleoli. Mitoses are rare, but vascular invasion is common.[61] The PRCC-TFE3 cases are more likely to have a nested to acinar pattern with clear to eosinophilic cytoplasm. Nuclei are similar in appearance to ASPSCR1-fused tumors and vascular invasion is less common. Both genetic variants result in grossly unencapsulated tumors. The morphologies of these 2 fusion subtypes overlap extensively and may also overlap with other subtypes of RCC, thus morphology alone cannot predict translocation partner[62] (Fig. 5).

A less common, but well-characterized, group of tRCCs contain fusion of MALAT1 on chromosome 11 (previously known as alpha) with TFEB on chromosome 6. TFEB-MALAT1 cases have a more solid to nested growth pattern and classic cases are described as being biphasic, with epithelioid tumor cells with abundant eosinophilic granular or clear cytoplasm and nuclei similar to the TFE3-rearranged tumors and a second population of smaller cells with denser chromatin clustered around hyaline basement membrane material. Again, the features of these tumors may overlap significantly with other categories of RCC.[63,64]

TFE3-positive tumors generally stain for PAX8, RCC, and CD10 and are variably positive for cytokeratins and cathepsin K. Some cases are positive for melanocytic markers, including HMB45 and

---

Box 4
Molecular features and their clinical impact in translocation renal cell carcinoma

- Molecular alterations:
  - TFE3 fusions most common: primary partners are ASPSCR1 and PRCC; others described
  - TFEB fusions with MALAT1 less common
- Clinicopathologic features:
  - Histology moderately correlates with fusion type, but extensive overlap with other tRCCs and fusion-negative RCCs
  - IHC available for TFE3 and TFEB but sensitivity and specificity affected by tissue, antibody, and technical factors
- Diagnostic molecular testing:
  - Most fusions can be detected by karyotype or FISH, but uncommon TFE3 fusion partners show cryptic inversions not detected by FISH
  - Consider NGS-based RNA testing of patients with morphologic features of tRCC, but with negative IHC and FISH

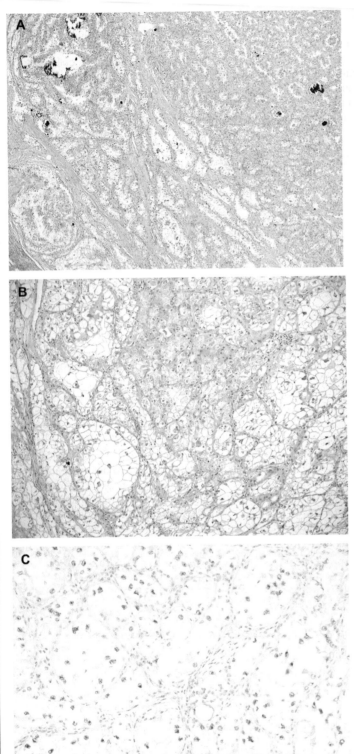

Fig. 5. tRCC. (*A*) TFE3-rearranged RCC showing papillary to nested architecture and psammoma bodies (hematoxylin-eosin, original magnification ×100). (*B*) Tumor cells with voluminous clear and granular cytoplasm (hematoxylin-eosin, original magnification ×200). (*C*) TFE3 immunohistochemistry (IHC) showing nuclear staining in tumor cells (TFE3 IHC, original magnification ×200).

melan-A (MART-1).[61,62,65,66] In contrast, *TFEB*-positive tumors are generally negative for cytokeratins and often positive for HMB45, melan-A, and cathepsin K. CD10 and RCC are focal to negative.[63–65,67]

Immunohistochemical staining has been developed that takes advantage of the overexpression of TFE3 and TFEB in the respective tumors. Positive staining is nuclear (see **Fig. 5**), and early studies of the antibodies showed a very high sensitivity and specificity.[63,68] However, it has become clear with additional experience that performance may vary widely depending on the antibody used, manual versus automated processing, fixation times, and other technical features.[64,69,70]

MOLECULAR PATHOLOGY FEATURES AND DIAGNOSIS

As with many fusion-driven tumors, broad use of NGS has expanded the known spectrum of fusions in tRCC. To date, at least 19 partners have been described for *TFE3*, with *ASPSCR1* and *PRCC* remaining the most common.[67,71–73] These now even include a case with an *EWSR1* fusion.[72] *SPFQ* (previously *SPF*) is the next most commonly described partner, which may be associated with an evolving category of melanotic renal and soft tissue tumors of mesenchymal differentiation.[74–76] TFE3 immunostaining, FISH, and/or karyotyping remain the most commonly used diagnostic modalities; however, immunostaining has limitations, as mentioned previously. In addition, strong nuclear TFE3 positivity is reported in *ALK*-fused RCCs, which represent an unrelated class of RCCs with very different morphology, and TFEB positivity may be seen in *TFEB*-amplified RCC, which is an aggressive tumor seen in adults.[67,77] Some of the more recently described fusions are inversions of the X chromosome, including those where *TFE3* partners with *NONO*, *RBM10*, and *GRIPAP1*. Because of the close proximity between the 2 genes involved in the inversion, the standard FISH break-apart probes for *TFE3* may not produce a sufficiently split signal for accurate interpretation.[78–83] Particularly in cases with the morphologic appearance of a tRCC, but with negative TFE3 and TFEB immunostaining and FISH, NGS-based fusion analysis may be considered to identify uncommon and technically challenging-to-detect fusions.

CLINICAL FEATURES

The MiT family of RCCs are seen in a wide spectrum of ages, from early childhood to late adulthood. Although they represent more than 40% of cases of RCC in the pediatric and young adult population, they account for a much lower proportion of RCCs in adults, closer to 1% to 4%.[66,83–85] However, because RCC is so much more common in adults, the numbers of tRCCs are much higher in the adult population. In patients less than 30 years of age, *TFE3*-rearranged cases account for approximately 93% of cases, whereas *TFEB*-rearranged cases account for the remainder.[67] Most cases present at stage III or IV, but, even in cases with lymph node metastases, survival is greater than 70%.[59,67,86,87] Cases of late recurrence many years after definitive therapy have been reported.[88–90] Prior chemotherapy has been identified as an environmental risk factor, with up to 15% of patients having a relevant history.[91]

CLEAR CELL SARCOMA OF THE KIDNEY

INTRODUCTION

Clear cell sarcoma of the kidney (CCSK) is a rare, but often diagnostically challenging, tumor of children. Although the diagnosis continues to be based primarily on histologic features, understanding of the molecular basis of this tumor has evolved rapidly in the past 5 years (**Box 5**).

CLINICAL FEATURES

CCSK accounts for approximately 5% of pediatric renal tumors and is one of the more aggressive pediatric renal tumors, with an overall survival of approximately 70%. Hilar lymph nodes are the most common site of metastasis at diagnosis, whereas bone, lung, and abdominal metastasis may be seen at relapse. There is also potential for late relapse, up to 10 years after initial diagnosis. The median age of diagnosis is 3 years, but CCSK can be seen in infants to teenagers.[92]

GROSS AND MICROSCOPIC FEATURES

Grossly, CCSK arises from the medulla and is often large at the time of diagnosis (**Fig. 6**). The microscopic appearance can be variable, but is classically described as having sheets, nests, or cords of tumor cells arranged around delicate so-called chicken-wire capillaries (see **Fig. 6**). Tumor cell nuclei are ovoid to spindled with fine chromatin and a clear appearance. Nucleoli are indistinct. Several patterns have been described with a range of cellularity, microcystic components, and extracellular matrices, lending to the potential for a broad differential diagnosis. Immunohistochemical staining is notable for cyclin D1 (see **Fig. 6**) and BCOR positivity, which were initially identified because of gene expression

---

Box 5
Molecular features and their clinical impact in clear cell sarcoma of the kidney

- Molecular alterations:
  - Most tumors have an internal tandem duplication of the *BCOR* gene
  - Minority of tumors have a *YWHAE-NUTM2B* fusion; rare tumors have *BCOR-CCNB3* fusions
- Clinicopathologic features:
  - Common molecular alterations and morphology links CCSK with undifferentiated round cell sarcomas, primitive myxoid mesenchymal tumor of infancy, and other tumors
- Diagnostic molecular testing:
  - Fusions can be detected by karyotype, FISH, RT-PCR, or RNA-based NGS technologies
  - *BCOR* ITD may be detected by PCR-based fragment analysis or by DNA or RNA-based NGS technologies but may require specific analysis pipeline considerations

---

data.[93,94] Cyclin D1 is nonspecific and can be seen in several tumors, including Ewing sarcoma, neuroblastoma, and other round cell sarcomas.[94–97] BCOR staining is also strong and diffuse but may also be positive in synovial sarcoma, which may be in the differential for CCSK.[97–100] A more recently described marker, NGFR, is also very sensitive, but not entirely specific.[101] BCL2, CD56, and TLE1 are also positive, whereas PAX8, desmin, CD34, and cytokeratins are generally negative.[92,99]

MOLECULAR PATHOLOGY FEATURES

A recurrent translocation between the long arm of chromosome 10 and the short arm of chromosome 17 was first identified in CCSK more than 20 years ago and was later found to represent a fusion between *YWHAE* and *NUTM2B*, previously known as *FAM22B*.[102–104] However, this fusion is only present in approximately 12% of cases.[104] More recently, most fusion-negative cases were found to have a recurrent internal tandem duplication in the *BCOR* gene.[93,105–107] This internal tandem duplication occurs at the end of the last exon of the gene and is always in frame.[105] This alteration seems to be specific for CCSK within a large sampling of other pediatric renal tumors and is mutually exclusive with the *YWHAE-NUTM2B* fusion.[105,106,108,109] The histologic and clinical characteristics of fusion-positive and internal tandem duplication (ITD)–positive cases are similar.[110]

Interestingly, gene expression profiling in the *BCOR* ITD cases shows marked overlap with *BCOR-CCNB3*–fused undifferentiated sarcomas.[92] Rare *YWHAE-NUTM2B* fusions were also reported in undifferentiated round cell sarcomas, leading to additional work to clarify the relationship between undifferentiated round cell sarcomas and CCSK. Similar *BCOR* ITD mutations were found in patients with the clinicopathologically similar tumors of CCSK, undifferentiated round cell sarcoma, and primitive myxoid mesenchymal tumor of infancy.[111] As may be expected based on these relationships, cases of CCSK with *BCOR-CCNB3* fusions have also been reported and may be seen in a slightly older patient population.[99,112,113] Additional tumors that share these molecular features now include a subset of high-grade brain tumors and uterine sarcomas.[114–116]

MOLECULAR PATHOLOGY DIAGNOSIS

Pathologic work-up of CCSK may vary depending on institutional resources and often relies on histologic features. Some of the more useful antibodies for immunohistochemical evaluation, such as NGFR, cyclin D1, and BCOR, may not be widely available. Because of the variability in molecular alterations, a molecular work-up may require testing by multiple modalities. FISH for the *YWHAE* rearrangement and the *BCOR-CCNB3* fusion is available, but the *BCOR* ITD cannot be detected by cytogenetics or by FISH. The *BCOR* ITD is exonic and can be detected by both DNA-based and RNA-based NGS methods, although, because of its location at the end of the last exon, bioinformatic analysis may require additional steps. If sending a tumor for sequencing, the ability of the laboratory to detect these alterations should be verified. RNA-based sequencing that can detect both the fusions and the *BCOR* ITD is the single most effective molecular test for the diagnosis of CCSK. The duplication can also be detected by techniques like capillary gel electrophoresis that analyze the size of the region.

RHABDOID TUMOR OF THE KIDNEY

INTRODUCTION

Rhabdoid tumors of the kidney are the most aggressive of the pediatric renal neoplasms.

Fig. 6. CCSK. (*A*) Large tumor with areas of necrosis and hemorrhage. (*B*) Sheets of small tumor cells with vesicular nuclei and scant cytoplasm with delicate, branching vasculature in the background (hematoxylin-eosin, original magnification ×200). (*C*) Cyclin D1 IHC showing strong nuclear positivity in tumor within a renal sinus vessel (cyclin D1 IHC, original magnification ×100).

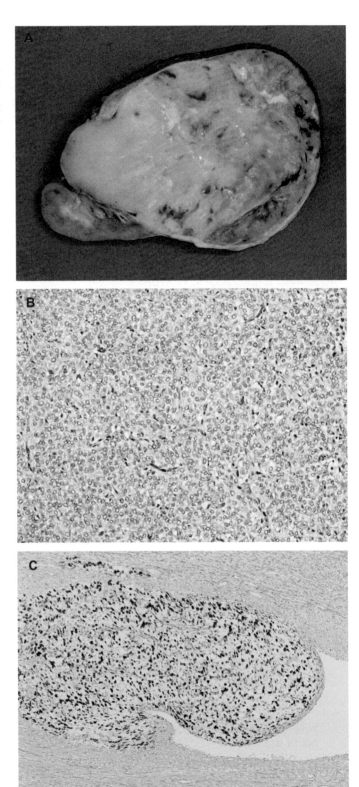

Although the role of *SMARCB1* mutations as the oncogenic driver in rhabdoid tumors is well-described in the literature, the functions and downstream interactions of the SMARCB1/INI1 protein are now leading investigations to new therapeutic options (**Box 6**).

CLINICAL FEATURES

Rhabdoid tumors most commonly present between birth and 3 years of age and often at an advanced stage.[117–119] Survival has remained poor over the past 30 years and continues to hover around 20% to 25%.[117,118] Increasing age and complete resection in the absence of metastatic disease are positive prognostic indicators, but survival remains poor even in that population.[117–119]

GROSS AND MICROSCOPIC FEATURES

Grossly, rhabdoid tumors present as bulky masses that often replace the kidney (**Fig. 7**). Microscopically, they are characterized by sheets of monotonous-appearing tumor cells with prominent nucleoli and vesicular chromatin (see **Fig. 7**). The abundant eosinophilic cytoplasm contains inclusions composed of intermediate filaments. Mitotic activity is high, but pleomorphism is only mild to moderate. The overall cellular pattern may vary between epithelioid, spindled, microcystic, or pseudoglandular. Tumors show aggressive invasion of the surrounding kidney and beyond.[117,120]

The hallmark immunohistochemical feature of rhabdoid tumors is the loss of nuclear SMARCB1/INI1 expression, which is universally present in normal tissues (see **Fig. 7**).[121,122] Vimentin strongly stains the cytoplasmic inclusions.[117,123] Epithelial markers, including pan-cytokeratin, EMA, and CAM 5.2, are positive in slightly more than half of cases. Variable staining is also reported for muscle-specific actin, CD99, NSE, and S100. Desmin and CD34 are generally negative, as are myogenic markers MyoD1 and myogenin.[123,124] Of note, a minority may be positive for WT1, perhaps providing clues to the underlying cell of origin for at least a subset of these tumors.[125]

MOLECULAR PATHOLOGY FEATURES AND DIAGNOSIS

Following multiple reports of deletions of the long arm of chromosome 22, the common overlapping regions were mapped to the *SMARCB1* gene, previously known as *BAF47*, *hSNFS*, *SNF5*, and *INI1*.[126] Additional loss-of-function mutations were also identified, resulting in biallelic loss or inactivation of the gene in both renal and extrarenal rhabdoid tumors, and a role for *SMARCB1* as a tumor suppressor gene was recognized.[126,127] Germline mutations were identified in a subset of cases, leading to the description of the rhabdoid tumor predisposition syndrome, type 1. The syndrome is associated with earlier presentation, bilateral primary renal tumors, and rhabdoid tumors at other sites.[118,127–130] About one-third of patients have an underlying germline mutation, with a large deletion, monosomy of chromosome 22, or copy-neutral loss of heterozygosity as the second hit.[130–134] The rhabdoid tumor

---

Box 6
Molecular features and their clinical impact in rhabdoid tumors of the kidney

- Molecular alterations:
  - Somatic or germline *SMARCB1* mutations
  - Overall very low tumor mutational burden
- Clinicopathologic features:
  - Morphologic and molecular overlap with rhabdoid tumors of other sites
  - Germline mutations are associated with rhabdoid tumor predisposition syndrome
  - Loss of SMARCB1/INI1 IHC nuclear staining is characteristic of rhabdoid tumors
  - Potential role for SMARCB1/INI1 in epigenetic regulation of other genes is a target for new therapeutic strategies
- Diagnostic molecular work-up:
  - Tumor diagnosis usually confirmed by IHC, without need for molecular testing
  - Identification of germline mutations may involve sequencing of tumor and germline specimens
  - Larger deletion events or LOH may require specific deletion/duplication technologies, like microarray or MLPA

Fig. 7. Rhabdoid tumor of the kidney. (*A*) Large tumor replacing the kidney and with extrarenal extension. (*B*) Sheets of irregular tumor cells with prominent nucleoli (hematoxylin-eosin, original magnification ×200).

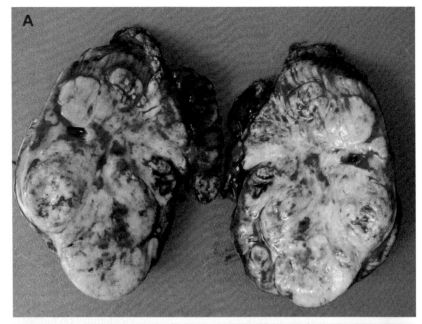

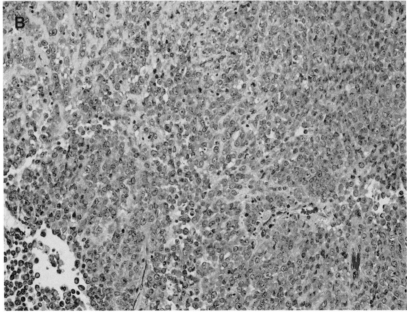

predisposition syndrome, type 2 is associated with mutations in the *SMARCA4* gene, but no cases with rhabdoid tumor of the kidney with *SMARCA4* mutations have been reported to date.[135] Published recommendations include molecular analysis of the tumor tissue for both mutations and deletions, followed by screening for the detected mutations in the blood, although, depending on the sequencing approach used, some mutations may not be detected.[134] Counseling for families is further complicated by the complexity of inheritance, with some mutations showing a low penetrance or variable expressivity and some showing confined gonadal mosaicism.[133] Some patients within an affected family may also present with schwannomatosis, usually without rhabdoid tumors, depending on the specific familial mutation.[134] Regular tumor surveillance by MRI is recommended for affected patients.[136]

Rhabdoid tumors are unusual and intriguing from a molecular perspective because of their general lack of additional mutational events beyond *SMARCB1*. Studies of tumor mutational burden have shown that rhabdoid tumors have

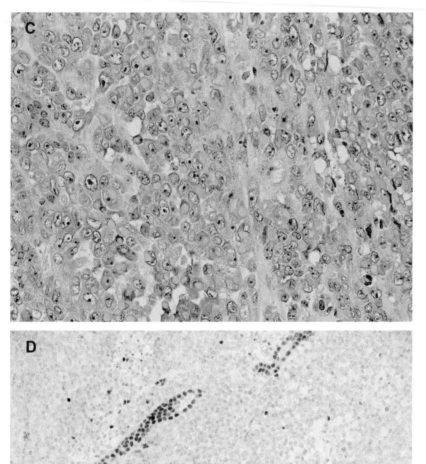

one of the lowest tumor mutational burdens of all cancer types, suggesting that SMARCB1 and its protein are the near-sole drivers of oncogenesis and tumor behavior.[137,138] The SMARCB1/INI1 protein is part of the SWI/SNF chromatin remodeling complex, which has an active role in transcriptional activation and repression. Via its role in this complex and the subsequent effects on epigenetic regulation of other genes, inactivation of SMARCB1/INI1 affects numerous critical cell pathways. Those pathways include cyclin D1 regulated cell cycle progression, sonic hedgehog, WNT/beta-catenin, RB, and MYC.[139] SMARCB1/INI1 and the SWI/SNF complex have a role in histone acetylation and, thus, transcriptional activation. The complex functions in opposition to the polycomb repressive complex 2 (PRC2), which includes EZH2 as its catalytic subunit, and is involved in histone methylation and transcriptional repression. Inactivation of *SMARCB1* leads to overexpression of *EZH2* and trimethylation of histone H3K27, causing transcriptional silencing of tumor suppressor genes.[139] The participation of so many cell pathways in the oncogenesis of rhabdoid tumors of the kidney and other sites has led to investigation of a variety of targeted therapies, including EZH2 inhibitors and immune checkpoint inhibitors.[140] These investigations remain in progress, with the hope of improving survival for patients with this devastating diagnosis.

DISCLOSURE

The author has no commercial or financial conflicts of interest to disclose.

REFERENCES

1. Joshi VV, Beckwith JB. Multilocular cyst of the kidney (cystic nephroma) and cystic partially differentiated nephroblastoma. Cancer 1989;64(2):466–79.
2. Manivel JC, Priest JR, Watterson J, et al. Pleuropulmonary blastoma. The so-called pulmonary blastoma of childhood. Cancer 1988;62:1516–26.
3. Delahunt B, Thompson KJ, Ferguson AF, et al. Familial cystic nephroma and pleuropulmonary blastoma. Cancer 1993;71:1338–42.
4. Priest JR, Watterson J, Strong L, et al. Pleuropulmonary blastoma: a marker for familial disease. J Pediatr 1996;128:220–4.
5. Lallier M, Bouchard S, DiLorenzo M, et al. Pleuropulmonary blastoma: a rare pathology with an even rarer presentation. J Pediatr Surg 1999;34:1057–9.
6. Ishida U, Kato K, Kigasawa H, et al. Synchronous occurrence of pleuropulmonary blastoma and cystic nephroma: possible genetic link in cystic lesions of the lung and the kidney. Med Pediatr Oncol 2000;35(1):85–7.
7. Hill DA, Ivanovich J, Priest JR. DICER1 mutations in familial pleuropulmonary blastoma. Science 2009;325(5943):965.
8. Bahubeshi A, Bal N, Frio TR. Germline DICER1 mutations and familial cystic nephroma. J Med Genet 2010;47(12):863–6.
9. Boman F, Hill DA, Williams GM, et al. Familial association of pleuropulmonary blastoma with cystic nephroma and other renal tumors: A report from the International Pleuropulmonary Blastoma Registry. J Pediatr 2006;149:850–4.
10. Doros LA, Rossi CT, Yang J. DICER1 mutations in childhood cystic nephroma and its relationship to DICER1-renal sarcoma. Mod Pathol 2014;27(9):1267–80.
11. Moch H, Humphrey PA, Ulbright TM, et al, editors. WHO classification of tumours of the urinary system and male genital organs. 4th edition. Lyon (France): International Agency for Research on Cancer; 2016.
12. Li Y, Pawel B, Hill DA, et al. Pediatric cystic nephroma are morphologically, immunohistochemically, and genetically distinct from adult cystic nephroma. Am J Surg Pathol 2017;41(4):472–81.
13. Cajaiba MM, Khanna G, Smigh EA, et al. Pediatric cystic nephromas: distinctive features and frequent DICER1 mutations. Hum Pathol 2016;48:81–7.
14. Foulkes WD, Priest JR, Duchaine TF. DICER1: mutations, microRNAs and mechanisms. Nat Rev Cancer 2014;14(10):662–72.
15. Schultz KAP, Williams GM, Kamihara J. DICER1 and associated conditions: identification of at-risk individual and recommended surveillance strategies. Clin Cancer Res 2018;24(10):2251–61.
16. Warren M, Hiemenz MC, Schmidt R. Expanding the spectrum of DICER1-associated sarcomas. Mod Pathol 2020;33:164–74.
17. Vujanic GM, Kelsey A, Perlman EJ, et al. Anaplastic sarcoma of the kidney: a clinicopathologic study of 20 cases of a new entity with polyphenotypic features. Am J Surg Pathol 2007;31:1459–68.
18. Wu MK, Vujanic GM, Fahiminiya S. Anaplastic sarcomas of the kidney are characterized by DICER1 mutations. Mod Pathol 2018;31(1):169–78.
19. Wu MK, Cotter MB, Pears J. Tumor progression in DICER1-mutated cystic nephroma – witnessing the genesis of anaplastic sarcoma of the kidney. Hum Pathol 2016;53:114–20.
20. Wu MK, Goudie C, Druker H. Evolution of renal cysts to anaplastic sarcoma of kidney in a child with DICER1 syndrome. Pediatr Blood Cancer 2016;63(7):1272–5.
21. Davis CJ, Barton JH, Sesterhenn IA, et al. Metanephric adenoma: clinicopathological study of fifty patients. Am J Surg Pathol 1995;19(10):1101–14.
22. Argani P, Beckwith BJ. Metanephric stromal tumor: report of 31 cases of a distinctive pediatric renal neoplasm. Am J Surg Pathol 2000;24(7):917–26.
23. Arroyo MR, Green DM, Perlman EJ, et al. The spectrum of metanephric adenofibroma and related lesions. Am J Surg Pathol 2001;25(4):433–44.
24. Palese MA, Ferrer F, Perlman E, et al. Metanephric stromal tumor: a rare benign pediatric mass. Urology 2001;58(3):462.
25. Hennigar RA, Bekwith JB. Nephrogenic Adenofibroma: a novel kidney tumor of young people. Am J Surg Pathol 1992;16(4):325–34.
26. Turner RM, Tomaszewski JJ, Fox JA, et al. Metanephric adenofibroma. Can J Urol 2013;20(2):6737–8.
27. Chami R, Yin M, Marrano P, et al. BRAF mutations in pediatric metanephric tumors. Hum Pathol 2015;46(8):1153–61.

28. Wobker S, Matoso A, Pratilas C, et al. Metanephric adenoma-epithelial Wilms tumor overlap lesions: an analysis of BRAF status. Am J Surg Pathol 2019;43(9):1157–69.

29. Muir TE, Cheville JC, Lager DJ. Metanephric adenoma, nephrogenic rests, and Wilms' tumor: a histologic and immunophenotypic comparison. Am J Surg Pathol 2001;25(10):1290–6.

30. Choueiri TK, Cheville J, Palescandolo E, et al. BRAF mutations in metanephric adenoma of the kidney. Eur Urol 2012;62(5):917–22.

31. Udager AM, Pan J, Magers MJ. Molecular and immunohistochemical characterization reveals novel BRAF mutations in metanephric adenoma. Am J Surg Pathol 2015;39(4):549–57.

32. Caliò A, Eble JN, Hes O, et al. Distinct clinicopathologic features in metanephric adenoma harboring BRAF mutation. Oncotarget 2016;8(33): 54096–105.

33. Ding Y, Wang C, Li X, et al. Novel clinicopathological and molecular characterization of metanephric adenoma: a study of 28 cases. Diagn Pathol 2018; 13(1):54.

34. Mangray S, Breese V, Jackson CL, et al. Application of BRAF V600E mutation analysis for the diagnosis of metanephric adenofibroma. Am J Surg Pathol 2015;39(9):1301–4.

35. Argani P, Lee J, Netto GJ, et al. Frequent BRAF V600E mutations in metanephric stromal tumor. Am J Surg Pathol 2016;40(5):719–22.

36. Marsden L, Jennings LJ, Gadd S, et al. BRAF exon 15 mutations in pediatric renal stromal tumors: prevalence in metanephric stromal tumors. Hum Pathol 2017;60:32–6.

37. Pinto A, Signoretti S, Hirsch MS, et al. Immunohistochemical staining for BRAF V600E supports the diagnosis of metanephric adenoma. Histopathology 2015;66(6):901–4.

38. Pan CC, Epstein JI. Detection of chromosome copy number alterations in metanephric adenomas by array comparative genomic hybridization. Mod Pathol 2010;23(12):1634–40.

39. Szponar A, Yusenko MV, Kovacs G. High-resolution array CGH of metanephric adenomas: lack of DNA copy number changes. Histopathology 2010;56(2): 212–6.

40. Toutain J, VuPhi Y, Doco-Fenzy M, et al. Identification of a complex 17q rearrangement in a metanephric stromal tumor. Cancer Genet 2011;204(6):340–3.

41. Gooskens SL, Houwing ME, Vujanic GM. Congenital mesoblastic nephroma 50 years after its recognition: a narrative review. Pediatr Blood Cancer 2017;64(7):1–9.

42. Vokuhl C, Nourkami-Tutdibi N, Furtwängler R, et al. ETV6-NTRK3 in congenital mesoblastic nephroma: A report of the SIOP/GPOH nephroblastoma study. Pediatr Blood Cancer 2018;65(4):1–6.

43. Bolande RP. Congenital mesoblastic nephroma of infancy. Perspect Pediatr Pathol 1973;1:227–50.

44. Pettinato G, Manivel JC, Wick MR, et al. Classical and cellular (atypical) congenital mesoblastic nephroma: a clinicopathologic, ultrastructural, immunohistochemical, and flow cytometric study. Hum Pathol 1989;20(7):682–90.

45. Furtwaengler R, Reinhard H, Leuschner I, et al. Mesoblastic nephroma – a report from the Gesellschaft fur Pädiatrische Onkologie und Hämatologie (GPOH). Cancer 2006;106(10):2275–83.

46. Jehangir S, Kurian JJ, Selvarajah D. Recurrent and metastatic congenital mesoblastic nephroma: where does the evidence stand? Pediatr Surg Int 2017;33:1183–8.

47. Rubin BP, Chen CJ, Morgan TW, et al. Congenital mesoblastic nephroma t(12;15) is associated with ETV6-NTRK3 gene fusion: cytogenetic and molecular relationship to congenital (infantile) fibrosarcoma. Am J Pathol 1998;153(5):1451–8.

48. Demellawy DE, Cundiff CA, Nasr A, et al. Congenital mesoblastic nephroma: a study of 19 cases using immunohistochemistry and ETV6-NTRK3 fusion gene rearrangement. Pathology 2016; 48(1):47–50.

49. Knezevich SR, Garnett MJ, Pysher TJ, et al. eTV6-NTRK3 gene fusions and trisomy 11 establish a histogenetic link between mesoblastic nephroma and congenital fibrosarcoma. Cancer Res 1998;58(22): 5046–8.

50. Argani P, Fritsch M, Kadkol SS, et al. Detection of the ETV6-NTRK3 chimeric RNA of infantile fibrosarcoma/cellular congenital mesoblastic nephroma in paraffin-embedded tissue: application to challenging pediatric renal stromal tumors. Mod Pathol 2000;13(1):29–36.

51. Anderson J, Gibson S, Sebire NJ. Expression of ETV6-NTRK in classical, cellular and mixed subtypes of congenital mesoblastic nephroma. Histopathology 2006;48(6):748–53.

52. Rudzinski ER, Lockwood CM, Stohr BA, et al. Pan-TRK immunohistochemistry identifies NTRK rearrangements in pediatric mesenchymal tumors. Am J Surg Pathol 2018;42(7):927–35.

53. Church AJ, Calicchio ML, Nardi V, et al. Recurrent EML4-NTRK3 fusions in infantile fibrosarcoma and congenial mesoblastic nephroma suggest a revised testing strategy. Mod Pathol 2018;31(3): 463–73.

54. Wegert J, Vokuhl C, Collord G, et al. Recurrent intragenic rearrangements of EGFR and BRAF in soft tissue tumors of infancy. Nat Commun 2018; 9(1):2378.

55. Antonescu CR, Dickson BC, Swanson D, et al. Spindle cell tumors with RET gene fusions exhibit a morphologic spectrum akin to tumors with

NTRK gene fusions. Oncogene 2020;39(6): 1361–77.

56. Davis JL, Vargas SO, Rudzinski ER, et al. Recurrent RET gene fusions in paediatric spindle mesenchymal neoplasms. Histopathology 2020;76(7): 1032–41.

57. Lei L, Stohr BA, Berry S, et al. Recurrent EGFR alterations in NTRK3 fusion negative congenital mesoblastic nephroma. Pract Lab Med 2020;21: e00164.

58. Albert CM, Davis JL, Federman N, et al. TRK fusion cancers in children: a clinical review and recommendations for screening. J Clin Oncol 2019; 37(6):513–24.

59. Geller JI, Ehrlich PF, Cost NG, et al. Characterization of adolescent and pediatric renal cell carcinoma: a report from the Children's Oncology Group Study AREN03B2. Cancer 2015;121(14): 2457–64.

60. Tomlinson GE, Nisen PD, Timmons CG, et al. Cytogenetics of a renal cell carcinoma in a 17-month old child. Evidence of Xp11.2 as a recurring breakpoint. Cancer Genet Cytogenet 1991;57(1):11–7.

61. Argani P, Antonescu CR, Illei PB, et al. Primary renal neoplasms with the ASPL-TFE3 gene fusion of alveolar soft part sarcoma: a distinctive tumor entity previously included among renal cell carcinomas of children and adolescents. Am J Pathol 2001;159(1):179–92.

62. Argani P, Antonescu CR, Couturier J. PRCC-TFE3 renal carcinomas: morphologic, immunohistochemical, ultrastructural, and molecular analysis of an entity associated with the t(X;1)(p11.2;q21). Am J Surg Pathol 2002;26(12):1553–66.

63. Argani P, Lae M, Hutchinson B, et al. Renal carcinomas with the t(6;11)(p21;q12): clinicopathologic features and demonstration of the specific alpha-TFEB gene fusion by immunohistochemistry, RT-PCR, and DNA PCR. Am J Surg Pathol 2005; 29(2):230–40.

64. Rao Q, Liu B, Cheng L, et al. Renal cell carcinomas with t(6;11)(p21;q12): A clinicopathologic study emphasizing unusual morphology, novel alpha-TFEB gene fusion point, immunobiomarkers, and ultrastructural features, as well as detection of the gene fusion by fluorescence in situ hybridization. Am J Surg Pathol 2012;36(9):1327–38.

65. Martignoni G, Pea M, Gobbo S, et al. Cathepsin-K immunoreactivity distinguishes MiTF/TFE family renal translocation carcinomas from other renal carcinomas. Mod Pathol 2009;22:1016–22.

66. Rao Q, Chen JY, Wang JD, et al. Renal cell carcinoma in children and young adults: clinicopathological, immunohistochemical, and VHL gene analysis of 46 cases with follow-up. Int J Surg Pathol 2011;19(2):170–9.

67. Cajaiba MM, Dyer L, Geller JI, et al. The classification of pediatric and young adult renal cell carcinomas registered on the children's oncology group (COG) protocol AREN03B2 after focused genetic testing. Cancer 2018;124(16):3381–9.

68. Argani P, Lal P, Hutchison B. Aberrant nuclear immunoreactivity for TFE3 in neoplasms with TFE3 gene fusions: a sensitive and specific immunohistochemical assay. Am J Surg Pathol 2003;27(6): 750–61.

69. Rao Q, Williamson SR, Zhang S, et al. TFE3 break-apart FISH has a higher sensitivity for Xp11.2 translocation-associated renal cell carcinoma compared with TFE3 or cathepsin K immunohistochemical staining alone: expanding the morphologic spectrum. Am J Surg Pathol 2013;37(6): 804–15.

70. Sharain RF, Gown AM, Greipp PT, et al. Immunohistochemistry for TFE3 lacks specificity and sensitivity in the diagnosis of TFE3-rearranged neoplasms: a comparative, 2-laboratory study. Hum Pathol 2019;87:65–74.

71. Caliò A, Segala D, Munari E, et al. MiT Family Translocation Renal Cell Carcinoma: from the Early Descriptions to the Current Knowledge. Cancers (Basel) 2019;11(8):1110.

72. Lang XP, Pan J, Yang CX, et al. A renal cell carcinoma with EWSR1-TFE3 fusion gene. Genes Chromosomes Cancer 2020;59(5):325–9.

73. Argani P, Zhang L, Sung YS, et al. A novel RBMX-TFE3 gene fusion in a highly aggressive pediatric renal perivascular epithelioid cell tumor. Genes Chromosomes Cancer 2020;59(1):58–63.

74. Rao Q, Shen Q, Xia QY, et al. PSF/SFPQ is a very common gene fusion partner in TFE3 rearrangement-associated perivascular epithelioid cell tumors (PEComas) and melanotic Xp11 translocation renal cancers: clinicopathologic, immunohistochemical, and molecular characteristics suggesting classification as a distinct entity. Am J Surg Pathol 2015;39(9):1181–96.

75. Argani P, Zhong M, Reuter VE, et al. TFE3-fusion variant analysis defines specific clinicopathologic associations among Xp11 translocation cancers. Am J Surg Pathol 2016;40:723–37.

76. Saleeb RM, Srigley JR, Sweet J, et al. Melanotic MiT family translocation neoplasms: Expanding the clinical and molecular spectrum of this unique entity of tumors. Pathol Res Pract 2017;213(11): 1412–8.

77. Argani P, Reuter VE, Zhang L, et al. TFEB-amplified Renal Cell Carcinomas: An Aggressive Molecular Subset Demonstrating Variable Melanocytic Marker Expression and Morphologic Heterogeneity. Am J Surg Pathol 2016;40(11):1484–95.

78. Hodge JC, Pearce KE, Wang X, et al. Molecular cytogenetic analysis for TFE3 rearrangement in

Xp11.2 renal cell carcinoma and alveolar soft part sarcoma: validation and clinical experience with 75 cases. Mod Pathol 2014;27(1):113–27.

79. Xia QY, Wang Z, Chen N, et al. Xp11.2 translocation renal cell carcinoma with NONO-TFE3 gene fusion: morphology, prognosis, and potential pitfall in detecting TFE3 gene rearrangement. Mod Pathol 2017;30(3):416–26.

80. Xia QY, Want XT, Zhan XM, et al. Xp11 Translocation Renal Cell Carcinomas (RCCs) With RBM10-TFE3 Gene Fusion Demonstrating Melanotic Features and Overlapping Morphology With t(6;11) RCC: Interest and Diagnostic Pitfall in Detecting a Paracentric Inversion of TFE3. Am J Surg Pathol 2017;41(5):663–76.

81. Classe M, Maloug GG, Su X, et al. Incidence, clinicopathological features and fusion transcript landscape of translocation renal cell carcinomas. Histopathology 2017;70(7):1089–97.

82. Wang XT, Xia QY, Zhou XJ, et al. Comment on "Incidence, clinicopathological features and fusion transcript landscape of translocation renal cell carcinomas. Histopathology 2017;71(5):835–6.

83. Classe M, Maloug GG, Su X, et al. Reply to "Incidence, clinicopathological features and fusion transcript landscape of translocation renal cell carcinomas. Histopathology 2017;71(5):836–7.

84. Komai Y, Fujiwara M, Fujii Y, et al. Adult Xp11 translocation renal cell carcinoma diagnosed by cytogenetics and mmunohistochemistry. Clin Cancer Res 2009;15:1170–6.

85. Zhong M, Osborne L, Merino MJ, et al. The study ofXp11 translocation renal cell carcinoma (RCC) in adults by TMA,IHC and FISH. Mod Pathol 2010;23(S1):232A.

86. Geller JI, Dome JS. Local lymph node involvement does not predict poor outcome in pediatric renal cell carcinoma. Cancer 2004;101:1575–83.

87. Malouf GG, Camparo P, Molinie V, et al. Transcription factor E3 and transcription factor EB renal cell carcinomas: clinical features, biological behavior and prognostic factors. J Urol 2011;185:24–9.

88. Dal Cin P, Stas M, Sciot R, et al. Translocation (X;1) reveals metastasis 31 years after renal cell carcinoma. Cancer Genet Cytogenet 1998;101:58–61.

89. Rais-Bahrami S, Drabick JJ, De Marzo AM, et al. Xp11 translocation renal cell carcinoma: delayed but massive and lethal metastases of a chemotherapy-associated secondary malignancy. Urology 2007;70:178.

90. Wu A, Kunju LP, Shah RB. Renal cell carcinoma in children and young adults: analysis of clinicopathological, immunohistochemical and molecular characteristics with an emphasis on the spectrum of Xp11.2 translocation-associated and unusual clear cell subtypes. Histopathology 2008;53(5):533–44.

91. Argani P, Laé M, Ballard ET, et al. Translocation carcinomas of the kidney after chemotherapy in childhood. J Clin Oncol 2006;24(10):1529–34.

92. Argani P, Perlman EJ, Berslow NE, et al. Clear cell sarcoma of the kidney: a review of 351 cases from the National Wilms Tumor Study Group Pathology Center. Am J Surg Pathol 2000;24(1):4–18.

93. Roy A, Kumar V, Zorman B, et al. Recurrent internal tandem duplications of BCOR in clear cell sarcoma of the kidney. Nat Commun 2015;6:8891.

94. Mirkovic J, Calicchio M, Fletcher CD, et al. Diffuse and strong cyclin D1 immunoreactivity in clear cell sarcoma of the kidney. Histopathology 2015;67:306–12.

95. Magro G, Salvatorelli L, Alaggio R, et al. Diagnostic utility of cyclin D1 in the diagnosis of small round blue cell tumor in children and adolescents. Hum Pathol 2017;60:58–65.

96. Creytens D, Ferdinande L, van Dorpe J. Diagnostic utility of cyclin D1 in the diagnosis of small round blue cell tumors in children and adolescents: beware of cyclin D1 expression in clear cell sarcoma of the kidney and CIC-DUX4 fusion–positive sarcomas. Comment on Magro et al (2016). Hum Pathol 2017;67:225–8.

97. Magro G, Salvatorelli L, Alaggio R, et al. Diagnostic utility of cyclin D1 in the diagnosis of small round blue cell tumors in children and adolescents: beware of cyclin D1 expression in clear cell sarcoma of the kidney and CIC-DUX4 fusion–positive sarcomas. Comment on Magro et al (2016) – reply. Hum Pathol 2017;67:225–8.

98. Kao YC, Sung YS, Zhang L, et al. BCOR overexpression is a highly sensitive marker in round cell sarcomas with BCOR genetic alterations. Am J Surg Pathol 2016;40(12):1670–8.

99. Argani P, Kao YC, Zhang L, et al. Primary renal sarcomas with BCOR-CCNB3 gene fusion: a report of 2 cases showing histologic overlap with clear cell sarcoma of kidney, suggesting further link between BCOR-related sarcomas of the kidney and soft tissue. Am J Surg Pathol 2017;41(12):1702–12.

100. Argani P, Pawel B, Szabo S, et al. Diffuse strong BCOR immunoreactivity is a sensitive and specific marker for clear cell sarcoma of the kidney (CCSK) in pediatric renal neoplasia. Am J Surg Pathol 2018;42(8):1128–31.

101. Arva NC, Bonadio J, Perlman E, et al. Diagnostic utility of PAX8, PASX2, and NGFR immunohistochemical expression in pediatric renal tumors. Appl Immunohistochem Mol Morphol 2018;26(10):721–6.

102. Punnett HH, Halligan GE, Zaeri N, et al. Translocation 1;17 in clear cell sarcoma of the kidney: a first report. Cancer Genet Cytogenet 1989;41(1):123–8.

103. Rakheja D, Weinberg AG, Tomlinson GE, et al. Translocation (10;17)(q22;p13): a recurring translocation in clear cell sarcoma of kidney. Cancer Genet Cytogenet 2004;154(2):175–9.

104. O'Meara E, Stack D, Lee CH, et al. Characterization of the chromosomal translocation t(10;17)(q22;p13) in clear cell sarcoma of kidney. J Pathol 2012;227:72–80.

105. Ueno-Yokohata H, Okita H, Nakasato K, et al. Consistent in-frame internal tandem duplications of BCOR characterize clear cell sarcoma of the kidney. Nat Genet 2015;47(8):861–3.

106. Karlsson J, Valind A, Gisselsson D. BCOR internal tandem duplication and YWHAE-NUTM2B/E fusion are mutually exclusive events in clear cell sarcoma of the kidney. Genes Chromosomes Cancer 2016; 55(2):120–3.

107. Astolfi A, Melchiona F, Perotti D, et al. Whole transcriptome sequencing identifies BCOR internal tandem duplication as a common feature of clear cell sarcoma of the kidney. Oncotarget 2015; 6(38):40934–9.

108. Gooskens SL, Gadd S, van den Heuvel-Eibrink MM, et al. BCOR internal tandem duplications in clear cell sarcoma of the kidney. Genes Chromosomes Cancer 2016;55(6):549–50.

109. Kenny C, Bausenwein S, Lazaro A, et al. Mutually exclusive BCOR internal tandem duplications and YWHAE-NUTM2 fusions in clear cell sarcoma of kidney: not the full story. J Pathol 2016;238(5): 617–20.

110. Gooskens SL, Kenny C, Lazaro A, et al. The clinical phenotype of YWHAE-NUTM2B/E positive pediatric clear cell sarcoma of the kidney. Genes Chromosomes Cancer 2016;55:143–7.

111. Kao YC, Sung YS, Zhang L, et al. Recurrent BCOR internal tandem duplication and YWHAE-NUTM2B fusions in soft tissue undifferentiated round cell sarcoma of infancy – overlapping genetic features with clear cell sarcoma of kidney. Am J Surg Pathol 2016;40(8):1009–20.

112. Wong MK, Ng CCY, Kuick CH. Clear cell sarcomas of the kidney are characterized by BCOR gene abnormalities, including exon 15 internal tandem duplications and BCOR-CCNB3 gene fusion. Histopathology 2018;72(2):320–9.

113. Han H, Betrannd KC, Patel KR, et al. BCOR-CCNB3 fusion-positive clear cell sarcoma of the kidney. Pediatr Blood Cancer 2019;26:e28151.

114. Mariño-Enriquez A, Lauria A, Przybyl J, et al. BCOR Internal Tandem Duplication in High-grade Uterine Sarcomas. Am J Surg Pathol 2018;42(3):335–41.

115. Yoshida Y, Nobusawa S, Nakata S, et al. CNS high-grade neuroepithelial tumor with BCOR internal tandem duplication: a comparison with its counterparts in the kidney and soft tissue. Brain Pathol 2018;28(5):710–20.

116. Astolfi A, Fiore M, Melchionda F, et al. BCOR involvement in cancer. Epigenomics 2019;11(7): 835–55.

117. Weeks DA, Beckwith JB, Mierau GW, et al. Rhabdoid tumor of kidney. A report of 111 cases from the National Wilms' Tumor Study Pathology Center. Am J Surg Pathol 1989;13(6):439–58.

118. Thomlinson GE, Breslow NE, Dome J, et al. Rhabdoid tumor of the kidney in the National wilms' Tumor Study: age at diagnosis as a prognostic factor. J Clin Oncol 2005;23:7641–5.

119. van den Heuvel-Eibrink MM, Grundy P, Graf N, et al. Characteristics and survival of 750 children diagnosed with a renal tumor in the first seven months of life: A collaborative study by the SIOP/GPOH/SFOP, NWTSG, and UKCCSG Wilms tumor study groups. Pediatr Blood Cancer 2008;50(6): 1130–4.

120. Schmidt D, Harms D, Zieger G. Malignant rhabdoid tumor of the kidney. Histopathology, ultrastructure and comments on differential diagnosis. Virchows Arch A Pathol Anat Histopathol 1982;398(1):101–8.

121. Hoot AC, RussoP, Judkins A, et al. Immunohistochemical analysis of hSNF5/INI1 distinguishes renal and extra-renal malignant rhabdoid tumors from other pediatric soft tissue tumors. Am J Surg Pathol 2004;28(11):1485–91.

122. Sigauke E, Rakheja D, Maddox DL, et al. Absence of expression of SMARCB1/INI1 in malignant rhabdoid tumors of the central nervous system, kidneys and soft tissue: an immunohistochemical study with implications for diagnosis. Mod Pathol 2006; 19(5):717–25.

123. Vujanic GM, Sandstedt B, Harms D, et al. Rhabdoid tumour of the kidney: a clinicopathological study of 22 patients from the International Society of Paediatric Oncology (SIOP) nephroblastoma file. Histopathology 1996;28:333–40.

124. Fanburg-Smith JC, Hengge M, Hengge UR, et al. Extra-renal rhabdoid tumors of soft tissue: a clinicopathologic and immunohistochemical study of 18 cases. Ann Diagn Pathol 1998;2:351–62.

125. Satoh F, Tsutsumi Y, Yokoyama S, et al. Comparative immunohistochemical analysis of developing kidneys, nephroblastomas and related tumors: considerations on their histogenesis. Pathol Int 2000;50(6):458–71.

126. Versteege I, Sévenet N, Lange J. Truncating mutations of hSNF5/INI1 in aggressive paediatric cancer. Nature 1998;394(6689):203–6.

127. Biegel JA, Zhou JY, Rorke LB, et al. Germ-line and acquired mutations of INI1 in atypical teratoid and rhabdoid tumors. Cancer Res 1999;59(1):74–9.

128. Sevenet N, Lellouch-Tubiana A, Schofield D, et al. Spectrum of hSNF5/INI1 somatic mutations in human cancer and genotype-phenotype correlations. Hum Mol Genet 1999;8:2359–68.

129. Lee HY, Yoon CS, Sevenet N. Rhabdoid tumor the kidney is a component of the rhabdoid predisposition syndrome. Pediatr Dev Pathol 2002;5(4): 395–9.

130. Geller JI, Roth JJ, Biegel JA. Biology and treatment of rhabdoid tumor. Crit Rev Oncog 2015;20(3–4): 199–216.

131. Biegel JA. Molecular genetics of atypical teratoid/rhabdoid tumors. Neurosurg Focus 2006;20(1): E11.

132. Kordes U, Gesk S, Fruhwald MC, et al. Clinical and molecular features in patients with atypical teratoid rhabdoid tumor or malignant rhabdoid tumor. Genes Chromosomes Cancer 2010;49:176–81.

133. Eaton KW, Tooke LS, Wainwright LM, et al. Spectrum of SMARCB1/INI1 mutations in familial and sporadic rhabdoid tumors. Pediatr Blood Cancer 2011;56(1):7–15.

134. Sredni ST, Tomita T. Rhabdoid tumor predisposition syndrome. Pediatr Dev Pathol 2015;18(1):49–58.

135. Pawel BR. SMARCB1-deficient tumors of childhood: a practical guide. Pediatr Dev Pathol 2017; 21(1):6–28.

136. Foulkes WD, Kamihara J, Evans DGR. Cancer surveillance in Gorlin syndrome and rhabdoid tumor predisposition syndrome. Clin Cancer Res 2017; 23(12):e62–7.

137. Lee RS, Stewar C, Carter SL. A remarkably simple genome underlies highly malignant pediatric rhabdoid cancers. J Clin Invest 2012;122(8):2983–8.

138. Abro B, Kaushal M, Chen L, et al. Tumor mutation burden, DNA mismatch repair status and checkpoint immunotherapy markers in primary and relapsed malignant rhabdoid tumors. Pathol Res Pract 2019;215(6):152395.

139. Kalimuthu SN, Chetty R. Gene of the month: SMARCB1. J Clin Pathol 2016;69:484–9.

140. Nemes K, Frühwald MC. Emerging therapeutic targets for the treatment of malignant rhabdoid tumors. Expert Opin Ther Targets 2018;22(4):365–79.

Newcomers in Vascular Anomalies

Alyaa Al-Ibraheemi, MD

KEYWORDS

• Vascular anomalies • Overgrowth • FAVA • Hemangioma • Lymphangiomatosis • PROS

Key points

- Vascular anomalies are classified as tumors and malformations.

- Diagnosis of vascular anomalies can be challenging due to overlapping clinical, radiologic, and morphologic features.

- For optimal treatment and follow-up, these patients should be cared for a by a multidisciplinary group with special interest and expertise in the field of vascular anomalies.

- Recent genetic studies have advanced our understanding of the mechanisms involved in the pathogenesis of vascular tumors and malformations.

- The mammalian target of Rapamycin inhibitor sirolimus has proved to be safe and efficacious in vascular anomalies.

ABSTRACT

Vascular anomalies are composed of tumors and malformations and with overlapping histologies, thus are often misdiagnosed or labeled with imprecise terminology. Lesions are common and usually diagnosed during infancy or childhood; the estimated prevalence is 4.5%. Vascular tumors rapidly enlarge postnatally and demonstrate endothelial proliferation. Malformations are errors in vascular development with stable endothelial turnover; they are typically named based on the primary vessel that is malformed (capillary, arterial, venous, lymphatic). This article reviews the pathologic and molecular genetic characteristics for select recently described vascular anomalies.

OVERVIEW

Vascular anomalies are disorders of the endothelium that can affect each part of the vasculature (capillaries, arteries, veins, or lymphatics). Lesions are usually diagnosed during infancy or childhood and are common, with an estimated prevalence of 4.5%. Although nearly always benign, vascular anomalies can involve any anatomic structure and can result in psychological morbidity caused by disfigurement. Vascular anomalies are composed of tumors and malformations that can be difficult to distinguish given overlapping histologic appearance and therefore they often are misdiagnosed or labeled with imprecise terminology.[1] Vascular tumors rapidly enlarge postnatally and demonstrate endothelial proliferation. Malformations are errors in vascular development with stable endothelial turnover; lesions are typically named based on the primary vessel that is malformed (capillary, arterial, venous, lymphatic). Significant progress in understanding vascular anomalies has been made during the past quarter century and classification of vascular anomalies continues to expand and has become more precise as the knowledge of these lesions evolves.[2] In this article, we review the pathologic and molecular genetic characteristics for select recently described vascular anomalies. For the complete list of vascular anomalies and their associated genes, please review the International Society for

Department of Pathology, Boston Children's Hospital, 300 Longwood Avenue, BCH 3027, Boston, MA 02115, USA

E-mail address: Alyaa.al-ibraheemi@childrens.harvard.edu

Surgical Pathology 13 (2020) 719–728
https://doi.org/10.1016/j.path.2020.08.008

surgpath.theclinics.com

the Study of Vascular Anomalies classification of 2018 (ISSVA) document (https://www.issva.org/UserFiles/file/ISSVA-Classification-2018.pdf).

CATALYTIC SUBUNIT OF PHOSPHATIDYLINOSITOL-3-KINASE–RELATED OVERGROWTH SPECTRUM

Congenital overgrowth syndromes are characterized by excessive proliferation of an organ or region of the body. These may be focal or diffuse and symmetric or asymmetric. A subset of these syndromes is associated with vascular anomalies (**Fig. 1**). The recently updated 2018 ISSVA classification groups most of these syndromes as vascular malformations associated with other anomalies with phosphatase and tensin homolog (PTEN) hamartoma of soft tissue and fibroadipose vascular anomalies (FAVA) classified as provisionally unclassified vascular anomalies.[3] Most overgrowth syndromes with vascular anomalies demonstrate a somatic mutation in the affected area or tissue only (mosaicism) with a small minority showing evidence of a hereditary germline mutation. Many overgrowth syndromes are traced to mutations in the phosphatidylinositol-3-kinase (PI3K)/protein kinase B (AKT)/mammalian target of Rapamycin (mTOR) cell signaling pathway, which is a major regulator in cell signaling and angiogenesis.[4–6] Somatic mutations that occur specifically in PIK3CA (the catalytic subunit of PI3K); account for a large subset of this group and result in syndromes under the umbrella term: PIK3CA-related overgrowth spectrum (PROS). PROS disorders include hyperplasia or hypertrophy of a body part often because of lipomatous overgrowth. In addition, slow-flow vascular malformations accompany the limb overgrowth with skin changes that serve as a hallmark of an underlying vascular malformation. Klippel-Trenaunay, CLOVES (congenital lipomatous overgrowth, vascular malformations, epidermal nevi, and scoliosis/skeletal/spine anomalies) syndrome, and FAVA are hallmarks of PROS.[3–5,7] Imaging studies

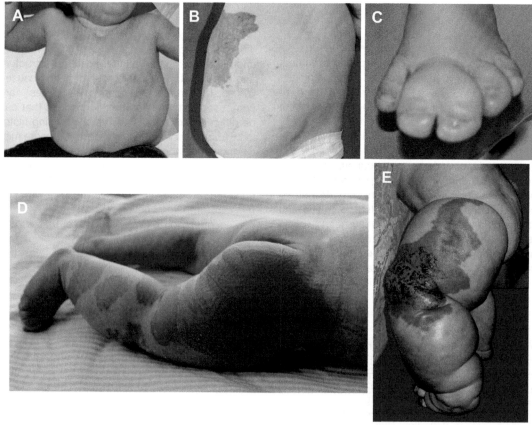

Fig. 1. Syndromes associated with overgrowth. (*A–C*) Patient with CLOVES with fatty of growth of trunk (*A, B*), overlying capillary stain (*B*) and toe abnormalities (*C*). (*D*) Patient with Parkes Weber syndrome with lower extremity overgrowth and cutaneous stain. (*E*) Patient with KTS with lower limb overgrowth, capillary stain, and lymphatic vesicles.

Table 1
Overview of overgrowth syndromes associated with vascular anomalies

Syndrome	ISSVA Classification	Genetic Mutation
Klippel-Trenaunay (KTS)	CM + VM −/+ LM + limb overgrowth	PIK3CA
CLOVES	LM + VM + CM −/+ AVM + limb overgrowth	PIK3CA
FAVA	Provisionally unclassified vascular anomaly	PIK3CA
CLAPO	Lower lip CM + face and neck LM + asymmetry and partial/generalized overgrowth	PIK3CA
MCAP	Megalencephaly + CM	PIK3CA
Parkes Weber (PWS)	CM + AVF + limb overgrowth	RASA1
PTEN Hamartoma and Bannayan-Riley-Ruvalcaba (BRR)	Provisionally unclassified vascular anomaly (PTHS); AVM + VM + macrocephaly, lipomatous overgrowth (BRR)	PTEN
Proteus syndrome	CM, VM, and/or LM + asymmetrical somatic overgrowth	AKT

Abbreviations: AVF, arteriovenous fistula; AVM, arteriovenous malformation; CLAPO, capillary malformation of the lower lip (C), lymphatic malformation of the face and neck (L), asymmetry of the face and limbs (A), and partial/generalized overgrowth (PO); CM, capillary malformation; LM, lymphatic malformation; MCAP, megalencephaly-polymicrogyria-polydactyly-hydrocephalus; VM, venous malformation.

are important in these lesions to determine the flow characteristics of a malformation while also providing information on lesion size and depth. Plain radiography can help to distinguish soft tissue and/or osseous overgrowth when present. MRI and MR angiography (MRA) are considered the gold standard for evaluating overgrowth syndromes to characterize the nature of the vascular malformation.

CLOVES syndrome is a noninherited rare disorder that was recently found to be associated with a somatic mutation of PIK3CA (see **Fig. 1**). Affected individuals may experience a wide array of complications, including recurrent infections, benign and malignant tumors, venous thromboembolism associated with ectatic veins, and limb and spinal abnormalities. Treatment with sirolimus has been beneficial in some patients, particularly in those with a lymphatic component.[8] Klippel-Trenaunay Syndrome (KTS) is characterized by a capillary lymphatic venous malformation and variable overgrowth of soft tissue and bone (see **Fig. 1**). Somatic mutations of PIK3CA also have been identified in patients with KTS. Patients with this syndrome can have chronic debilitating pain, a coagulopathy with risk for bleeding and thrombosis, orthopedic issues, pulmonary hypertension, disfigurement, recurrent infections, and progressive disease. Sirolimus therapy has been reported to improve pain, function, coagulopathy, and quality of life; benefits seem to be greatest in individuals with a significant lymphatic component.[9]

PTEN is an inhibitor of PI3K and helps to mediate tissue growth. Mutations that occur in PTEN allow for the unregulated activation of PI3K. PTEN hamartoma and Bannayan-Riley-Ruvalcaba syndromes are the 2 major PTEN syndromes that feature concomitant vascular anomalies in their phenotypes. Mutations in AKT and RASA1 promote angiogenesis and tissue growth through the upregulation of mTOR and PI3K, respectively. AKT mutations result in the Proteus syndrome, which results in an ever-changing phenotype after a normal phenotypic appearance at birth. RASA1 mutations are seen in capillary malformation-arteriovenous malformations, with Parkes Weber syndrome presenting as a manifestation of this disorder. **Table 1** provides a summary of overgrowth syndromes associated with vascular anomalies.[3,9]

MICROSCOPIC FEATURES

Biopsies are rarely performed for these lesions. Resection specimens typically result from debulking procedures (**Fig. 2**). There is significant overlap in morphology, and the vascular malformation in patients with PROS typically shows combined capillary-lymphatico-venous malformation with soft tissue and bony overgrowth. They tend to involve skin and subcutaneous tissue, sometimes extending to underlying skeletal muscle. Pure lymphatic malformation can also be seen. The lymphatic component is composed of thin-walled channels containing clear fluid and often blood. Frequently, there is evidence of ulceration, infection, inflammation, intralesional hemorrhage, and thrombosis. The deeply located channels are

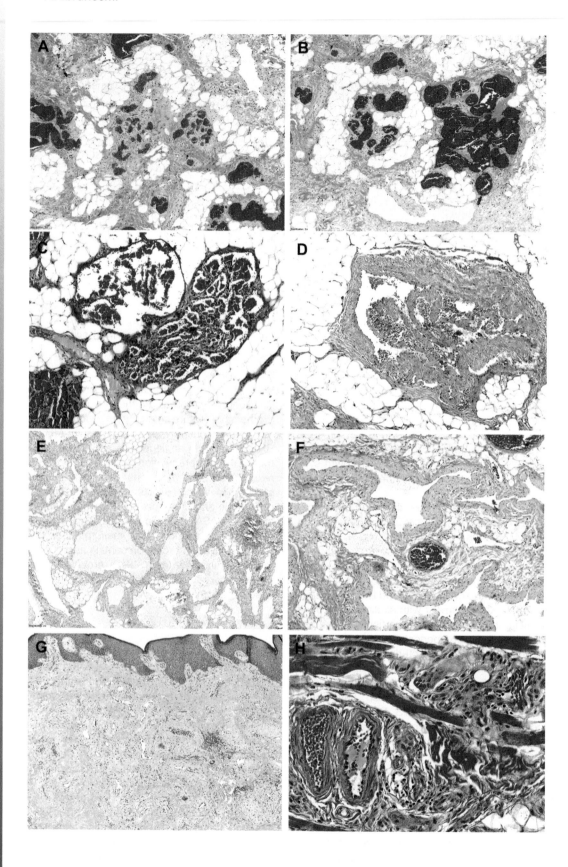

thicker, muscular, and frequently larger. The intervening stroma tends to be fibrous with abundant adipose tissue and may contain collections of lymphocytes. The venous component consists of abnormal tortuous, thick-walled channels dispersed or in back-to-back clusters. In Parkes Weber syndrome or in high-flow lesions, features of arteriovenous shunting are typically present and consist of larger arteries, large veins with intimal and medial thickening, and a small vessel component. The cutaneous stain is typically capillary-venous morphology in the papillary and reticular dermis.

PROGNOSIS AND THERAPY

Vascular anomalies may cause clinical problems such as disfigurement, acute and chronic pain, coagulopathy, bleeding, thrombosis, organ and musculoskeletal dysfunction, and death. These disorders, especially the most severe, are progressive and have lifelong complications. Several multidisciplinary vascular anomalies centers now serve as regional, national, or international referral sites. A multidisciplinary team that includes medical, surgical, pathology, and radiology experts is frequently essential in the long-term management of these complex patients. Currently, management of these lesions is highly individualized and depends on the patient's symptoms along with lesion location and morphology. A combination of surgery, cryotherapy, sclerotherapy, and medical therapy may be used.[10–12]

FIBROADIPOSE VASCULAR ANOMALY

CLINICAL PRESENTATION AND RADIOLOGIC FEATURES

FAVA is a recently defined lesion of the extremities that typically presents in childhood and adolescence. The distinct clinical, radiological, and histologic features of FAVA were first defined by Alomari and colleagues.[13] FAVA is an intramuscular vascular malformation commonly occurring in adolescent girls. The classic clinical presentation is an asymmetric lump, typically involving the lower extremity.[13–15] Patients present with complex symptoms including intractable pain, discomfort, functional impairment, and contracture. The lesion is seen to arise from one predominant muscle or a musculo-fascial compartment, but can extend into adjacent compartments, neurovascular structures, periosteum, and skin. The FAVA lesion is typically a slow-flow anomaly characterized by phlebectasia without discrete cutaneous findings. Ultrasound appearance is typically an echogenic, solid, fibrofatty mass with phlebectasia. MRI/MRA will show characteristics of a fibrofatty lesion replacing the muscle with T1 and T2 hyperintense and heterogeneous signal relative to muscle, with avid postcontrast enhancement.[13]

GROSS FEATURES

Macroscopic examination shows a poorly marginated and usually predominantly fatty mass with a variable number of rounded red vascular nodules approximately 1 cm in diameter (**Fig. 3**).

HISTOLOGY

Microscopically, the nodules consist of thin-walled back-to-back blood-filled sacs that sometimes seem to emanate as diverticula from larger abnormal centrally placed venous channels (veno-diverticular complexes) (see **Fig. 3**). Abnormal small and medium-sized veins also can be present. Dense fibrous tissue is a prominent component and tends toward a perivascular distribution. Nerves are often surrounded by dense fibrous tissue and sometimes have internal abnormal vascular channels. Lymphoplasmacytic nodules are invariably present. Other findings in some lesions include foci of abnormal lymphatic vessels, clusters of channels of indeterminate nature with thick hypermuscularized walls and small lumens, bone, and perineurial hyperplasia. Unlike PTEN hamartoma of soft tissue, FAVA is a slow-flow lesion and does not have arteriovenous communication. The skeletal muscle usually

Fig. 2. Histologic features of debulking specimens from patients with overgrowth spectrum shows vascular malformation with mixed phenotypes with abundant adipose tissue [hematoxylin-eosin, original magnification ×40 (A); hematoxylin-eosin, original magnification ×100 (B)] (A, B). The venous component is composed of cluster of thin-walled veins, some with organizing thrombi [hematoxylin-eosin, original magnification ×200] (C, D). The lymphatic component is composed of networks of irregularly dilated lymphatic channels of variable wall thickness, some with muscular wall [hematoxylin-eosin, original magnification ×40 (E); hematoxylin-eosin, original magnification ×200 (F)] (E, F). The arteriovenous malformation in a patient with Parkes Weber syndrome shows variable-size vessels with abnormal arteries involving the dermis [hematoxylin-eosin, original magnification ×100] (G) and extending to underlying skeletal muscle [hematoxylin-eosin, original magnification ×400] (H). (A, B) Resections from patients with KTS, (C–F) resections from patient with CLOVES, (G, H) resections from patient with Parkes Weber syndrome.

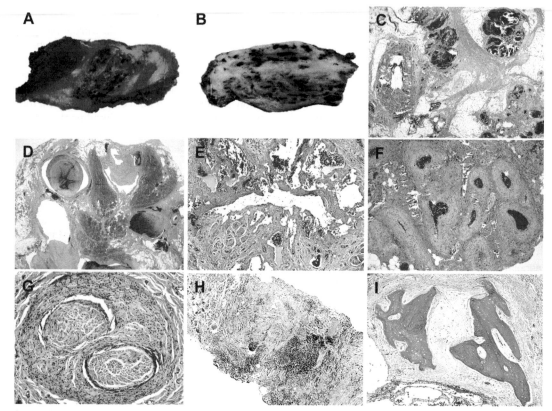

Fig. 3. Macroscopic examination of FAVA shows predominantly fatty mass with a variable number of rounded red vascular nodules involving skeletal muscle (*A*, *B*). Microscopically, FAVA is composed of clusters thin-walled back-to-back blood-filled sacs, abnormal veins, and fibrous and adipose tissue [hematoxylin-eosin, original magnification ×40] (*C*). Dilated veins can have organizing thrombi [hematoxylin-eosin, original magnification ×40] (*D*), and sometimes seem to emanate as diverticula from larger abnormal centrally placed venous channels [hematoxylin-eosin, original magnification ×200] (*E*). Other findings include clusters of channels of indeterminate nature with thick, hypermuscularized walls [hematoxylin-eosin, original magnification ×200] (*F*), perineurial hyperplasia [hematoxylin-eosin, original magnification ×200] (*G*), stromal lymphocytic infiltrate [hematoxylin-eosin, original magnification ×100] (*H*), and metaplastic bone [hematoxylin-eosin, original magnification ×100] (*I*).

shows some degree of atrophy and regenerating fibers. In patients who have undergone sclerotherapy, findings included fibrous obliteration of venous lumens, perivascular fibrosis, and foreign material with a foreign body giant cell response.

DIAGNOSIS

The diagnosis of FAVA is chiefly made based on the clinical and radiologic features. Biopsies are rarely performed.

TREATMENT AND PROGNOSIS

Resection has been the treatment of choice. Endovascular and sclerotherapy treatment of FAVA can control symptoms, but likelihood of recurrence of the lesion is high. Cryoablation may also serve as a viable therapeutic option in the treatment of FAVA lesions.[16] On the basis of targeting the activating mutations in PIK3CA in

FAVA, mTOR inhibition with sirolimus has been recently reported as beneficial in 8 patients with FAVA. Sirolimus, an inhibitor of mammalian target of rapamycin, is an important mediator of the phosphoinositide 3-kinase signaling pathway, and has been shown to improve a range of other vascular anomalies.[8,13–18]

Key Points

- Distinctive intramuscular slow-flow vascular malformation with abundant fibrous and adipose tissue.

- More common in adolescent girls.

- Commonly occurs in the lower extremity with gastrocnemius muscle being the most frequently affected muscle.

- The diagnosis is chiefly made based on the clinical and radiologic features.
- Patients present with complex symptoms including intractable pain, discomfort, functional impairment, and contracture.
- Microscopically, it consists of nodules of thin-walled back-to-back blood-filled sacs in a background of fibroadipose tissue and skeletal muscle.
- Treatment is combination of surgical resection, cryoablation, and medical therapy.
- It harbors the PIK3CA mutation.

KAPOSIFORM LYMPHANGIOMATOSIS

CLINICAL PRESENTATION AND RADIOLOGIC FEATURES

Kaposiform lymphangiomatosis (KLA), a newly described entity, is an aggressive lymphatic anomaly that has features of both tumor and malformation.[19,20] KLA is clinically heterogeneous and typically affects children and young adults. It most commonly involves the thoracic cavity, bone, skin, and spleen, and is associated with a life-threatening coagulopathy characterized by severe hypofibrinogenemia, thrombocytopenia, and bleeding. KLA has overlapping imaging features with central conducting lymphatic anomaly and

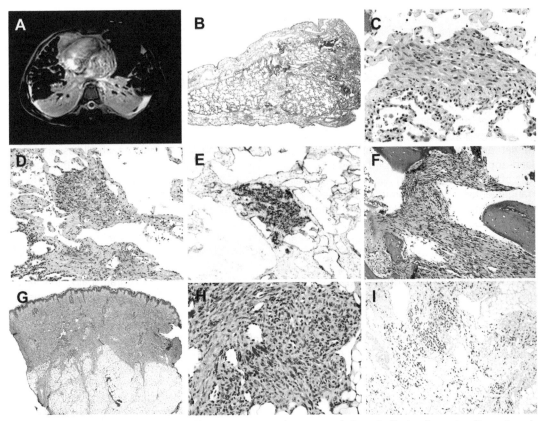

Fig. 4. MRI of a patient with KLA shows bilateral lung involvement and pleural effusion [hematoxylin-eosin, original magnification ×20] (A). KLA involving the lung shows pleural thickening and expansion by lymphatic channels [hematoxylin-eosin, original magnification ×20] (B). Within the lymphatic channels, there are poorly canalized foci of spindle cells [hematoxylin-eosin, original magnification ×200 (C); hematoxylin-eosin, original magnification ×200 (D)] (C, D), also highlighted by D240 stain [D240 Immunohistochemistry X100] (E). KLA involving bone [hematoxylin-eosin, original magnification ×200] (F) showing areas of spindle cell proliferation occupying marrow spaces. KLA involving the skin shows dilated lymphatics with areas of spindling resembling kaposiform hemangioendothelioma [hematoxylin-eosin, original magnification ×20 (G); hematoxylin-eosin, original magnification ×200 (H)] (G, H). PROX1 immunostain is positive in the spindle cell proliferation supporting lymphatic phenotype [PROX-1 immunohistochemistry x 100] (I).

generalized lymphatic anomaly. The presence of mediastinal or retroperitoneal enhancing and infiltrative soft tissue disease along the lymphatic distribution should favor a diagnosis of KLA. Somatic NRAS mutation is a recurrent alteration in KLA.[21,22]

GROSS FEATURES

Grossly, lesions show dilated lymphatic channels, sometimes filled with blood, and hemorrhage.

MICROSCOPIC FEATURES

Histologic evaluation reveals focal areas of spindle cells with lymphatic disease similar to kaposiform hemangioendothelioma (KHE) but the spindle cell component is more dispersed and arranged in poorly defined clusters or anastomosing strands/sheets (**Fig. 4**). In general, the histopathology of the affected tissues show a lymphatic anomaly, characterized by dilated and irregular lymphatic channels of varying size with variable wall thickness, sometimes muscularized. The lumens contain pale proteinaceous material or blood with sparse lymphocytes and macrophages. The endothelial cells are flat and exhibit multifocal proliferation of bland-appearing spindle-shaped cells along the walls of the lymphatic channels, often in parallel arrangement. Intracytoplasmic hemosiderin can be seen. In the lungs, pleura and interlobar septa can be thickened and contain abnormal lymphatic channels. Splenic involvement can show marked sinusoidal dilatation lined by plaques of spindle cells. In some cases, the spindle cell proliferation can be pronounced, mimicking kaposiform hemangioendothelioma. By immunohistochemistry, these lesions have a lymphatic phenotype and show immunoreactivity to D240 and PROX1, in addition to other endothelial markers such as CD34, CD31, and ERG.

PROGNOSIS AND THERAPY

Disease progression is common, with hemorrhage and pleural/pericardial effusions causing the most significant morbidity. Outcomes are poor, with a reported 5-year survival of 51%. It requires a multimodal approach to control or ameliorate symptoms. Current therapy is supportive with sirolimus, frequently in combination with steroids and/or vincristine.[8]

Key Points

- Aggressive lymphatic anomaly typically affects children and young adults
- It most commonly involves the thoracic cavity, bone, skin, and spleen
- It is associated with coagulopathy
- It has overlapping imaging features with central conducting lymphatic anomaly and generalized lymphatic anomaly
- Histologically: KLA is characterized by the presence of variably abundant foci of spindled endothelial cells accompanying abnormal lymphatic channels of varying size
- Associated with somatic activating mutation of NRAS gene
- Requires multidisciplinary approach

INTRAMUSCULAR FAST-FLOW VASCULAR ANOMALY

CLINICAL AND RADIOLOGIC FEATURES

Intramuscular hemangioma, small vessel or capillary type, was originally described by Allen and Enzinger in 1972.[23] These are solitary, benign, painless vascular tumors that primarily affect skeletal muscle. The median age at diagnosis is 25 years and as many as 25% of patients are in the pediatric age group. Affected areas include the extremities (38%), trunk (32%), and head/neck (30%).[24] Skin overlying the affected muscle is grossly normal. Radiographically, the lesions are well-defined heterogeneous intramuscular solid soft tissue masses with increased arterial flow (fast-flow), enhancement with contrast, and intralesional fat.[24] The lesion is recognized to have overlapping clinical and radiologic features with arteriovenous malformation (AVM) and has been considered in the same differential diagnosis. The term of intramuscular fast-flow vascular anomaly has been recently proposed by Goss and colleagues,[25] given the discovery of MAP2K1 and KRAS mutations in these lesions.

GROSS FEATURES

Intramuscular fast-flow vascular anomaly lesions are typically nonencapsulated lesions with red vascular components admixed with fat and skeletal muscle.

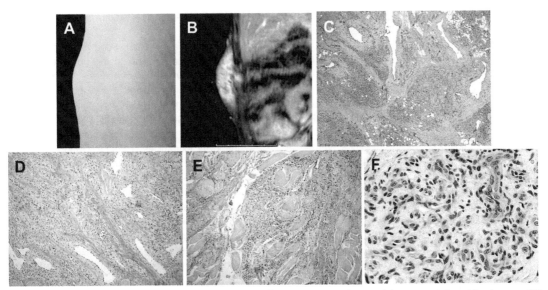

Fig. 5. Intramuscular fast-flow vascular anomaly typically presents as a lump without overlying skin changes (A), computed tomography with contrast shows well-defined enhanced soft tissue mass, (B). Histologically, intramuscularfast-flow vascular anomaly is composed of lobules of small capillarous vessels within skeletal muscle [[hematoxylin-eosin, original magnification ×40 (C); [hematoxylin-eosin, original magnification ×100 (D-E)] (C–E). The lobules contain small vessels lined by flat to plump endothelial cells, surrounded by thin layer of basement membrane [hematoxylin-eosin, original magnification ×400] (F).

MICROSCOPIC FEATURES

Lesions vary in appearance and histologic fields also vary (Fig. 5). The most characteristic feature is the presence of lobules or sheets of capillaries with plump endothelial cells. Large arteries and veins and a number of vessels that are indeterminate in lineage can be seen. Arteries show focal dissolution of their internal elastic lamina with neointimal cushions and veins show thickened walls with neointimal hyperplasia.

PROGNOSIS AND THERAPY

Treatment options include embolization and/or resection when lesions become symptomatic; however, 20% of tumors recur after excision.

- soft tissue masses with increased arterial flow (fast-flow)
- Approximately 25% of patients are in the pediatric age group
- Typical locations include the extremities, trunk, and head/neck
- Histologically, the most characteristic feature is the presence of lobules or sheets of capillaries with plump endothelial cells dispersed throughout skeletal muscle
- MAP2K1 and KRAS mutations have been identified in these lesions.
- Resection is the preferred treatment of choice

Key Points

- Also known as intramuscular hemangioma, small vessel type
- Has overlapping features with arteriovenous malformation radiologically and histologically
- Radiographically, the lesions are well-defined, heterogeneous, intramuscular, solid

DISCLOSURE

The authors declare that they have nothing to disclose.

REFERENCES

1. Wassef M, Blei F, Adams D, et al. Vascular anomalies classification: recommendations from the International Society for the Study of Vascular Anomalies. Pediatrics 2015;136(1):e203–14.

2. Adams DM. Practical genetic and biologic therapeutic considerations in vascular anomalies. Tech Vasc Interv Radiol 2019;22(4):100629.

3. ISSVA. ISSVA classificatiob. Available at: https://www.issva.org/UserFiles/file/ISSVA-Classification-2018.pdf. Accessed August 7, 2020.

4. Hughes M, Hao M, Luu M. PIK3CA vascular overgrowth syndromes: an update. Curr Opin Pediatr 2020;32(4):539–46.

5. Keppler-Noreuil KM, Rios JJ, Parker VE, et al. PIK3CA-related overgrowth spectrum (PROS): diagnostic and testing eligibility criteria, differential diagnosis, and evaluation. Am J Med Genet A 2015; 167a(2):287–95.

6. Mirzaa G, Conway R, Graham JM Jr, et al. PIK3CA-related segmental overgrowth. In: Adam MP, Ardinger HH, Pagon RA, et al, editors. GeneReviews(®). Seattle (WA): University of Washington; 1993. Seattle Copyright © 1993-2020, University of Washington, Seattle. GeneReviews is a registered trademark of the University of Washington, Seattle. All rights reserved.

7. Keppler-Noreuil KM, Sapp JC, Lindhurst MJ, et al. Clinical delineation and natural history of the PIK3CA-related overgrowth spectrum. Am J Med Genet A 2014;164a(7):1713–33.

8. Lackner H, Karastaneva A, Schwinger W, et al. Sirolimus for the treatment of children with various complicated vascular anomalies. Eur J Pediatr 2015;174(12):1579–84.

9. Martinez-Lopez A, Salvador-Rodriguez L, Montero-Vilchez T, et al. Vascular malformations syndromes: an update. Curr Opin Pediatr 2019;31(6):747–53.

10. Adams DM, Brandão LR, Peterman CM, et al. Vascular anomaly cases for the pediatric hematologist oncologists—an interdisciplinary review. Pediatr Blood Cancer 2018;65(1). https://doi.org/10.1002/pbc.26716.

11. Adams DM, Ricci KW. Vascular anomalies: diagnosis of complicated anomalies and new medical treatment options. Hematol Oncol Clin North Am 2019;33(3):455–70.

12. Hori Y, Ozeki M, Hirose K, et al. Analysis of mTOR pathway expression in lymphatic malformation and related diseases. Pathol Int 2020;70(6):323–9.

13. Alomari AI, Spencer SA, Arnold RW, et al. Fibro-adipose vascular anomaly: clinical-radiologic-pathologic features of a newly delineated disorder of the extremity. J Pediatr Orthop 2014;34(1):109–17.

14. Cheung K, Taghinia AH, Sood RF, et al. Fibroadipose vascular anomaly in the upper extremity: a distinct entity with characteristic clinical, radiological, and histopathological findings. J Hand Surg Am 2020;45(1):68.e1–13.

15. Wang KK, Glenn RL, Adams DM, et al. Surgical management of fibroadipose vascular anomaly of the lower extremities. J Pediatr Orthop 2020;40(3): e227–36.

16. Shaikh R, Alomari AI, Kerr CL, et al. Cryoablation in fibro-adipose vascular anomaly (FAVA): a minimally invasive treatment option. Pediatr Radiol 2016; 46(8):1179–86.

17. Erickson J, McAuliffe W, Blennerhassett L, et al. Fibroadipose vascular anomaly treated with sirolimus: successful outcome in two patients. Pediatr Dermatol 2017;34(6):e317–20.

18. Adams DM, Trenor CC 3rd, Hammill AM, et al. Efficacy and safety of sirolimus in the treatment of complicated vascular anomalies. Pediatrics 2016; 137(2):e20153257.

19. Croteau SE, Kozakewich HP, Perez-Atayde AR, et al. Kaposiform lymphangiomatosis: a distinct aggressive lymphatic anomaly. J Pediatr 2014;164(2): 383–8.

20. Fernandes VM, Fargo JH, Saini S, et al. Kaposiform lymphangiomatosis: unifying features of a heterogeneous disorder. Pediatr Blood Cancer 2015;62(5):901–4.

21. Barclay SF, Inman KW, Luks VL, et al. A somatic activating NRAS variant associated with kaposiform lymphangiomatosis. Genet Med 2019;21(7): 1517–24.

22. Ozeki M, Aoki Y, Nozawa A, et al. Detection of NRAS mutation in cell-free DNA biological fluids from patients with kaposiform lymphangiomatosis. Orphanet J Rare Dis 2019;14(1):215.

23. Allen PW, Enzinger FM. Hemangioma of skeletal muscle. An analysis of 89 cases. Cancer 1972;29(1):8–22.

24. Yilmaz S, Kozakewich HP, Alomari AI, et al. Intramuscular capillary-type hemangioma: radiologic-pathologic correlation. Pediatr Radiol 2014;44(5): 558–65.

25. Goss JA, Konczyk DJ, Smits PJ, et al. Intramuscular fast-flow vascular anomaly contains somatic MAP2K1 and KRAS mutations. Angiogenesis 2019; 22(4):547–52.

Challenges in the Diagnosis of Pediatric Spindle Cell/Sclerosing Rhabdomyosarcoma

Sonja Chen, MBBS[a],*, Erin R. Rudzinski, MD[b],
Michael A. Arnold, MD, PhD[c]

KEYWORDS

• Spindle cell • Sclerosing • Rhabdomyosarcoma • Pediatric

Key points

• Spindle cell/sclerosing rhabdomyosarcoma is a variant of rhabdomyosarcoma, which frequently harbors recurrent genetic alterations that are associated with unique clinical and prognostic features.

• *MYOD1* mutant spindle cell/sclerosing rhabdomyosarcoma is associated with high mortality and overall poor outcome.

• *VGLL2* or *NCOA2* fusion-related spindle cell rhabdomyosarcoma is associated with an excellent prognosis.

• A subset of spindle cell/sclerosing rhabdomyosarcoma lack defined molecular alterations as yet and may represent a spindle cell predominant pattern of embryonal rhabdomyosarcoma.

• Histologic mimics of spindle cell/sclerosing rhabdomyosarcoma can be identified using a panel of immunohistochemical and molecular markers.

ABSTRACT

Rhabdomyosarcoma (RMS) is the most common pediatric soft tissue sarcoma, representing approximately 40% of all pediatric soft tissue sarcomas. The spindle cell/sclerosing subtype of RMS (SSRMS) accounts for roughly 5% to 10% of all cases of adult and pediatric RMS. Historically, SSRMS were described as paratesticular tumors with an excellent outcome. However, more recent studies have identified unique molecular subgroups of SSRMS, including those with *MYOD1* mutations or *VGLL2/NCOA2* fusions, which have widely disparate outcomes. The goal of this article is to better describe the biological heterogeneity of SSRMS, which may allow the pathologist to provide important prognostic information.

OVERVIEW

Rhabdomyosarcoma (RMS) is the most common pediatric soft tissue sarcoma, representing approximately 40% of all pediatric soft tissue sarcomas[1] with an incidence of 400 to 500 new cases per year in the United States.[2] Historically, RMS has been divided into 3 major subtypes: embryonal, alveolar, and pleomorphic, based on histologic features and immunohistochemistry.

---

[a] Warren Alpert Medical School of Brown University, Lifespan Academic Medical Center, Rhode Island Hospital, 593 Eddy Street APC12-115, Providence, RI 02903, USA; [b] Seattle Children's Hospital and University of Washington Medical Center, 4800 Sand Point Way Northeast, Seattle, WA 98105, USA; [c] Children's Hospital Colorado, University of Colorado, Anschutz Medical Campus, Aurora, 13123 East 16th Avenue, Aurora, CO 80045, USA
* Corresponding author.
E-mail address: sonja.chen@lifespan.org

Surgical Pathology 13 (2020) 729–738
https://doi.org/10.1016/j.path.2020.08.010

Because ancillary techniques have increasingly become incorporated into pathology, molecular findings have served to subdivide these groups further, allowing for identification of diagnostic and prognostic markers. One such subtype with a distinct morphology, which underwent major changes within the last 20 years, is spindle cell/sclerosing rhabdomyosarcoma.

Once classified as a histologic variant of embryonal rhabdomyosarcoma (ERMS), spindle cell/sclerosing rhabdomyosarcoma became a stand-alone entity in 2013 in the fourth edition of the World Health Organization (WHO) Classification of Tumors of Soft Tissue and Bone.[3] This subtype of RMS accounts for roughly 5% to 10% of all cases of adult and pediatric RMS. Spindle cell RMS was first described in 1995, as a paratesticular tumor occurring in pediatric patients, associated with a superior prognosis.[4] In 2002, sclerosing RMS, a hyalinizing, matrix-rich variant, was initially described in adult patients[5] and subsequently recognized as a challenging diagnosis in pediatric patients.[6] These entities were grouped together in the 2013 WHO,[3] as in some cases both morphologies are seen in the same tumor, particularly in older patients who had poor outcomes. Further investigation resulted in the recognition of distinct morphologic, molecular, and prognostic features that currently correspond to at least 3 subgroups of molecular features in the spindle cell/sclerosing subtype of RMS (SSRMS) morphologic category: (1) MYOD1 mutated, (2) VGLL2/NCOA2 fused, (3) TFCP2 gene fusions, and (4) tumors (no known genetic abnormalities).

CLINICAL FEATURES

Each of the subgroups of SSRMS have characteristic clinical features that may aid in diagnosis. SSRMS with MYOD1 mutations most commonly arise in the head and neck (parameningeal) region when in children, followed by the extremities. In contrast, SSRMS with VGLL2/NCOA2 fusions usually occur in the chest wall/paravertebral region and are rare in the extremities. RMS with TFCP2 gene fusions is an emerging group with spindle and epithelioid features that frequently involves the craniofacial skeleton. SSRMS without known molecular alterations most frequently arise in sites common to embryonal RMS, including the paratestis and retroperitoneum.

Similarly, these subgroups occur at different ages. SSRMS with VGLL2/NCOA2 fusions can be considered congenital/infantile SSRMS. To date, these tumors have not been described in children younger than 2 years. In contrast, SSRMS with MYOD1 mutations occur more frequently in adolescents/young adults, although rare cases have been described in children as young as 2 years of age. The limited number of RMS cases with TFCP2 gene fusions has been described in a wide range of ages, including children. SSRMS without known molecular alterations tend to occur in children aged 0 to 10 years, overlapping the age distribution of embryonal RMS.

GROSS FEATURES

Gross examination typically reveals a firm, relatively well-demarcated, and unencapsulated lesion with an average size of 4 to 6 cm (range, 2–35 cm). In pediatric patients, the largest recorded size is 16 cm, occurring in the lower extremity.[7] The cut surface typically reveals a nodular pattern with a gray-white, whorled appearance that can overlap with the gross appearance of ERMS[5,8] (**Fig. 1**).

MICROSCOPIC FEATURES

The microscopic features of each molecular subgroup of SSRMS have subtle differences. SSRMS with MYOD1 mutations may have spindled and/or sclerosing morphology. The spindle cell pattern is characterized by long fascicles of spindled cells with inconspicuous nucleoli, eosinophilic cytoplasm, and distinct cellular borders, whereas the sclerosing pattern has round to oval cells in small nests or cords within sclerotic stroma (**Fig. 2**). These cells may cling to the stroma and separate, giving a microalveolar appearance. These components can be seen in varied proportions, with either pattern predominating. Classic rhabdomyoblasts are rare in these tumors. RMS with MYOD1 mutations may have weak to absent myogenin and weak desmin staining, but MYOD1 staining is strong and diffuse.

In contrast, SSRMS with VGLL2 or NCOA2 gene fusions have a purely spindled morphology, with fascicles of monomorphic spindled cells having indistinct cell borders. Rhabdomyoblasts with cytoplasmic cross-striations are often observed in a subset of tumor cells (see **Fig. 2**).[5,9] These tumors have weak to moderate myogenin and desmin staining, similar to the pattern expected in embryonal RMS.

SSRMS that lack recurrent genetic alterations are predominantly spindled but may be admixed with areas of more typical embryonal RMS. The proportion of sclerosis or spindled cell components necessary to designate a tumor as the SSRMS variant is not currently established, but in general one or both of these patterns should comprise most of the tissue sample. This group

Fig. 1. Gross appearance of embryonal rhabdomyosarcoma. This paratesticular tumor is sharply demarcated and separated from the testicle (*center*). The cut surface is vaguely nodular with a yellow-tan color and foci of hemorrhage. (*Courtesy of* Dr. Mark Lovell, Children's Hospital Colorado, Aurora, CO.)

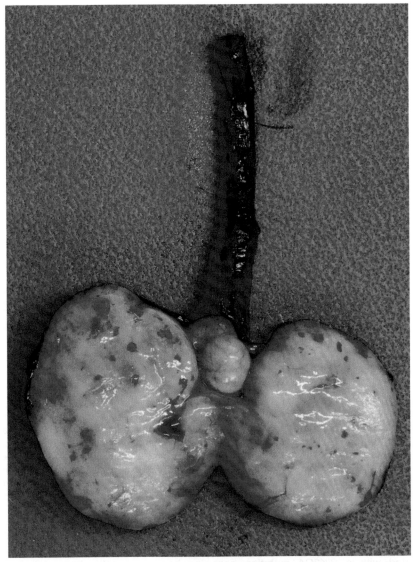

of SSRMS has expression of muscle markers similar to that seen in embryonal RMS.

DIAGNOSIS

The diagnosis of spindle cell/sclerosing RMS largely rests on the histologic and immunohistochemical findings. Molecular analysis, discussed earlier, predominately provides prognostic information.

MOLECULAR PATHOLOGY AND PROGNOSIS

MYOD1 MUTANT SPINDLE CELL/SCLEROSING RHABDOMYOSARCOMA

MYOD1 encodes a myogenic basic-helix-loop-helix transcription factor with critical roles in muscle development.[10,11] A recurrent somatic point mutation of Leu122Arg (p.L122R) in *MYOD1*[12,13] was initially described in the subset of RMS cases without alveolar histology that have subsequently been recategorized as associated with spindle cell/sclerosing RMS. This preliminary study demonstrated that none of the spindle cell/sclerosing RMS cases were *FOXO1* fusion positive. Outcomes were also noted to be poor in these cases. Further study has demonstrated that the p.L122 R *MYOD1* mutation is the most common genetic abnormality in pediatric spindle cell/sclerosing rhabdomyosarcoma, and in one series half of the cases occurred in children 2 years of age or younger.[14] In addition, there may be accompanying *PIK3CA* mutations, seen in up to one-third of the cases.[7] *MYOD1*-mutated tumors tend to follow a highly aggressive course with a high mortality (83%) despite multimodality therapy, similar to

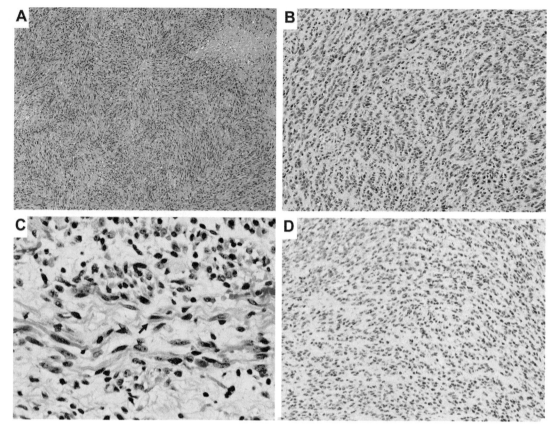

Fig. 2. Spindle cell/sclerosing rhabdomyosarcoma. Spindle cell rhabdomyosarcoma can show fascicles that range from storiform (*A*, 10x objective magnification) to elongated. Sclerosing rhabdomyosarcoma is characterized by sclerotic stroma that divides the round to oval tumor cells into small nests (*B*, 20x objective magnification). Rhabdomyoblasts with cross-striations (*C, arrow,* 60x objective magnification) can be seen in embryonal rhabdomyosarcoma or spindle cell/sclerosing rhabdomyosarcoma. In spindle cell/sclerosing rhabdomyosarcoma, *MYOD1* immunohistochemistry (*D,* 20x objective magnification) typically shows strong and diffuse nuclear staining.

alveolar RMS.[14,15] In addition, a single case of heterozygous *MYOD1* p.E118 K mutation not associated with a *PIK3CA* mutation has also been identified in pediatric spindle cell/sclerosing RMS.[7]

SPINDLE CELL RHABDOMYOSARCOMA WITH *NCOA2/VGLL2* GENE FUSIONS

These tumors have emerged as unique biological subtype based on the presence of gene fusions that activate critical transcriptional activators of muscle-specific genes, such as *VGLL2*, *TEAD1*, and *SRF* (**Fig. 3**).[14] *VGLL2* (vestigial-like 2, a.k.a. *VGL2* or *VITO1*) is a key cofactor of TEF-1and MEF2 family members in regulating muscle-specific gene transcription in skeletal muscle, and these genes are essential for muscle development.[16–18] *VGLL2* is expressed in differentiating somites and branchial arches during embryogenesis and is exclusively expressed in skeletal

muscle in the adult.[19] *VGLL2* gene rearrangement located at 6q22 locus is the most common (64%) genetic abnormality in congenital/infantile SRMS, being fused to either *NCOA2* on 8q13.3 or *CITED2* on 6q23.3.[20] Both *NCOA2* and *CITED2* share a CBP/p300 interaction domain, which is known to be a transcriptional/epigenetic regulator of tumorigenesis.[20] Other partners of *VGLL2* or *NCOA2* include *TEAD1,* a key molecule of muscle development, transactivating multiple target genes involved in cell proliferation and differentiation pathways;[21] *SRF* (serum response factor), which is highly expressed in skeletal muscle and controls skeletal muscle–specific gene expression (*dystrophin, muscle creatine kinase, MYOD1*).[22] Both *SRF* and *TEAD1* have been shown to be involved in the control of muscle-specific gene transcription.

In general, techniques used in the identification of molecular alterations typically include karyotype and fluorescence in situ hybridization (FISH) with specific gene probes to either *VGLL2* or *NCOA2*.

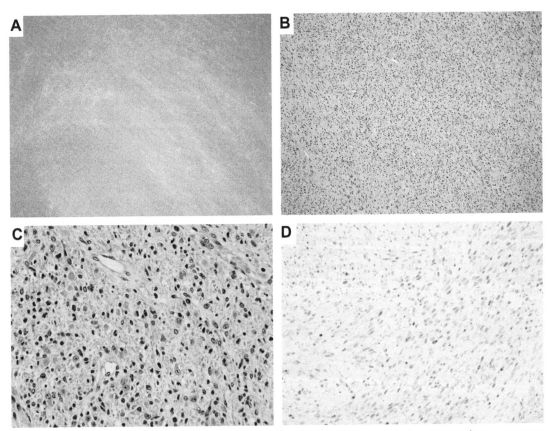

Fig. 3. Infantile spindle cell rhabdomyosarcoma with *VGLL2* or *NCOA2* fusions. At low power, these tumors can show variable cellularity, reminiscent of ERMS (*A*, 4x objective magnification). At higher power, the cells are seen to be arranged in intersecting fascicles (*B*, 10x objective magnification). The cells have round to oval nuclei with some variation in nuclear size, and occasional cells have rhabdoid cytology (*C*, 40x objective magnification). Similar to other spindle cell/sclerosing rhabdomyosarcomas, MYOD1 immunohistochemistry is often diffuse (*D*, 20x objective magnification).

In addition, next-generation sequencing (NGS), which casts a wider net, can be used to identify novel fusion partners. Although karyotype requires fresh tissue, FISH and NGS can be performed on formalin-fixed paraffin-embedded tissue, provided that there is enough viable tumor with good-quality genetic material.

This subset of patients tends to have a favorable clinical outcome, without metastatic potential and are free of disease at long-term follow-up (median of 7 years).[14]

RHABDOMYOSARCOMA WITH *TFCP2* GENE FUSIONS

To date, this very rare group is composed of 18 reported cases, which includes 6 patients aged 18 years and younger.[23–25] These aggressive tumors were initially described in young women (age range 16–38 years) and developed in bony sites including the pelvis, chest wall, and sphenoid, with overall survival in the initial report of less than 5 months.[23] A fourth case arising in the mandible of an adult male was identified.[24] Subsequently, 14 additional reported cases also showed bone involvement, especially involving craniofacial bones, with poor survival.[25] Histologically, these tumors demonstrate epithelioid, round cell, or sclerosing features arranged in small sheets or short fascicles with variable amounts of fibrous stroma and prominent nucleoli. By immunohistochemistry, they are positive for desmin, MYOD1, and myogenin.[23] In addition, ALK overexpression by immunohistochemistry, without an underlying *ALK1* gene fusion, has also been seen. ALK upregulation is frequently associated with an internal deletion at genomic level.[25] This may yet prove to be an actionable therapeutic target.

SPINDLE CELL/SCLEROSING RHABDOMYOSARCOMA LACKING RECURRENT GENETIC ALTERATIONS

This group of tumors lacks any identifiable recurrent genetic abnormalities and presents with a predilection for the genitourinary or intraabdominal location. Histologic findings include minute foci of anaplasia.[14] Although the data were limited, these patients seemed to follow a more favorable course compared with *MYOD1* mutant cases.[14]

DIFFERENTIAL DIAGNOSIS

The differential of spindle cell/sclerosing rhabdomyosarcoma can vary depending on whether the tumor is more round cell/sclerosing or spindled. However, the diagnosis can usually be made based on histology and molecular analysis.

EMBRYONAL RHABDOMYOSARCOMA

ERMS often presents as a mass occurring in the genitourinary tract, head and neck, or abdomen of infants and children younger than 5 years. The conventional type is associated with a 5-year survival of 66%. Histologically, it is composed of variably cellular sheets of rhabdomyoblasts with varying epithelioid appearance and cross-striations present in the cytoplasm of at least a subset of tumor cells. By immunohistochemistry, the tumor cells are variably positive with myogenin and desmin (**Fig. 4**). With the aforementioned spindle cell and sclerosing subtypes removed from this category, the only caveat is determining how much of these features are required in a tumor to reclassify it. It is recommended to pursue molecular analysis in any ERMS that has even limited spindle or sclerosing appearance in order to properly classify and prognosticate regarding these entities.

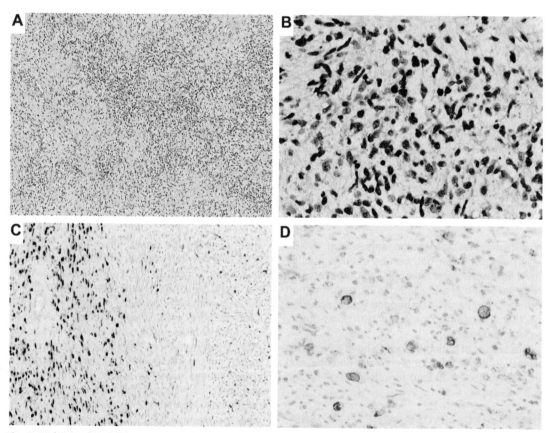

Fig. 4. Embryonal rhabdomyosarcoma. At low power, EMRS is often characterized by alternating darker and lighter areas reflecting variable cellularity (*A*, 10x objective magnification). At high power, the cells of ERMS are generally small with variation in size and shape and embedded in an eosinophilic to myxoid background (*B*, 60x objective magnification). Myogenin reactivity in ERMS is typically less than 50% of nuclei; however, significant variation can be seen within and between cases (*C*, 20x objective magnification). Desmin reactivity is variable within ERMS, most often seen in tumor cells with more abundant cytoplasm, reflecting greater skeletal muscle differentiation (*D*, 40x objective magnification).

ERMS has no known canonical genetic alterations that can aid in diagnosis. In addition, the presence of a *MYOD1* p.L122 R mutation is a poor prognostic finding, even in cases that do not share a spindle cell/sclerosing histology.[13]

ALVEOLAR RHABDOMYOSARCOMA

Alveolar RMS (ARMS) comprises roughly 20% of all pediatric rhabdomyosarcomas[3] and typically occurs in the extremities of older children and adolescents with a median age of 6.8 to 9 years.[26] Classically, these are cellular small round blue cell tumors with a distinct architectural pattern of nests with central dyscohesion imparting a characteristic "alveolar appearance," typically separated by fibrous septa. As a histologic mimic, SSRMS may histologically have a microalveolar pattern, with abundant collagen and pseudovascular spaces lined by tumor cells.[5,27,28] However, immunohistochemistry can be used to distinguish ARMS from SSRMS. Although ARMS has strong

and diffuse nuclear myogenin staining, SSRMS will show more variable staining in a patchy distribution. In addition, most of the ARMS cases have canonical fusions of *PAX3/7* to *FOXO1*.

INFANTILE FIBROSARCOMA AND OTHER *NTRK*-REARRANGED TUMORS

Infantile fibrosarcoma (also known as congenital fibrosarcoma) is a malignant tumor of infancy that classically presents as a rapidly enlarging mass in the extremity of a child younger than 2 years. Most of the cases are diagnosed within the first year of life.[29] Less commonly, they can present in the trunk or head and neck region. Grossly, they form a lobulated, poorly circumscribed mass with a firm grey-white cut surface with foci of hemorrhage and necrosis. Although the histology can be deceivingly variable, the classic form, composed of long fascicles of densely cellular spindle cells with a variable amount of collagenous stroma, is most likely to

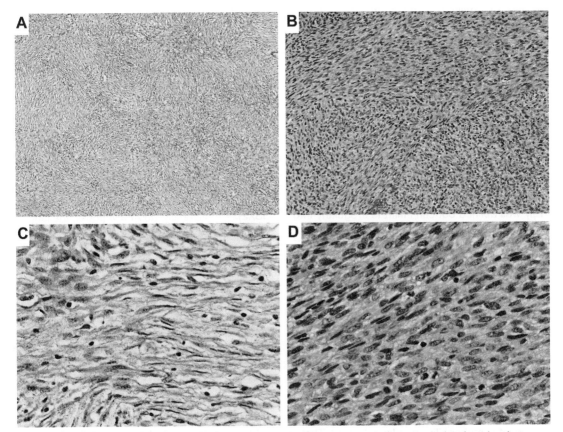

Fig. 5. Infantile fibrosarcoma. The spindle cells of infantile fibrosarcoma can be arranged in fascicles that range from short and storiform (*A*, 10x objective magnification) to long, broad fascicles (*B*, 10x objective magnification). At high magnification, the nuclei of the spindle cells can range from thin and elongated (*C*, 60 X objective magnification) to plump and ovoid (*D*, 60x objective magnification).

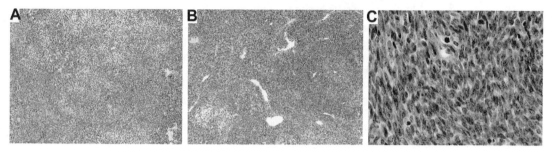

Fig. 6. Synovial sarcoma. The varied histology of synovial sarcoma is capable of mimicking the histology of ERMS with variable light and dark areas at low power (*A*, 10x objective magnification). In many cases, distinctive hemangiopericytic vessels can be identified in synovial sarcoma (*B*, 10x objective magnification). At high power, the nuclei of synovial sarcoma are ovoid and extremely monotonous, often overlapping each other (*C*, 60x objective magnification).

enter the differential for spindle cell/sclerosing RMS (**Fig. 5**). However, variable mitoses, apoptosis, and areas of necrosis as well as a scattered mononuclear inflammatory infiltrate are frequently present in infantile fibrosarcoma, unlike spindle cell/sclerosing RMS.[30] The clinical outcome is generally favorable, with rare metastases and a mortality rate of less than 5%. Recurrence rates are up to 50% of patients treated with a combination of chemotherapy and surgery.[31] Recurrent *ETV6–NTRK3* translocations are reported in approximately 70% of cases.[32]

SYNOVIAL SARCOMA

Synovial sarcoma is a malignant mesenchymal neoplasm with variable epithelial differentiation, with a propensity to occur in adolescents and young adults and that can arise at almost any site. Grossly the lesions are multinodular ranging from 1 to 15 cm in diameter. They can seem relatively well defined but can infiltrate irregularly into the surrounding soft tissues and may be adherent to an adjacent tendon or neurovascular bundle.[33] The cut surface may be solid, firm, and fleshy to smooth and glistening to tan, gritty, and calcified. Although calcification is common, it can be difficult to discern grossly. Occasionally, there is cyst formation, with often multiple smooth walled cysts, containing mucoid fluid or blood.[33]

Monophasic synovial sarcoma, spindle cell type, is the most common subtype of synovial sarcoma. It is composed of hypercellular arrays of relatively small spindle cells with uniform, ovoid, short, or elongated vesicular nuclei with evenly dispersed chromatin, inconspicuous nuclei, and very scanty amphophilic cytoplasm (**Fig. 6**). There is typically little intervening collagenous stroma, and a characteristic feature is the tightly packed nature of the cells with indistinct cell borders,

giving the appearance of nuclear overlapping. However, collagenous/hyalinized stroma that can sometimes be extensive, rarely with amianthoid fibers, has been described.[9,34]

Although morphologically, monophasic synovial sarcoma may resemble spindle cell/sclerosing RMS, the immunohistochemical and molecular findings will assist in its correct classification. By immunohistochemistry, the lesional cells of monophasic synovial sarcoma are positive for EMA, keratin, and TLE1, with recent evidence of positivity for SS18-SSX fusion-specific antibody as well as SSX antibody, with greater than 95% sensitivity and specificity of both of the latter stains. These lesional cells are negative or weakly/rarely positive for desmin, myogenin, and SMA.[35,36] Finally, the canonical t(X;18) (p11.2;q11.2) translocation is seen in more than 90% of these lesions, involving the SS18 (formerly SYT) gene on chromosome 18 and one of several synovial sarcoma X (*SSX*) genes on chromosome X (usually *SSX1* or *SSX2*).[36]

SUMMARY

Spindle cell/sclerosing RMS is a unifying histologic category for at least 3 biologically distinct subtypes of rhabdomyosarcoma, which each have age-dependent and prognostically significant genetic alterations. *MYOD1* mutations impart a poor prognosis, occur in patients older than 2 years and may have spindled or sclerosing morphology. *VGLL2* or *NCOA2* gene fusions have a good prognosis and occur almost exclusively in patients younger than 2 years. There is a subset of tumors that has no identifiable genetic alteration, which may represent spindle cell predominant embryonal RMS, but more study is needed.

CLINICS CARE POINTS

MYOD1 mutant RMS

- Head and neck/extremity—most common sites
- Most common in adolescents/young adults (range: 2–82 years)
- Spindle cell and/or sclerosing morphology
  - Differentiated rhabdomyoblasts are typically rare
- Weak to absent myogenin, but strong diffuse MYOD1 staining
- Poor outcome

VGLL2/NCOA2 fusion RMS

- Chest wall/paravertebral—most common site
- Almost exclusively occurs in those younger than 2 years
- Pure spindle morphology
  - Variable presence of differentiated rhabdomyoblasts
- Excellent outcome

Other

- Paratesticular and retroperitoneal—most common sites
- Wide age range
- Spindle cell morphology most common
- Excellent outcome
- May represent a spindle cell predominant pattern of embryonal RMS

DISCLOSURE

The authors have nothing to disclose.

REFERENCES

1. Ognjanovic S, Linabery AM, Charbonneau B, et al. Trends in childhood rhabdomyosarcoma incidence and survival in the United States, 1975-2005. Cancer 2009;115(18):4218–26.
2. Society AC. Key statistics for rhabdomyosarcoma. 2020. Available at: https://www.cancer.org/cancer/rhabdomyosarcoma/about/key-statistics.html#references. Accessed February 17th, 2020.
3. World Health Organization (WHO) Classification of Tumours Editorial Board. Soft Tissue and Bone Tumours. WHO Classification of tumours. Lyon International Agency for Research on Cancer. 5th edition, Vol. 3. 2020.
4. Leuschner I, Newton WA, Schmidt D, et al. Spindle cell variants of embryonal rhabdomyosarcoma in the paratesticular region. Am J Surg Pathol 1993; 17(3):221–30.
5. Folpe AL, McKenney JK, Bridge JA, et al. Sclerosing rhabdomyosarcoma in adults. Am J Surg Pathol 2002;26(9):1175–83.
6. Zambrano E, Pérez-Atayde AR, Ahrens W, et al. Pediatric sclerosing rhabdomyosarcoma. Int J Surg Pathol 2006;14(3):193–9.
7. Tsai JW, ChangChien YC, Lee JC, et al. The expanding morphological and genetic spectrum of MYOD1-mutant spindle cell/sclerosing rhabdomyosarcomas: a clinicopathological and molecular comparison of mutated and non-mutated cases. Histopathology 2019;74(6):933–43.
8. Nascimento AF, Fletcher CD. Spindle cell rhabdomyosarcoma in adults. Am J Surg Pathol 2005; 29(8):1106–13.
9. Cavazzana AO, Schmidt D, Ninfo V, et al. Spindle cell rhabdomyosarcoma. Am J Surg Pathol 1992; 16(3):229–35.
10. Sassoon D, Lyons G, Wright WE, et al. Expression of two myogenic regulatory factors myogenin and MyoDl during mouse embryogenesis. Nature 1989; 341(6240):303–7.
11. Kablar B, Asakura A, Krastel K, et al. MyoD and Myf-5 define the specification of musculature of distinct embryonic origin. Biochem Cell Biol 1998;76(6):1079–91.
12. Szuhai K, de Jong D, Leung WY, et al. Transactivating mutation of the MYOD1 gene is a frequent event in adult spindle cell rhabdomyosarcoma. J Pathol 2014;232(3):300–7.
13. Kohsaka S, Shukla N, Ameur N, et al. A recurrent neomorphic mutation in MYOD1 defines a clinically aggressive subset of embryonal rhabdomyosarcoma associated with PI3K-AKT pathway mutations. Nat Genet 2014;46(6):595–600.
14. Alaggio R, Zhang L, Sung YS, et al. A molecular study of pediatric spindle and sclerosing rhabdomyosarcoma: identification of novel and recurrent VGLL2-related fusions in infantile cases. Am J Surg Pathol 2016;40(2):224–35.
15. Agaram NP, LaQuaglia MP, Alaggio R, et al. MYOD1-mutant spindle cell and sclerosing rhabdomyosarcoma: an aggressive subtype irrespective of age. A reappraisal for molecular classification and risk stratification. Mod Pathol 2018;32(1):27–36.
16. Maeda T, Chapman DL, Stewart AFR. Mammalian vestigial-like 2, a cofactor of TEF-1 and MEF2 transcription factors that promotes skeletal muscle differentiation. J Biol Chem 2002; 277(50):48889–98.
17. Gunther S, Mielcarek M, Kruger M, et al. VITO-1 is an essential cofactor of TEF1-dependent muscle-specific gene regulation. Nucleic Acids Res 2004; 32(2):791–802.
18. Potthoff MJ, Arnold MA, McAnally J, et al. Regulation of skeletal muscle sarcomere integrity and postnatal muscle function by Mef2c. Mol Cell Biol 2007;27(23): 8143–51.

19. Yoshida T. MCAT elements and the TEF-1 family of transcription factors in muscle development and disease. Arterioscler Thromb Vasc Biol 2008;28(1):8–17.

20. Wang F, Marshall CB, Ikura M. Transcriptional/epigenetic regulator CBP/p300 in tumorigenesis: structural and functional versatility in target recognition. Cell Mol Life Sci 2013;70(21):3989–4008.

21. Qiu H, Wang F, Liu C, et al. TEAD1-dependent expression of the FoxO3a gene in mouse skeletal muscle. BMC Mol Biol 2011;12(1):1.

22. Pipes GC, Creemers EE, Olson EN. The myocardin family of transcriptional coactivators: versatile regulators of cell growth, migration, and myogenesis. Genes Dev 2006;20(12):1545–56.

23. Watson S, Perrin V, Guillemot D, et al. Transcriptomic definition of molecular subgroups of small round cell sarcomas. J Pathol 2018;245(1):29–40.

24. Dashti NK, Wehrs RN, Thomas BC, et al. Spindle cell rhabdomyosarcoma of bone with FUS-TFCP2 fusion: confirmation of a very recently described rhabdomyosarcoma subtype. Histopathology 2018;73(3):514–20.

25. Le Loarer F, Cleven AHG, Bouvier C, et al. A subset of epithelioid and spindle cell rhabdomyosarcomas is associated with TFCP2 fusions and common ALK upregulation. Mod Pathol 2020;33(3):404–19.

26. Newton WA Jr, Soule EH, Hamoudi AB, et al. Histopathology of childhood sarcomas, Intergroup Rhabdomyosarcoma Studies I and II: clinicopathologic correlation. J Clin Oncol 1988;6(1):67–75.

27. Mentzel T, Kuhnen C. Spindle cell rhabdomyosarcoma in adults: clinicopathological and immunohistochemical analysis of seven new cases. Virchows Arch 2006;449(5):554–60.

28. Rudzinski ER, Teot LA, Anderson JR, et al. Dense pattern of embryonal rhabdomyosarcoma, a lesion easily confused with alveolar rhabdomyosarcoma: a report from the soft tissue sarcoma committee of the children's oncology group. Am J Clin Pathol 2013;140(1):82–90.

29. Blocker S, Koenig J, Ternberg J. Congenital fibrosarcoma. J Pediatr Surg 1987;22(7):665–70.

30. Coffin CM, Jaszcz W, O'Shea PA, et al. So-called congenital-infantile fibrosarcoma: does it exist and what is it? Pediatr Pathol 1994;14(1):133–50.

31. Loh ML, Ahn P, Perez-Atayde AR, et al. Treatment of infantile fibrosarcoma with chemotherapy and surgery: results from the Dana-Farber cancer institute and children's hospital, Boston. J Pediatr 2002;24(9):722–6.

32. Knezevich SR, McFadden DE, Tao W, et al. A novel ETV6-NTRK3 gene fusion in congenital fibrosarcoma. Nat Genet 1998;18(2):184–7.

33. Fisher C. Synovial sarcoma. Ann Diagn Pathol 1998;2(6):401–21.

34. Orenstein JM. Amianthoid fibers in a synovial sarcoma and a malignant schwannoma. Ultrastruct Pathol 1983;4(2–3):163–76.

35. Pelmus M, Guillou L, Hostein I, et al. Monophasic fibrous and poorly differentiated synovial sarcoma. Am J Surg Pathol 2002;26(11):1434–40.

36. Baranov E, McBride MJ, Bellizzi AM, et al. A Novel SS18-SSX fusion-specific antibody for the diagnosis of synovial sarcoma. Am J Surg Pathol 2020;44(7):922–33.

Pediatric and Infantile Fibroblastic/ Myofibroblastic Tumors in the Molecular Era

Jessica L. Davis, MD[a],*, Erin R. Rudzinski, MD[b]

KEYWORDS

- Fibroblastic • Myofibroblastic • Nodular fasciitis • Myofibroma • Fibromatosis
- Infantile fibrosarcoma • Receptor tyrosine kinases

Key points

- Fibroblastic/myofibroblastic tumors in the pediatric population can be diagnostically challenging; however, morphology can be extremely helpful to guide testing.
- Most of these tumors have molecular drivers, many are alterations in receptor tyrosine kinase pathways.
- Knowing which ancillary tests are available to confirm diagnoses and/or for prognosis or predictive testing can help guide clinical management.

ABSTRACT

Pediatric fibroblastic/myofibroblastic tumors are rare but include a wide variety of benign to malignant tumors. Given their uncommon frequency, they may present as a diagnostic dilemma. This article is focused on using clinical and pathologic clues in conjunction with the increasingly relevant and available molecular techniques to classify, predict prognosis, and/or guide treatment in these tumors.

kinases. In the age of molecular pathology and targeted therapies, knowing which ancillary tests are available is often key to support diagnosis, predict prognosis, and/or guide therapy.

OVERVIEW

Fibroblastic/myofibroblastic tumors in the pediatric population include a range of benign, intermediate risk, and frankly malignant tumors that can be diagnostically challenging; however, morphology is the first step in diagnosis and can be extremely helpful to guide complementary testing. An increasing number of tumors in this category have recurrent molecular drivers, many of which are alterations in receptor tyrosine

Pediatric Myofibroblastic Tumors

Nodular/cranial fasciitis

Classic myofibroma/myofibromatosis

Cellular myofibroma

Fibrous hamartoma of infancy

Calcifying aponeurotic fibroma

Lipofibromatosis

Inclusion body fibromatosis

Gardner fibroma/desmoid fibromatosis

Inflammatory myofibroblastic tumor

Infantile fibrosarcoma

Other receptor tyrosine kinase fused spindle cell tumors

a Department of Pathology, Oregon Health & Science University, L-471, Portland, OR 97239, USA;
b Department of Laboratories, Seattle Children's Hospital, OC.8.720, Seattle, WA 98105, USA
* Corresponding author.
E-mail address: davisjes@ohsu.edu

Surgical Pathology 13 (2020) 739–762
https://doi.org/10.1016/j.path.2020.08.009
1875-9181/20/© 2020 Elsevier Inc. All rights reserved.

surgpath.theclinics.com

NODULAR FASCIITIS/CRANIAL FASCIITIS

OVERVIEW

Nodular fasciitis is considered an example of "transient" neoplasia. As such, it can demonstrate many worrisome features, including rapid growth. Nodular fasciitis most commonly involves the upper extremities and head and neck; however, it can occur in a wide range of sites. Cranial fasciitis is a distinct subtype of nodular fasciitis typically affecting young children (younger than 2 years), which may extend into the underlying skull.[1] Regardless of site, most cases are centered within the subcutaneous tissue and superficial fascia; rare cases involve deeper tissues, intraarticular, or intravascular locations.[2–4] One-quarter of cases of nodular fasciitis affect children. There is no sex predilection for nodular or intravascular fasciitis; however, cranial fasciitis occurs more frequently in boys.[1,2]

GROSS FEATURES

Nodular fasciitis is well-circumscribed with a myxoid to fibrous cut surface. Size typically are ≤2 cm and nearly always ≤5 cm.

MICROSCOPIC FEATURES

Nodular fasciitis is composed of loose fascicles of bland myofibroblasts that often have a "tissue-culture" appearance and are arranged in broad, intersecting fascicles (Fig. 1A). Early lesions have abundant myxoid stroma and may have microcyst formation (Fig. 1B). Cellularity may be high and mitotic figures numerous. Extravasated red blood cells are common, as are osteoclast-type giant cells (see Fig. 1B). There are varying degrees of admixed inflammation. Older lesions have increasing collagenous stroma, sometimes with keloidal-type collagen. Nodular fasciitis is usually positive for smooth muscle actin in a myofibroblastic (tram-track) pattern.

MOLECULAR FEATURES

Nodular and cranial fasciitis (as well as the related entities of aneurysmal bone cyst, fasciitis-like fibroma of tendon sheath, myositis ossificans, and others) are characterized by *USP6* gene rearrangements. Fluorescence in situ hybridization (FISH) for USP6 rearrangements is an easily accessible confirmatory test, but the test is subject to false negative results and only has an approximately 70% detection rate.[5,6] RNA sequencing platforms may also be used to confirm the diagnosis, if needed.[7,8]

DIAGNOSIS AND DIFFERENTIAL DIAGNOSIS

The differential diagnosis includes benign fibrous histiocytoma, myofibroma, and desmoid fibromatosis. Fibrous histiocytomas are dermal-based lesions, rather than involving the fascial planes. These lesions are rarely myxoid, and lack microcystic change. Myofibroma, classically, is biphasic with peripheral collagenized/chondroid regions. A hemangiopericytomatous vasculature is often present in myofibroma, in contrast to the delicate vessels and extravasated red blood cells typical of nodular fasciitis. Older lesions of nodular fasciitis may mimic desmoid fibromatosis, and both lesions may have extravasated red blood cells; however, desmoid tumors are characterized by long fascicles of spindled cells with curvilinear vascular pattern. Nuclear staining for beta-catenin is positive in most desmoid tumors and not seen in nodular fasciitis.[9]

PROGNOSIS

Simple excision is adequate therapy, and tumors often spontaneously regress. Recurrence of nodular fasciitis is rare.

 Key Features

Loose, intersecting fascicles of plump myofibroblasts (see Fig. 1A)

Myxoid stroma with microcysts, extravasated red blood cells (see Fig. 1B)

Older lesions may be collagenous (keloidal)

 Pitfalls

! "Pseudosarcomatous" with high mitotic rate and increased cellularity in early lesions

! May invade into adjacent normal structures (cranial fasciitis with skull invasion)

CLASSIC MYOFIBROMA/MYOFIBROMATOSIS

OVERVIEW

Myofibroma (classic) is a benign myofibroblastic and/or pericytic tumor which typically presents in

Fig. 1. Nodular fasciitis is a well-circumscribed lesion composed of zonally arranged, loose fascicles of spindled cells (*A*) (original magnification ×20). There is frequent myxoid stroma with microcystic degeneration and scattered extravasated red blood cells (*B*) (original magnification ×100).

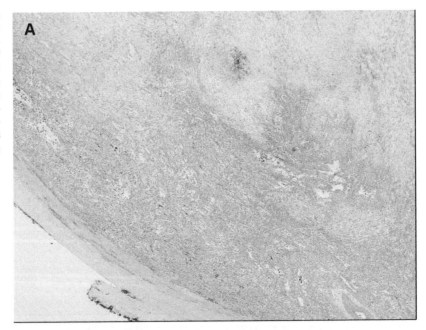

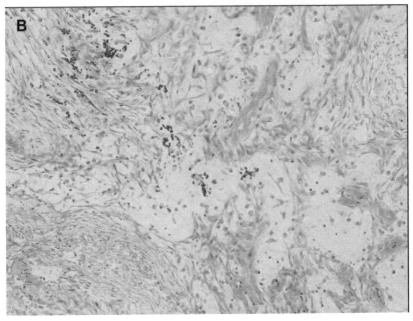

early childhood (most <2 years); approximately 30% are congenital.[10] In the infantile population, nearly one-fourth of cases are multifocal (myofibromatosis), whereas the adult type is typically solitary.[10,11] There is a close relationship between myofibroma and myopericytoma, which represent slight morphologic variations of the same entity. There is a male sex predilection (2:1). Extremities and the head and neck region are most commonly involved; other sites of involvement include the trunk, and rarely bone. In multifocal disease, visceral involvement may be present.[11]

GROSS FEATURES

Grossly, myofibromas are well-circumscribed lesions with a fibrous cut surface. Superficial nodules are usually ≤2 cm, although some deep lesions may be large. Necrosis and calcification may be present in large tumors.

MICROSCOPIC FEATURES

Myofibromas are nodular, relatively well-circumscribed masses with a characteristic biphasic appearance. The center of the mass is

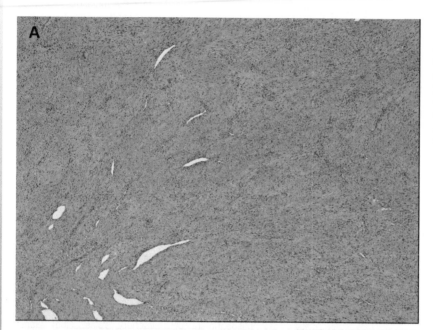

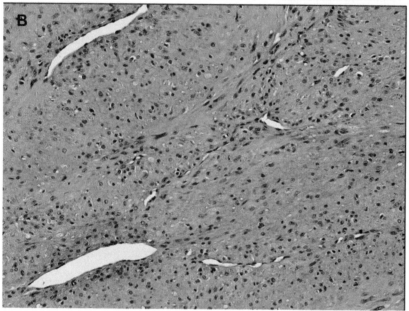

Fig. 2. (A) Classic myofibroma shows dilated, hemangiopericytic blood vessels centrally, with more myxoid change peripherally. (B) A pseudochondroid matrix is common, with tumor cells pushing into dilated vascular spaces.

highly cellular, composed of immature, plump, spindle cells with admixed hemangiopericytoma (HPC)-like vessels (**Fig. 2**A, B), whereas the periphery of the nodule demonstrates variably myoid-appearing spindle cells with more eosinophilic cytoplasm, hyalinization, and often a chondromyxoid stroma (see **Fig. 2**A, B). This pattern of zonation may be reversed in older children or adults, and these masses may occasionally be calcified.[12] Central necrosis and frequent mitoses may be present, without prognostic significance.

There is often a protrusion or outpouching of cells into large vascular spaces, a finding that may be confused for vascular invasion (see **Fig. 2**B). By immunohistochemistry, classic myofibroma(tosis) expresses diffuse smooth muscle actin (SMA), without concurrent desmin expression.[12]

MOLECULAR FEATURES

Genetically, myofibroma(tosis) contains a variety of activating *PDGFRB* mutations including point mutations, insertions and deletions.[13,14] These changes are best detected by DNA-based sequencing assays that can detect both point mutations as well as larger structural alterations, but they will be missed by most FISH or RNA-based techniques.

DIAGNOSIS AND DIFFERENTIAL DIAGNOSIS

A diagnosis of myofibroma is usually straightforward, but the differential diagnosis can include nodular fasciitis, leiomyoma, desmoid fibromatosis, or infantile fibrosarcoma (IFS). Nodular fasciitis is generally less well circumscribed and has a looser arrangement of cells with a myxoid background, extravasated red blood cells, inflammation and osteoclast-type giant cells. Leiomyomas are rare in the pediatric population. This differential could be considered if a sample lacks zonation and is diffusely myoid; however, leiomyomas should express diffuse desmin. Desmoid fibromatosis contains long fascicles of spindled cells, without the zonation seen in myofibroma. Additionally, desmoid fibromatosis shows nuclear staining for beta-catenin. IFS may have hemangiopericytic vasculature, but usually has a high mitotic rate and lacks the zonal appearance of myofibroma.[15] In some circumstances, genetic testing may be useful for diagnostic confirmation.

PROGNOSIS

Myofibromas are benign lesions, and one-third of pediatric cases spontaneously regress; however, multifocal disease with visceral involvement is associated with poor prognosis and can be lethal.[10] Given the presence of activating *PDGFRB* mutations, patients with visceral involvement, a large tumor burden, or tumor involvement of critical structures may be treated with PDGFRB inhibitors.

Key features

Biphasic neoplasm

Central cellular regions, often with hemangiopericytic vascular pattern (see **Fig. 2**A, B)

Peripheral myoid nodules often have chondroid/hyalinized stroma (see **Fig. 2**A, B)

Tumor nodules may protrude into large vessels

Strong, diffuse SMA staining

Pitfall

! Children with multiple lesions should be screened for visceral involvement

CELLULAR MYOFIBROMA

OVERVIEW

Cellular/atypical myofibroma typically occurs in adolescents and adults (median age 14 years). It may arise in a broad range of anatomic sites including the trunk, extremities, head and neck, or viscera. There is a slight female predominance in the few published cases.[16,17]

GROSS FEATURES

Cellular myofibroma may be well-circumscribed, but more often has a multinodular or infiltrative growth pattern. Tumor size ranges from 2 to 7 cm, with an average of 4 cm in greatest dimension.

MICROSCOPIC FEATURES

Two morphologic patterns are described in cellular myofibroma. The first consists of oval to round cells in a syncytial or nested pattern around a rich capillary network (**Fig. 3**A, B). The second demonstrates monomorphic spindle cells in intersecting fascicles. As with classic myofibroma, there is often a protrusion or outpouching of cells into large vascular spaces (see **Fig. 3**A). Masses may show one or both patterns. Mitotic activity is usually low, but may be brisk with a few cases showing more than 10 mitoses per 10 high power fields. Tumor necrosis is not described, but calcification may be present. By immunohistochemistry, these tumors can coexpress SMA and desmin (**Fig. 3**C), which can be a pitfall in misdiagnosis of a smooth muscle tumor.[17]

MOLECULAR FEATURES

The tumors harbor *SRF*-gene fusions, most commonly *SRF-RELA*. Rare cellular myoid tumors have been described with *SRF-ICA1L* gene fusion with a similar morphology, which express SMA and calponin, but lack desmin and caldesmon expression.[18] FISH studies using probes to *SRF* are available, or RNA sequencing can be used to confirm the diagnosis, if necessary. Care should

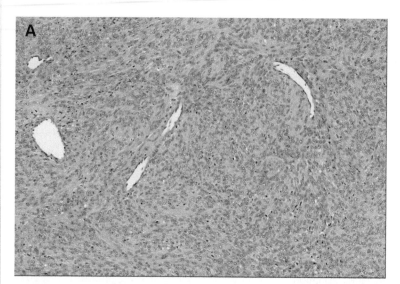

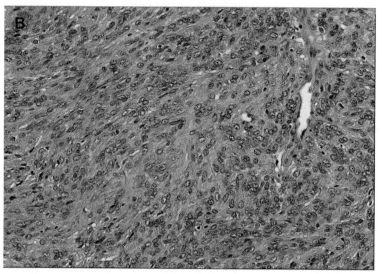

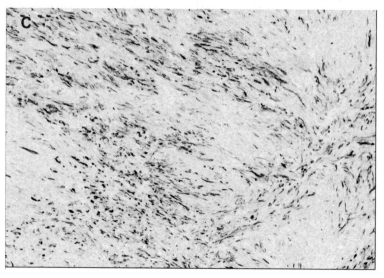

Fig. 3. (*A*) Cellular myofibroma is characterized by sheets of spindled cells, with the same hemangiopericytomatous vascular pattern as classic myofibroma. (*B*) Cellular myofibroma may have groups of round to ovoid cells. (*C*) Desmin expression may present diagnostic confusion with myogenic tumors.

be taken to note which gene partner is on an RNA panel to ensure that *SRF* variant gene fusions can be detected.

PROGNOSIS

Despite the atypical features in cellular myofibroma, including mitotic activity and diffuse hypercellularity, most cases reported to date have a benign course with rare local recurrences.[16,17] A single patient with *SRF-ICA1L* fusion has been reported to develop metastatic disease.[18]

Key features

Hypercellular tumor with intersecting fascicles of myoid cells or nested groups of ovoid cells resembling myopericytoma (see Fig. 3A, B)

Low risk of local recurrence

Rare cases of metastatic disease described

Pitfalls

! Desmin expression may cause diagnostic confusion with myogenic tumors (see Fig. 3C)

! Atypical features including high cellularity and mitotic activity may prompt concern for a sarcoma (see Fig. 3A, B)

FIBROUS HAMARTOMA OF INFANCY

OVERVIEW

As the name suggests, fibrous hamartoma of infancy (FHI) is a tumor of young children; typically presenting at ≤2 years of age.[19–21] Tumors typically arise in the axilla, shoulder, or upper arm, although the groin and thigh region may also be affected. FHI involves the superficial subcutaneous tissues and dermis.[19–21]

GROSS FEATURES

FHI is a poorly circumscribed lesion that may appear mostly fatty, with variable amounts of fibrous tissue, including less commonly mostly fibrous. Tumors may be large, but average 3 cm.

MICROSCOPIC FEATURES

FHI is composed of 3 discrete components, including mature adipose tissue, mature myofibroblastic proliferation with spindled cells arranged in collagenous stroma, and nodules of primitive round to stellate cells in a myxoid background, in various proportions (Fig. 4A, B). In older lesions, the myofibroblastic component often becomes pseudoangiomatous (Fig. 4C).[20,21]

MOLECULAR FEATURES

FHI is characterized by *EGFR* exon 20 insertion/duplication mutations.[22] Although molecular confirmation is rarely needed, these mutations can be detected with a variety of DNA sequencing approaches.

DIAGNOSIS AND DIFFERENTIAL DIAGNOSIS

The differential diagnosis includes lipofibromatosis, occasionally more newly described entities with receptor tyrosine kinase fusions (eg, *NTRK*-rearranged spindle cell tumors), and/or giant cell fibroblastoma depending on classic or alternative histologic pattern. Lipofibromatosis may be distinguished from FHI based on site of involvement (typically the hand or foot in lipofibromatosis vs the limb-girdles or proximal limbs in FHI) and the lack of a primitive, myxoid component in lipofibromatosis. In some cases, *NTRK*-rearranged/spindle cell mesenchymal tumors may mimic FHI. These tumors can be distinguished based on their frequent coexpression of CD34 and S100, as well as the lack of the distinctive triphasic configuration.

PROGNOSIS

FHI is a benign tumor that has no metastatic potential. It may locally recur if incompletely excised.

Key features

Triphasic tumor with (1) mature myofibroblastic proliferation of spindled cells in a collagenous background, (2) nodules of primitive cells in a myxoid stroma, and (3) mature adipose tissue (see Fig. 4A, B)

Older lesions may acquire a pseudoangiomatous appearance (see Fig. 4C)

Typically involves the limb girdle regions (axilla, shoulder, upper arm, groin, thigh)

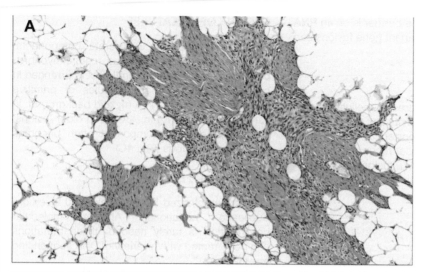
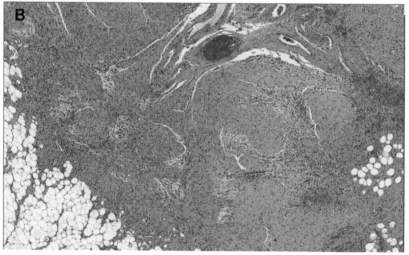
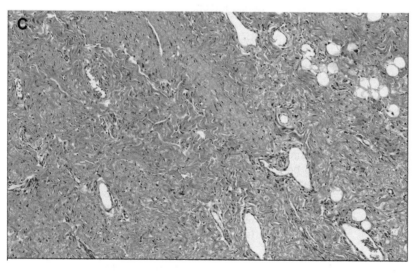

Fig. 4. FHI is a triphasic tumor composed of mature adipose tissue admixed with spindled, fibroblastic cells as well as islands of primitive mesenchymal cells (*A*) (original magnification ×100). FHI may be variably cellular and some tumors may be dominated by the spindle cell component (*B*) (original magnification ×50). Older lesions may become less cellular and acquire a pseudoangiomatous appearance (*C*) (original magnification ×100).

Pitfalls

! When primitive mesenchyme not prominent may overlap with lipofibromatosis

! When pseudoangiomatous pattern predominates may overlap with giant cell fibroblastoma (see Fig. 4C)

CALCIFYING APONEUROTIC FIBROMA

OVERVIEW

The peak incidence of calcifying aponeurotic fibroma is the second decade, although it can occur over a wide age range. Most cases arise in the hands and feet. The lesions are deeply seated adjacent to fascia or tendons.[23,24]

GROSS FEATURES

Calcifying aponeurotic fibroma is a poorly circumscribed lesion, often with a gritty cut surface corresponding to the degree of calcification. Most cases measure 1 to 3 cm.

MICROSCOPIC FEATURES

Calcifying aponeurotic fibroma is composed of sheets of myofibroblastic cells in a collagenous background with admixed, coarse calcification (Fig. 5A). The calcified regions are often associated with rounded, chondrocytelike cells (Fig. 5B). Occasional osteoclast-type giant cells may be seen. In young children, cases may be more cellular, with long fascicles of myofibroblasts (see Fig. 5A).[23,24]

MOLECULAR FEATURES

Calcifying aponeurotic fibroma is associated with *FN1:EGF* fusions.[25] These fusions can be detected with FISH or RNA sequencing platforms.

DIAGNOSIS AND DIFFERENTIAL DIAGNOSIS

The differential diagnosis includes lipofibromatosis, myofibroma, and desmoid fibromatosis. Lipofibromatosis is characterized by spindled cells that infiltrate into adipose tissue. These lesions lack calcification or a chondroid appearance; however, some studies of lipofibromatosis have shown recurrent *FN1:EGF* fusions.[26] Some cases of lipofibromatosis have also been reported to have recurred with the morphologic appearance of calcifying aponeurotic fibroma, raising the possibility that early lesions of calcifying aponeurotic fibroma may have a lipofibromastosis-like morphologic pattern. The relationship between these 2 entities is unclear and this remains an evolving topic. Myofibromas may be calcified, but they lack the rounded chondrocytes of calcifying aponeurotic fibroma. In addition, diffuse SMA staining supports a diagnosis of myofibroma. Desmoid fibromatosis lacks calcifications and chondroid foci; nuclear beta-catenin staining supports a diagnosis of desmoid tumor.

PROGNOSIS

Calcifying aponeurotic fibroma recurs locally in approximately one-half of cases, sometimes repeatedly. There is no risk of metastasis.

Key features

Sheets of bland, spindled cells with coarse calcification (see Fig. 5A)

Chondroid foci with rounded chondrocytes (see Fig. 5B)

Usually involves the hands and feet

High rate of local recurrence

Pitfall

! Early lesions may resemble lipofibromatosis

LIPOFIBROMATOSIS

OVERVIEW

Lipofibromatosis is a rare pediatric soft tissue tumor of early childhood with half of cases occurring by age 1 year, and 20% present congenitally. The median age of diagnosis is 3 years. There is a 2:1 male predominance. Cases occur almost exclusively in the hands and feet.[26,27]

GROSS FEATURES

Lipofibromatosis is a poorly circumscribed mass composed of variable amounts of adipose tissue

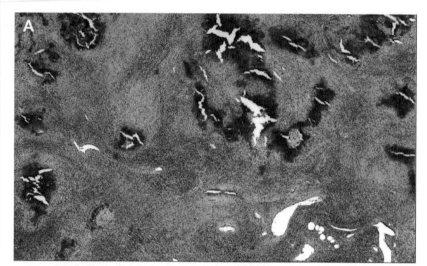

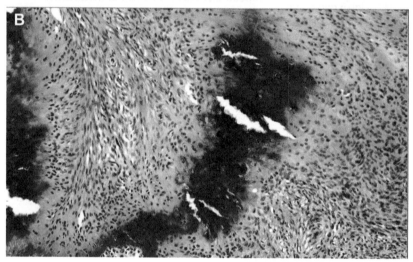

Fig. 5. Calcifying aponeurotic tumor is composed of short fascicles of spindled cells with patchy calcification (*A*) (original magnification ×20). Cells associated with the calcifications may become chondroid with round nuclei and increased stroma (*B*) (original magnification ×100).

and fibrous tissue. Most tumor are small, ranging from 1 to 7 cm.

MICROSCOPIC FEATURES

Lipofibromatosis is composed of mature adipocytes admixed with long fascicles of bland spindle cells (fibroblastic cells) (**Fig. 6**A). Fat typically comprises most of the mass. Collections of univacuolated cells mimicking lipoblasts may be present adjacent to the fibroblastic component (**Fig. 6**B).[26,27] The tumor is infiltrative and may entrap adjacent skeletal muscle. By immunohistochemistry, lipofibromatosis has variable expression of SMA and CD34.

MOLECULAR FEATURES

Gene fusions involving a variety of epidermal growth factor (EGF) receptor ligands (*EGF,*

HBEGF, TGFA) and receptor tyrosine kinases (*EGFR, PDGFRB, RET,* and *ROS1*) have been described.[26] The only recurrent fusion to date has been *FN1-EGF*, which is also commonly present in calcifying aponeurotic fibromas.[26] Given the breadth of fusion partners involved, RNA sequencing platforms that allow a wide variety of genes to be analyzed with a partner agnostic approach are recommended for any additional molecular profiling.

DIAGNOSIS AND DIFFERENTIAL DIAGNOSIS

The differential diagnosis includes desmoid fibromatosis, palmar/plantar fibromatosis, calcifying aponeurotic fibroma and FHI. Superficial palmar/plantar fibromatosis and calcifying aponeurotic fibroma are both common to the hands and feet. As mentioned previously, some cases of lipofibromatosis have recurred with the appearance of

Fig. 6. (*A*) Lipofibromatosis consists of predominantly mature adipose tissue with fibrous septae expanded by a proliferation of bland ovoid to spindled cells. (*B*) Microfat, simulating lipoblasts, may be seen at the edges of these fibrous septae.

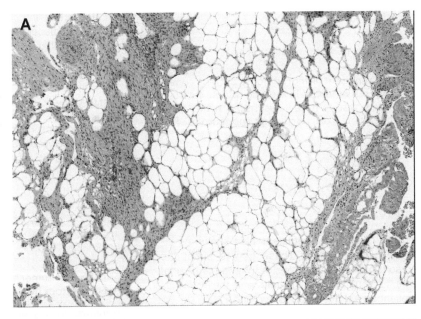

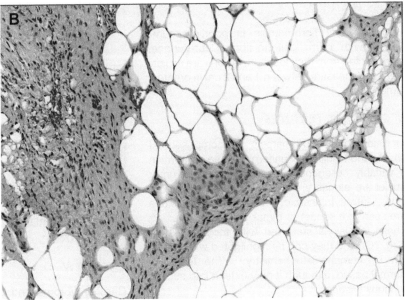

calcifying aponeurotic fibroma, suggesting that lipofibromatosis may simply represent recurrent morphologic pattern in these infiltrative tumors of the extremities rather than a common diagnosis.[26] Superficial and desmoid fibromatoses are characterized by sweeping fascicles of spindled cells and are usually more cellular than lipofibromatosis, without the prominent adipocytic component. FHI does not typically involve the hands and feet, and it demonstrates nodules of primitive cells in a myxoid matrix which are lacking in lipofibromatosis.

PROGNOSIS

Lipofibromatosis has a high risk of local recurrence (70%) but no metastatic potential.

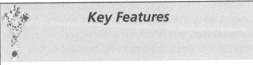

Key Features

Disorganized fascicles of spindled cells infiltrating through mature adipose tissue (see Fig. 6A, B)

INCLUSION BODY FIBROMATOSIS

OVERVIEW

Inclusion body fibromatosis is also known as infantile digital fibroma. These tumors affect the dorsum of fingers and toes in infants (<1 year of age). Lesions may be multiple, and they typically present as a dome-shaped swelling.[28,29]

GROSS FEATURES

Inclusion body fibromatosis is poorly circumscribed with a firm, uniform fibrous cut surface. As expected from their location, lesions are usually small and measure between 1 and 2 cm in greatest dimension.

MICROSCOPIC FEATURES

Inclusion body fibromatosis is composed of sheets and fascicles of uniform spindle cells within a variably collagenous stroma (**Fig. 7**A). Tumor nuclei are elongate, with fine chromatin. Perinuclear, intracytoplasmic, eosinophilic inclusions are seen in a subset of tumor cells (**Fig. 7**B).[28–30] These inclusions stain red with trichrome stain (**Fig. 7**C), and they can be highlighted with calponin by immunohistochemistry.[30] The lesion is dermal based, although it may extend into subcutaneous tissues.

MOLECULAR FEATURES

No recurrent molecular alterations have been described in inclusion body fibromatosis to date.

DIAGNOSIS AND DIFFERENTIAL DIAGNOSIS

The differential diagnosis includes other fibromatoses arising in the hands and feet. Palmar/plantar fibromatoses are relatively rare in young children, arise in the deep aponeurotic tissues rather than within the dermis, and lack inclusion bodies. Desmoid fibromatosis is similarly a tumor of deep tissues rather than the dermis, and it is composed of long fascicles of spindle cells with nuclear

beta-catenin staining. Calcifying aponeurotic fibroma arises adjacent to deep tendons or aponeuroses and is characterized by calcification and chondroid foci rather than intracytoplasmic inclusions.

PROGNOSIS

Inclusion body fibromatosis has a high rate of local recurrence, between 50% and 75%, and may multiply recur. It does not have metastatic potential.

GARDNER FIBROMA/DESMOID FIBROMATOSIS

OVERVIEW

Gardner fibroma and desmoid fibromatosis are related entities that may present as a manifestation of familial adenomatous polyposis.[31,32] Gardner fibroma most often presents in children, with 80% of cases occurring in the first decade.[31] In contrast, desmoid fibromatosis presents most often is adults, but desmoids are also a relatively common myofibroblastic tumor in children and rare cases may be congenital. There is no sex predilection.[33] Gardner fibroma typically involves the back and paraspinal soft tissue, followed by the chest wall, abdomen, head and neck, and extremities. The latter sites are also typical of desmoid fibromatosis. Desmoid fibromatoses are deep-seated tumors that occur along fascial planes, between muscle bundle, or within the abdomen. A

Fig. 7. Inclusion body fibromatosis is located beneath acral skin of the digits (*A*) (original magnification ×20). The tumor is composed of plump, spindled cells separated by collagenous stroma (*B*) (original magnification ×400). Eosinophilic inclusions may be seen on hematoxylin-eosin stain (*arrows*, *B*), but are more easily highlighted as fuschinophilic on trichrome stain (*C*) (original magnification ×400).

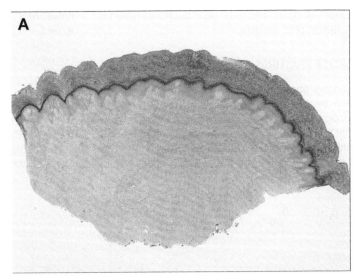

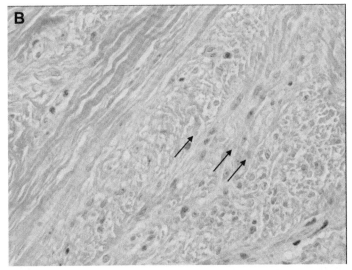

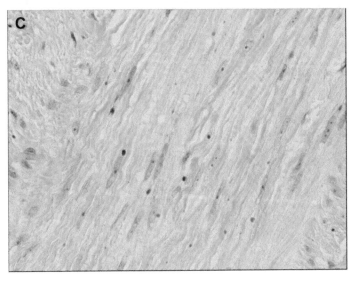

subset of desmoids may be induced by trauma, including prior surgery.[33]

GROSS FEATURES

Gardner fibromas are poorly demarcated lesions, with thickened fibrous plaques that may not be recognizable as a discrete mass. Desmoid fibromatoses appear deceptively well-circumscribed, with a firm, whorled, fibrous cut surface. The size range is widely variable, with most lesions measuring between 3 and 10 cm in greatest extent.

MICROSCOPIC FEATURES

Gardner fibromas are characterized by thickened, sclerotic collagen with intralesional "cracks" (**Fig. 8**A, B). This process may entrap adjacent normal structures, such as muscle and nerves. Gardner fibroma is positive for CD34 and negative

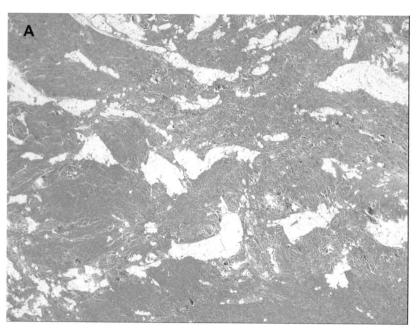

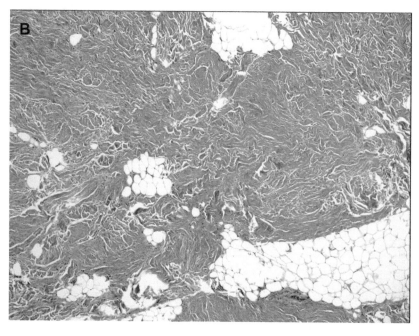

Fig. 8. Gardner fibroma demonstrates plaquelike, dense collagen that often entraps native nerves and vessels (*A*) (original magnification ×40). The tumor is notably hypocellular and the collagen often gives a "cracked-earth" appearance (*B*) (original magnification ×100). (*Courtesy* of Michael A. Arnold, MD, PhD, Aurora, CO.)

for SMA. Nuclei may be positive for beta-catenin.[31]

Desmoid fibromatosis is composed of long fascicles of spindled cells, often infiltrative into fibroadipose tissue or skeletal muscle (**Fig. 9A, B**). The tumor cells are bland, with uniform, ovoid nuclei having fine chromatin and inconspicuous nucleoli (see **Fig. 9B**). Thin-walled, "curvilinear" blood vessels are often present with mild perivascular edema (see **Fig. 9B**). Extravasated red blood cells and keloidal collagen may be present. Occasional tumors, particularly those in young children or arising in the mesentery, may have a myxoid stroma.[33] By immunohistochemistry, desmoid tumors show patchy SMA expression with at least scattered cells demonstrating nuclear staining for beta-catenin (~80% of cases).[34,35]

MOLECULAR FEATURES

Desmoid fibromatosis harbors mutations in the *CTNNB1* or less frequently the *APC* gene, whereas 70% of Gardner fibromas are associated with germline *APC* mutations. When associated with *APC* mutations, appropriate screening for colonic polyps should be perused as clinically appropriate.[31–35] Both *CTNNB1* and *APC* mutations may be detected by DNA sequencing.

DIAGNOSIS AND DIFFERENTIAL DIAGNOSIS

The differential diagnosis includes hypertrophic scar and nodular fasciitis. Scar tissue may be suggested by the presence of fat necrosis, hemosiderin, or other signs of prior trauma. Scar tissue lacks nuclear beta-catenin staining, although it may have patchy expression of other markers of Wnt pathway activation, such as Lef1. Nodular fasciitis has a more typically myxoid stroma with microcysts, intersecting broad fascicles of spindled cells, and lacks prominent thin-walled perifascicular blood vessels.

PROGNOSIS

Gardner fibroma may recur as desmoid fibromatosis. Desmoid tumors have a high rate of local recurrence, and systemic therapies are often used as a therapeutic adjunct to control tumor growth. Treatment options include watchful waiting, with attempts at resection based on symptoms and the ability to achieve wide margins. Chemotherapeutic regimens have included cyclooxygenase 2 inhibitors, and more recent studies suggest sorafenib may be useful in medically refractory cases. Other clinical trials including agents that target the beta-catenin pathway are being investigated.[36]

Gardner fibroma

Key Features

Hypocellular spindle cell lesion with sclerotic, "cracked" collagen (see Fig. 8A, B)

70% associated with germline *APC* mutations

Pitfall

!May recur as desmoid fibromatosis

Desmoid fibromatosis

Key Features

Long infiltrative fascicles of bland spindle cells (see Fig. 9A)

Curvilinear vessels with perivascular edema (see Fig. 9B)

May have extravasated red blood cells

Myxoid stroma present in rare cases, often in young children or at mesenteric sites

Pitfalls

! Myxoid cases may mimic nodular fasciitis

! May be difficult to distinguish from scar

! Nuclear beta-catenin staining may be weak/focal

INFLAMMATORY MYOFIBROBLASTIC TUMOR

OVERVIEW

Inflammatory myofibroblastic tumor is a fibroblastic/myofibroblastic tumor of low-malignant potential. It most commonly occurs in children and young adults, with a slight female predominance. Tumors can occur throughout the body; however, classic sites include intra-abdominal, retroperitoneal, lung, bladder, and uterus.[37–39] The clinical presentation varies depending on site involved, but approximately one-third of patients can have "B-symptoms" including fever, weight loss, fatigue, and laboratory abnormalities, including anemia, thrombocytosis, and elevated erythrocyte sedimentation rate/C-reactive protein.[37–40]

GROSS FEATURES

Inflammatory myofibroblastic tumor is often circumscribed, with a variably fibrous to myxoid cut surface. Tumors may range from 1 to 20 cm, with an average size of 6 cm.

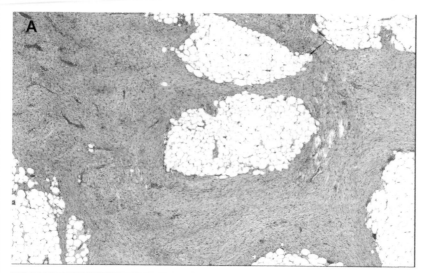

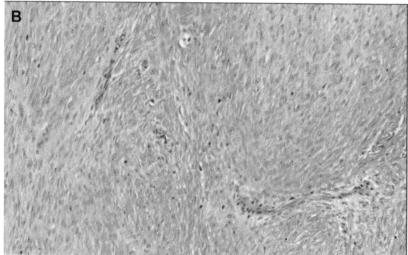

Fig. 9. Desmoid fibromatosis is composed of long fascicles of bland spindled cells; here shown infiltrating into mature adipose tissue (*A*) (original magnification ×40). Curvilinear vessels with mild perivascular edema are helpful diagnostic clues (*B*) (original magnification ×1000); these can become ectatic in area of increased collagen.

MICROSCOPIC FEATURES

Inflammatory myofibroblastic tumor may show a range of morphologic patterns. Most commonly, tumors are characterized by plump spindle cells in a myxoid to collagenized background with a dense inflammation including plasma cells, lymphocytes, and eosinophils (Fig. 10A, B). Other areas may show a more compact hypercellular spindle cell population arranged in fascicles (Fig. 10A). Less often, tumors are hyalinized (sclerotic) with a hypocellular spindle cell population and sparse inflammation. The epithelioid variant of inflammatory myofibroblastic tumor epithelioid inflammatory myofibroblastic sarcoma occurs almost exclusively intra-abdominally and is associated with a more aggressive biologic behavior.[38]

By immunohistochemistry, inflammatory myofibroblastic tumors consistently express SMA; those with anaplastic lymphoma kinase (ALK)-rearrangements will show ALK expression.

MOLECULAR FEATURES

Inflammatory myofibroblastic tumors in children and young adults are largely driven by receptor tyrosine kinase fusions, most commonly *ALK* gene fusions that are present in approximately 60% of cases. *ALK* may be fused to a variety of gene partners, and in some cases the partner may predict overall behavior (eg, *ALK-RANBP2* is associated with epithelioid morphology and an aggressive behavior). Other less frequent receptor tyrosine kinase fusions identified in inflammatory myofibroblastic tumor include *ROS1, RET,* or *PDGFRB. ALK* or other tyrosine kinase gene rearrangements are infrequent in inflammatory myofibroblastic tumors occurring in adults older than

40.[40,41] FISH for *ALK* rearrangements may be considered as a diagnostic adjunct. For cases lacking evidence of an *ALK* rearrangement by immunohistochemistry or FISH, a larger RNA sequencing panel may be useful.

DIAGNOSIS AND DIFFERENTIAL DIAGNOSIS

The differential diagnosis of inflammatory myofibroblastic tumor can be quite broad, and it is dependent on the anatomic site. For instance, in tumors involving the gastrointestinal tract, gastrointestinal stromal tumor may be considered. Gastrointestinal stromal tumors have a more uniform fascicular architecture, lack the prominent inflammatory infiltrate, and are positive for CD117 and DOG1. Similarly, desmoid fibromatosis may be considered, particularly at mesenteric sites where these tumors are more often myxoid. However, nuclear beta-catenin staining may differentiate these tumors from the more commonly ALK-positive inflammatory myofibroblastic tumor. In the retroperitoneum, de-differentiated liposarcoma may be a histologic concern, although this tumor type is exceedingly rare in the pediatric population. IFS may rarely occur intra-abdominally, but in intra-abdominal or retroperitoneal cases this can be a particularly challenging differential diagnosis in young children. There is extensive overlap morphologically between inflammatory myofibroblastic tumor and IFS, and ALK negative cases of inflammatory myofibroblastic tumor should be tested thoroughly for alternative receptor tyrosine kinase fusions including *NTRK*.

PROGNOSIS

Approximately 25% of inflammatory myofibroblastic tumors recur, but distant metastasis are rare (~5%). Patients with *ALK* rearrangements may be eligible with targeted therapy with pan-tyrosine kinase inhibitors and/or ALK-inhibitors.[40,41] New drugs targeting many of the other receptor tyrosine kinases described as variant gene fusions are becoming increasingly available, as well.

> **Key features**
>
> Tumors typically involves mesentery, lung and retroperitoneum and infrequently occurs in subcutaneous tissues
>
> Prominent inflammatory infiltrate including plasma cells and lymphocytes (**Fig. 10B**)
>
> 60% of cases are ALK positive (**Fig. 10C**)

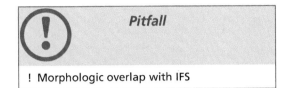
> **⚠ Pitfall**
>
> ! Morphologic overlap with IFS

INFANTILE FIBROSARCOMA

OVERVIEW

IFS is a malignant fibroblastic tumor. It most commonly presents in the first 2 years of life (~80% to 90%) with approximately one-third arising congenitally; other cases have been reported later in life. IFS has a predilection for the superficial and deep soft tissues of the extremities, trunk and head/neck regions; rare cases have been described in visceral locations.[42–44] Analogous tumors in the kidney are designated cellular congenital mesoblastic nephroma.[45]

GROSS FEATURES

IFS presents as a poorly circumscribed mass, with infiltrative borders which may extend into adjacent normal tissues. Although some tumors may have a thin pseudo-capsule. Tumors range in size from 1 to 15 cm, with a median size of 5 to 6 cm.

MICROSCOPIC FEATURES

IFS displays a broad morphologic spectrum. The most common morphologic patterns are those of a cellular neoplasm with spindled to ovoid cells, scant cytoplasm and angulated nuclei, which are arranged in long "herringbone" fascicles (**Fig. 11A, B**) or haphazardly (**Fig. 11C, D**). The background stroma varies from myxoid to collagenized (see **Fig. 11**). A prominent HPC-like vascular pattern is often present. Mitoses and necrosis are not of prognostic significance. By immunohistochemistry, tumors show variable expression of SMA, CD34, S100 and rarely desmin. IFSs with *NTRK* gene rearrangements demonstrate expression for panTRK antibody.[46] Those with *NTRK1/2* fusions have cytoplasmic expression, whereas those with *NTRK3* fusions have nuclear expression.[46]

MOLECULAR FEATURES

IFS and cellular congenital mesoblastic nephroma are driven by oncogenic activation of kinase

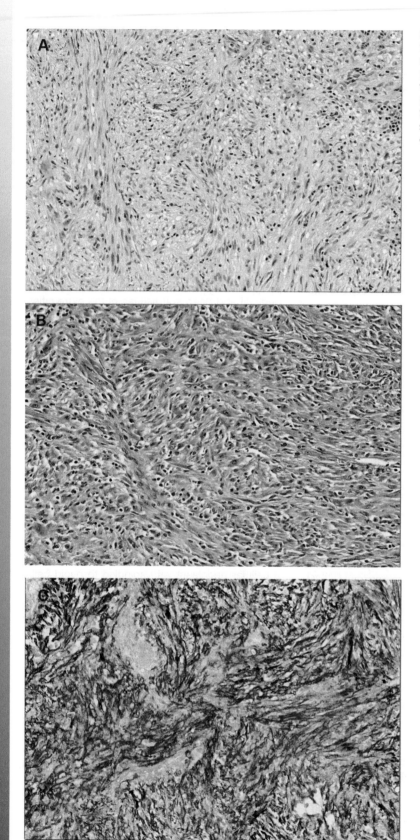

Fig. 10. (*A*) Inflammatory myofibroblastic tumor demonstrates intersecting fascicles of plump, spindled cells. (*B*) Most tumors show admixed lymphoplasmacytic inflammation. (*C*) Sixty percent of tumors demonstrate immunohistochemical expression for ALK.

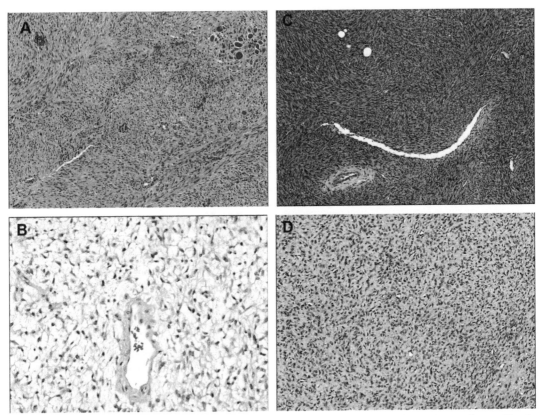

Fig. 11. IFS is classically a hypercellular tumor composed of fascicles of spindled cells (*A*) (original magnification ×100, *TPR:NTRK1*). The tumor often infiltrates skeletal muscle. Another common/classic pattern is primitive stellate cells in a myxoid stroma (*B*) (original magnification ×200x, *ETV6:NTRK3*). Tumors may have a prominent HPC-like vascular network (*C*) (original magnification ×100, *ETV6:NTRK3*). Some tumors are the round cell variant/pattern (*D*) (original magnification ×100, *EML4:NTKR3*).

signaling (fusions or activating mutations). The most frequent alteration is the canonical *ETV6:NTRK3* fusion, which can be detected by FISH for *ETV6* rearrangements.[43] Alterative fusions/mutations involving other kinases or downstream effector molecules also occur, including in *NTRK1, NTRK2, BRAF, MET, RET*, and alternative *NTRK3* fusions.[43,48–50] Each of these receptor tyrosine kinases may fuse with a variety of gene partners, making a partner agnostic RNA sequencing methodology the test of choice for confirming the diagnosis of *ETV6* negative tumors. Rarely, tumors may harbor point mutations or insertions in *BRAF* or *EGFR*, and additional DNA sequencing may be useful in cases lacking identifiable gene fusions.

DIAGNOSIS AND DIFFERENTIAL DIAGNOSIS

The differential diagnosis includes inflammatory myofibroblastic tumor, myofibroma/myofibromatosis, primitive myxoid mesenchymal tumor of infancy, and spindle cell rhabdomyosarcoma. IFS and inflammatory myofibroblastic tumor may show marked morphologic overlap, including the presence of lymphoplasmacytic inflammation. In contrast to IFS, inflammatory myofibroblastic tumors typically involve older patients and spare the limbs and subcutaneous tissues. Classically, inflammatory myofibroblastic tumor is associated with *ALK* gene rearrangements, whereas IFS is associated with *ETV6:NTRK3* fusion. However, given the presence of a wide variety of actionable receptor tyrosine kinase fusions in both tumor types, identification of the underlying molecular alteration may be the most clinically useful data the pathologist can contribute. IFS may occasionally have decreased cellularity and increased collagen, sometimes with patchy SMA staining, and resemble myofibromatosis. Multifocality favors the diagnosis of myofibromatosis, but in some cases identification of a *PDGFRB* mutation may be necessary for definitive diagnosis. Primitive myxoid mesenchymal tumor of infancy (and the related undifferentiated round cell sarcoma of infancy) is a rare tumor that may occasionally show morphologic overlap with IFS. Primitive myxoid mesenchymal tumor of infancy demonstrates a delicate, branching, curvilinear vascular pattern as opposed to the dilated, hemangiopericytic vessels seen in IFS. Primitive myxoid mesenchymal tumor of infancy is characterized by *BCOR* alterations, most often internal tandem duplications and rarely gene fusions. Of note, *BCOR*-internal tandem duplications are best detected by DNA sequencing methodologies and are not reliably detected with most RNA fusion panels. Spindle cell rhabdomyosarcoma may show overlap with the classic pattern of IFS, but the presence of nuclear myogenin or MyoD1 staining confirms the diagnosis of rhabdomyosarcoma.

PROGNOSIS

IFS is locally aggressive with a 25% to 40% risk of local recurrence. It metastasizes in frequently, with metastasis reported in 8% to 15% of cases. The prognosis is favorable with an overall 10-year survival of 90% with therapy. The advent of targeted tyrosine kinase inhibitors, including Food and Drug Administration (FDA)-approved TRK-inhibitors, may alter the prognosis and management of this disease.

Key features

Typically involves extremities of young children

Classically has fascicles of spindled cells in a herringbone arrangement (see **Fig. 11A, B**)

Often has hemangiopericytic vascular pattern

Pitfalls

! Morphologic overlap with inflammatory myofibroblastic tumor

! High mitotic rate and necrosis may raise possibility of a high-grade sarcoma

RECEPTOR TYROSINE KINASE (NEUROTROPHIC TYROSINE RECEPTOR KINASE AND OTHERS)–REARRANGED SPINDLE CELL TUMOR

OVERVIEW

This is an emerging category of rare, molecularly defined spindle cell tumors that encompass a wide range of morphologies. These tumors have been described under several different names including lipofibromatosis-like neural tumor, CD34/S100 positive spindle cell tumor, and *NTRK*-positive tumor resembling peripheral nerve sheath tumor.[51–53] Most tumors are described within the first 2 decades of life, with a median age of 13 years. However, there is a broad age range at presentation, which extends from infancy into late adulthood. Most published cases have arisen in the superficial tissues of extremities or trunk.[47,51–53]

GROSS FEATURES

There is little published to date on the macroscopic appearance of these tumors, but they may range from predominantly fatty and lipofibromatosis-like to large, fibromyxoid masses.

MICROSCOPIC FEATURES

This emerging diagnostic category has a broad spectrum of morphologies, including IFS-like, lipofibromatosis-like, inflammatory myofibroblastic tumor (IMT)-like, and some that resemble malignant peripheral nerve sheath tumor (MPNST).[47] Those with a lipofibromatosis-like appearance have a haphazard arrangement of monomorphic ovoid to spindle cells with indistinct cytoplasm and are highly infiltrative into subcutaneous fat. Mitotic activity is usually low. Those that are IFS or MPNST-like often consist of uniform spindle cells arranged in sheets, fascicles or patternless patterns (**Fig. 12A–C**). There may be distinctive stromal and/or perivascular hyalinization. Tumors may be variably cellular, merging with hypocellular regions having a myxoid background. In more cellular tumors, mitotic activity may be brisk and tumor necrosis can be seen. By immunohistochemistry, many tumors show coexpression of CD34 and S100 to variable degrees, with absence of Sox10 (**Fig. 12D, E**). In those tumors with *NTRK* gene fusions, panTRK expression is also present (**Fig. 12F**).

MOLECULAR FEATURES

Growing evidence has demonstrated *NTRK1/2/3*, *RAF1*, *BRAF*, and *RET* gene fusions in tumors within this morphologic and immunophenotypic spectrum.[51,53] Given the variety of fusions described to date, RNA panels with the ability to detect novel partners are recommended as first-line molecular testing in these tumors.

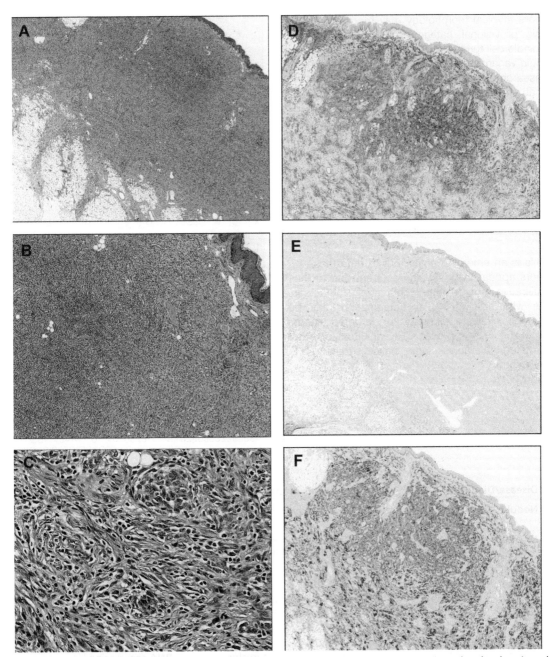

Fig. 12. Other receptor tyrosine kinase fused tumors are often superficial in location and involve the dermis and superficial subcutaneous tissue (A – 10x, B-40x). Like infantile fibrosarcoma, these tumors are often composed of fascicles of spindled cells with admixed lymphocytes (C – 400x). Many of these tumors show immunohistochemical expression for CD34 (D-20x) with or without S100 expression (E -20x). In those tumors with NTRK rearrangements, immunohistochemistry for panTRK is present, as seen in this NTRK1 rearranged tumor with strong, diffuse cytoplasmic staining for panTRK (F – 20x).

DIAGNOSIS AND DIFFERENTIAL DIAGNOSIS

The primary differential diagnosis is IFS. Some studies have suggested a relationship of IFS and this emerging category of neurotrophic tyrosine receptor kinase (NTRK)-rearranged spindle cell tumors; however, this is not yet well established. In general, classic IFS is a tumor of young children, involves the extremities, is most commonly associated with *ETV6-NTRK3* fusions, has a marked cellularity with brisk mitotic activity and lacks expression of S100 and CD34. Tumors with a more atypical morphology may represent IFS or this provisional category of *NTRK*-rearranged spindle cell tumors which may represent morphologic variants or spectrum of IFS. However, more research is needed to identify histologic features that allow definitive classification. For some patterns of *NTRK*-rearranged spindle cell tumor, lipofibromatosis may enter the differential diagnosis. Tumors harboring receptor tyrosine kinase fusions are generally more cellular and solid than lipofibromatosis, and although CD34 has been described in lipofibromatosis; S100 expression is typically not seen.[26,27,52]

PROGNOSIS

This is an emerging entity, but to date these tumors appear to be locally recurrent due to their infiltrative growth pattern, but rarely metastatic. As with IFS, molecular confirmation may be needed evaluate eligibility for targeted agents including FDA-approved TRK-inhibitors or other targeted therapies (eg, clinical trials RET-inhibitors).

Key features

Primitive spindled to ovoid cells arranged in sheets or poorly formed fascicles (see Fig. 12A–C)

Highly infiltrative into surrounding fat

Often show coexpression of CD34 and S100 (see Fig. 12D, E)

Pitfall

! Provisional and evolving entity with unclear biologic behavior and/or relationship to other RTK tumors (ie, IFS, IMT)

CLINICS CARE POINTS: WHICH TEST TO CHOOSE?

Disease/Diagnosis	Molecular Alteration	Confirmatory Molecular Testing
Nodular fasciitis	*USP6* rearrangements	FISH RNA sequencing
Myofibroma/myofibromatosis	*PDGFRB* point mutations, insertions, deletions	DNA sequencing
Cellular myofibroma	*SRF:RELA* fusions; rarely *SRF:other*	FISH RNA sequencing
Inflammatory myofibroblastic tumor	*ALK* rearrangements, less often *ROS, RET,* or *PDGFRB* rearrangements	FISH RNA sequencing
Infantile fibrosarcoma (and related tumors)	*ETV6:NTRK3* and a variety of other receptor tyrosine kinase rearrangements (*NTRK1,2,3; RET, MET*); rarely *BRAF* point mutations/duplications	FISH RNA sequencing DNA sequencing
Lipofibromatosis	Varied gene fusions	RNA sequencing
Calcifying aponeurotic fibroma	*FN1:EGF* fusions	FISH RNA sequencing
Fibrous hamartoma of infancy	*EGFR* exon 20 insertion/duplications	DNA sequencing
Inclusion body fibromatosis	Unknown	
Desmoid fibromatosis	*Beta-catenin* mutations; *APC* mutations	DNA sequencing

DISCLOSURE

The authors have nothing to disclose.

REFERENCES

1. Lauer DH, Enzinger FM. Cranial fasciitis of childhood. Cancer 1980;45(2):401–6.
2. Meister P, Bückmann FW, Konrad E. Extent and level of fascial involvement in 100 cases with nodular fasciitis. Virchows Arch A Pathol Anat Histol 1978; 380(2):177–85.
3. de Feraudy S, Fletcher CD. Intradermal nodular fasciitis: a rare lesion analyzed in a series of 24 cases. Am J Surg Pathol 2010;34(9):1377–81.
4. Patchefsky AS, Enzinger FM. Intravascular fasciitis: a report of 17 cases. Am J Surg Pathol 1981;5(1): 29–36.
5. Erber R, Agaimy A. Misses and near misses in diagnosing nodular fasciitis and morphologically related reactive myofibroblastic proliferations: experience of a referral center with emphasis on frequency of USP6 gene rearrangements. Virchows Arch 2018; 473(3):351–60.
6. Salib C, Edelman M, Lilly J, et al. USP6 gene rearrangement by FISH analysis in cranial fasciitis: a report of three cases. Head Neck Pathol 2019; 14(1):257–61.
7. Patel NR, Chrisinger JSA, Demicco EG, et al. USP6 activation in nodular fasciitis by promoter-swapping gene fusions. Mod Pathol 2017;30(11):1577–88.
8. Lam SW, Cleton-Jansen AM, Cleven AHG, et al. Molecular analysis of gene fusions in bone and soft tissue tumors by anchored multiplex PCR-based targeted next-generation sequencing. J Mol Diagn 2018;20(5):653–63.
9. Rakheja D, Cunningham JC, Mitui M, et al. A subset of cranial fasciitis is associated with dysregulation of the Wnt/beta-catenin pathway. Mod Pathol 2008; 21(11):1330–6.
10. Chung EB, Enzinger FM. Infantile myofibromatosis. Cancer 1981;48(8):1807–18.
11. Mentzel T, Dei Tos AP, Sapi Z, et al. Myopericytoma of skin and soft tissues: clinicopathologic and immunohistochemical study of 54 cases. Am J Surg Pathol 2006;30(1):104–13.
12. Beham A, Badve S, Suster S, et al. Solitary myofibroma in adults: clinicopathological analysis of a series. Histopathology 1993;22(4):335.
13. Agaimy A, Bieg M, Michal M, et al. Recurrent somatic PDGFRB mutations in sporadic infantile/solitary adult myofibromas but not in angioleiomyomas and myopericytomas. Am J Surg Pathol 2017; 41(2):195–203.
14. Cheung YH, Gayden T, Campeau PM, et al. A recurrent PDGFRB mutation causes familial infantile myofibromatosis. Am J Hum Genet 2013; 92(6):996–1000.
15. Alaggio R, Barisani D, Ninfo V, et al. Morphologic overlap between infantile myofibromatosis and infantile fibrosarcoma: a pitfall in diagnosis. Pediatr Dev Pathol 2008;11(5):355–62.
16. Linos K, Carter JM, Gardner JM, et al. Myofibromas with atypical features: expanding the morphologic spectrum of a benign entity. Am J Surg Pathol 2014;38(12):1649–54.
17. Antonescu CR, Sung YS, Zhang L, et al. Recurrent SRF-RELA fusions define a novel subset of cellular myofibroma/myopericytoma: a potential diagnostic pitfall with sarcomas with myogenic differentiation. Am J Surg Pathol 2017;41(5):677–84.
18. Suurmeijer AJ, Dickson BC, Swanson D, et al. Novel SRF-ICA1L fusions in cellular myoid neoplasms with potential for malignant behavior. Am J Surg Pathol 2019;44(1):55–60.
19. Enzinger FM. Fibrous hamartoma of infancy. Cancer 1965;18:241–8.
20. Saab ST, McClain CM, Coffin CM. Fibrous hamartoma of infancy: a clinicopathologic analysis of 60 cases. Am J Surg Pathol 2014;38(3):394–401.
21. Al-Ibraheemi A, Martinez A, Weiss SW, et al. Fibrous hamartoma of infancy: a clinicopathologic study of 145 cases, including 2 with sarcomatous features. Mod Pathol 2017;30(4):474–85.
22. Park JY, Cohen C, Lopez D, et al. EGFR exon 20 insertion/duplication mutations characterize fibrous hamartoma of infancy. Am J Surg Pathol 2016; 40(12):1713–8.
23. Allen PW, Enzinger FM. Juvenile aponeurotic fibroma. Cancer 1970;26(4):857–67.
24. Fetsch JF, Miettinen M. Calcifying aponeurotic fibroma: a clinicopathologic study of 22 cases arising in uncommon sites. Hum Pathol 1998;29(12): 1504–10.
25. Puls F, Hofvander J, Magnusson L, et al. FN1-EGF gene fusions are recurrent in calcifying aponeurotic fibroma. J Pathol 2016;238(4):502–7.
26. Al-Ibraheemi A, Folpe AL, Perez-Atayde AR, et al. Aberrant receptor tyrosine kinase signaling in lipofibromatosis: a clinicopathological and molecular genetic study of 20 cases. Mod Pathol 2019;32(3): 423–34.
27. Fetsch JF, Miettinen M, Laskin WB, et al. A clinicopathologic study of 45 pediatric soft tissue tumors with an admixture of adipose tissue and fibroblastic elements, and a proposal for classification as lipofibromatosis. Am J Surg Pathol 2000; 24(11):1491–500.
28. Bhawan J, Bacchetta C, Joris I, et al. A myofibroblastic tumor. Infantile digital fibroma (recurrent digital fibrous tumor of childhood). Am J Pathol 1979;94(1):19–36.

29. Laskin WB, Miettinen M, Fetsch JF. Infantile digital fibroma/fibromatosis: a clinicopathologic and immunohistochemical study of 69 tumors from 57 patients with long-term follow-up. Am J Surg Pathol 2009;33(1):1–13.

30. Henderson H, Peng YJ, Salter DM. Anti-calponin 1 antibodies highlight intracytoplasmic inclusions of infantile digital fibromatosis. Histopathology 2014; 64(5):752–5.

31. Coffin CM, Hornick JL, Zhou H, et al. Gardner fibroma: a clinicopathologic and immunohistochemical analysis of 45 patients with 57 fibromas. Am J Surg Pathol 2007;31(3):410–6.

32. Cates JM, Stricker TP, Sturgeon D, et al. Desmoid-type fibromatosis-associated Gardner fibromas: prevalence and impact on local recurrence. Cancer Lett 2014;353(2):176–81.

33. Zreik RT, Fritchie KJ. Morphologic spectrum of desmoid-type fibromatosis. Am J Clin Pathol 2016; 145(3):332–40.

34. Bhattacharya B, Dilworth HP, Iacobuzio-Donahue C, et al. Nuclear beta-catenin expression distinguishes deep fibromatosis from other benign and malignant fibroblastic and myofibroblastic lesions. Am J Surg Pathol 2005;29(5):653–9.

35. Bo N, Wang D, Wu B, et al. Analysis of β-catenin expression and exon 3 mutations in pediatric sporadic aggressive fibromatosis. Pediatr Dev Pathol 2012;15(3):173–8.

36. Kummar S, O'Sullivan Coyne G, Do KT, et al. Clinical activity of the γ-secretase inhibitor PF-03084014 in adults with desmoid tumors (aggressive fibromatosis). J Clin Oncol 2017;35(14):1561–9.

37. Coffin CM, Watterson J, Priest JR, et al. Extrapulmonary inflammatory myofibroblastic tumor (inflammatory pseudotumor). A clinicopathologic and immunohistochemical study of 84 cases. Am J Surg Pathol 1995;19(8):859–72.

38. Coffin CM, Hornick JL, Fletcher CD. Inflammatory myofibroblastic tumor: comparison of clinicopathologic, histologic, and immunohistochemical features including ALK expression in atypical and aggressive cases. Am J Surg Pathol 2007;31(4):509–20.

39. Haimes JD, Stewart CJR, Kudlow BA, et al. Uterine inflammatory myofibroblastic tumors frequently harbor ALK fusions with IGFBP5 and THBS1. Am J Surg Pathol 2017;41(6):773–80.

40. Gleason BC, Hornick JL. Inflammatory myofibroblastic tumours: where are we now? J Clin Pathol 2008;61(4):428–37.

41. Lovly CM, Gupta A, Lipson D, et al. Inflammatory myofibroblastic tumors harbor multiple potentially actionable kinase fusions. Cancer Discov 2014; 4(8):889–95.

42. Chung EB, Enzinger FM. Infantile fibrosarcoma. Cancer 1976;38:729–39.

43. Knezevich SR, McFadden DE, Tao W, et al. A novel ETV6-NTRK3 gene fusion in congenital fibrosarcoma. Nat Genet 1998;18(2):184–7.

44. Davis JL, Lockwood CM, Stohr B, et al. Expanding the spectrum of pediatric NTRK-rearranged mesenchymal tumors. Am J Surg Pathol 2019;43(4): 435–45.

45. Wegert J, Vokuhl C, Collord G, et al. Recurrent intragenic rearrangements of EGFR and BRAF in soft tissue tumors of infants. Nat Commun 2018;9(1):2378.

46. Rudzinski ER, Lockwood CM, Stohr BA, et al. Pan-Trk immunohistochemistry identifies NTRK rearrangements in pediatric mesenchymal tumors. Am J Surg Pathol 2018;42(7):927–35.

47. Davis JL, Lockwood CM, Albert CM, et al. Infantile NTRK-associated mesenchymal tumors. Pediatr Dev Pathol 2018;21(1):68–78.

48. Tannenbaum-Dvir S, Glade Bender JL, Church AJ, et al. Characterization of a novel fusion gene EML4-NTRK3 in a case of recurrent congenital fibrosarcoma. Cold Spring Harb Mol Case Stud 2015;1: a000471.

49. Kao YC, Fletcher CDM, Alaggio R, et al. Recurrent BRAF gene fusions in a subset of pediatric spindle cell sarcomas: expanding the genetic spectrum of tumors with overlapping features with infantile fibrosarcoma. Am J Surg Pathol 2018;42(1):28–38.

50. Davis JL, Vargas SO, Rudzinski ER, et al. Recurrent RET gene fusions in pediatric spindle mesenchymal neoplasms. Histopathology 2020;76(7):1032–41.

51. Suurmeijer AJH, Dickson BC, Swanson D, et al. A novel group of spindle cell tumors defined by S100 and CD34 co-expression shows recurrent fusions involving RAF1, BRAF, and NTRK1/2 genes. Genes Chromosomes Cancer 2018;57(12):611–21.

52. Agaram NP, Zhang L, Sung YS, et al. Recurrent NTRK1 gene fusions define a novel subset of locally aggressive lipofibromatosis-like neural tumors. Am J Surg Pathol 2016;40(10):1407–16.

53. Michal M, Ptáková N, Martínek P, et al. S100 and CD34 positive spindle cell tumor with prominent perivascular hyalinization and a novel NCOA4-RET fusion. Genes Chromosomes Cancer 2019;58(9): 680–5.

Round Cell Sarcomas
Newcomers and Diagnostic Approaches

Anita Nagy, MD, FRCPath[a],
Gino R. Somers, MBBS, PhD, FRCPA[b,c],*

KEYWORDS

- Ewing sarcoma • BCOR-rearranged sarcoma • CIC-rearranged sarcoma
- Non-ETS fused round cell sarcoma

Key points

- Ewing sarcoma is the prototypical round cell sarcoma of soft tissue and bone.
- New subtypes of round cell sarcomas have been recognized based on novel genetic alterations.
- These new entities are *CIC*-rearranged sarcomas, *BCOR*-rearranged sarcomas, and non–ETS-fused round cell sarcomas.
- Many of these newcomers have different chemosensitivities and clinical outcomes compared with traditional Ewing sarcoma, making diagnosis and subclassification clinically important.
- Novel immunohistochemical stains against chimeric fusion proteins and molecular tests to confirm the underlying gene rearrangements should be an integral part of the diagnostic workup of round cell sarcomas.

ABSTRACT

Undifferentiated sarcomas of soft tissue and bone have been defined as tumors with no identifiable morphologic, immunohistochemical, or molecular features indicating tumor cell origin. In young patients, these tumors frequently have a round or spindle cell morphology. Recently described recurrent translocations within this category have led to the recognition of new molecular subtypes of round cell sarcomas, and several of them have a more aggressive clinical course and less chemosensitivity. Because these "newcomers" are diagnosed based on their molecular characteristics, molecular investigation is key in the diagnosis and optimal treatment of these challenging tumors.

OVERVIEW

The majority of pediatric round cell tumors can be classified based on their morphologic, immunohistochemical and molecular features. The classical pediatric round cell sarcoma is Ewing sarcoma, which harbors characteristic rearrangements involving the *EWSR1* gene.[1] However, a small percentage of these highly aggressive malignant tumors show no diagnostic morphologic or immunohistochemical features, and molecular testing fails to detect any known genetic alteration.[1,2] These tumors have been variously called Ewing-like sarcomas, primitive round cells sarcomas, or undifferentiated round cell sarcomas. These tumors are usually treated with regimens similar to those used for Ewing sarcoma.

---

[a] Division of Pathology, Department of Paediatric Laboratory Medicine, Hospital for Sick Children, Burton Wing, 555 University Avenue, Toronto, Ontario M5G 1X8, Canada; [b] Pathology, Department of Paediatric Laboratory Medicine, Hospital for Sick Children, Burton Wing, 555 University Avenue, Toronto, Ontario, M5G 1X8, Canada; [c] Department of Laboratory Medicine and Pathobiology, University of Toronto, Toronto, Ontario, Canada
* Corresponding author.
E-mail address: gino.somers@sickkids.ca

Surgical Pathology 13 (2020) 763–782
https://doi.org/10.1016/j.path.2020.08.004
1875-9181/20/© 2020 Elsevier Inc. All rights reserved.

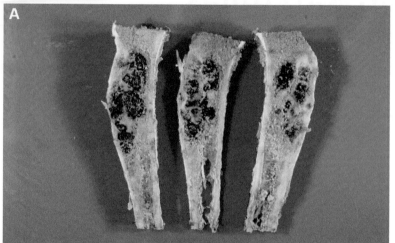

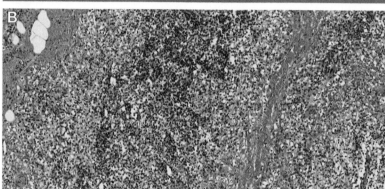

Fig. 1. Left proximal tibia with Ewing sarcoma. (*A*) Macroscopic appearance of the tumor after formalin fixation and decalcification. (*B*) Solid sheets of tumor cells with darkly and lightly stained cells (original magnification ×100; stain: hematoxylin and eosin).

In the last few years, molecular studies have detected recurrent translocations within the Ewing-like sarcoma group, helping to define new genetic subgroups, such as the *CIC*-rearranged sarcomas, *BCOR*-rearranged sarcomas, and sarcomas with fusion between *EWSR1* and other non-ETS genes. There is increasing evidence that these new entities have different outcomes than Ewing sarcoma and require different therapeutic approaches.

These new entities are listed under undifferentiated small round cell sarcomas of bone and soft tissue in the newest 2020 World Health Organization classification.[3] They show overlapping morphologic and immunohistochemical features, and their diagnosis requires molecular confirmation of the characteristic recurrent translocations.

This article summarizes our current knowledge of Ewing sarcoma and these new entities in pediatric patients, and focuses on new diagnostic tools that allow accurate diagnosis and subclassification.

EWING SARCOMA

Ewing sarcoma is the second most common bone tumor in children after osteosarcoma. The tumor is characterized by a monomorphic population of small round cells, membranous CD99 positivity, and recurrent translocations most frequently between the *EWRS1* (Ewing sarcoma breakpoint region 1) gene on 22q12 and the *FLI1* (Friend leukemia integration 1) gene on 11q24.

Most patients (80%) are younger than 20 years, and the peak incidence is in the second decade. There is a male predominance of 1.4 to 1.0.[1,3,4] It typically involves the metaphysis or diaphysis of long bones, pelvis and ribs. Less frequently affected bones are the skull, vertebra, or short bones of the hands and feet. Around 10% to 20% of cases of Ewing sarcoma are detected in extraskeletal sites and organs.[1,3] Extraskeletal Ewing sarcoma more frequently occurs in older children and adolescents.[5]

GROSS AND MICROSCOPIC FEATURES

The tumor usually has a multilobulated tan–grey appearance and is typically present in the medulla of the bone (**Fig. 1**A). It destructs the underlying structures and invades into the adjacent soft tissue.

Fig. 1. (continued). (*C*) Round nuclei with finely dispersed chromatin, inconspicuous nucleoli and small amounts of cytoplasm (original magnification ×400; stain: hematoxylin and eosin). (*D*) Immunohistochemical stain with CD99 show a membranous staining pattern (original magnification ×200).

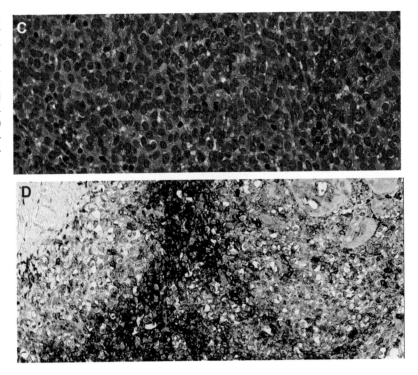

Histologically, Ewing sarcoma comprises densely cellular, patternless sheets of uniform small round or ovoid cells. There is a high nuclear to cytoplasmic ratio with darkly and lightly stained nuclei. The light cells contain round nuclei with finely dispersed chromatin and the dark cells have slightly irregular nuclei with more clumped chromatin. The cytoplasm is minimal and eosinophilic. Occasional cytoplasmic vacuoles are noted, which represent glycogen accumulation (demonstrated by periodic acid–Schiff staining) (Fig. 1B, C). The intervening stoma is minimal and reticulin staining is only seen around the vessels. Mitoses are usually abundant and the proliferation index is high. Some tumors may show a higher degree of neural differentiation (previously called primitive neuroectodermal tumor), such as Homer-Wright rosettes, but this feature has no prognostic significance.

Postchemotherapy resection specimens show a variable degree of chemotherapy-induced changes, such as necrosis, hemorrhage, and loose connective tissue.[3] Calcification is not typically seen. Margin status and viable tumor volume are important prognostic factors, similar to osteosarcoma, and should be documented in the pathology report.[6,7]

IMMUNOHISTOCHEMISTRY

Ewing sarcoma characteristically shows distinct membranous staining with CD99 (95%)[3]

(Fig. 1D). CD99 is a cell surface glycoprotein (product of MIC2 antigen) and not a chimeric protein of the gene fusion. It is highly sensitive for Ewing sarcoma, but not entirely specific, and can be expressed in other malignancies (Table 1). Negative staining, however, suggests another diagnosis (Box 1, Table 2). NKX2-2 (member of NK2 family of transcription factors) is a downstream target of *EWSR1-FLI1* fusion protein,[8,9] and has been reported to be a useful marker for Ewing sarcoma; however, can also be expressed in other *EWSR1* rearranged tumors.[10]

In sarcomas with *EWSR1-FLI1* fusion, the FLI1 protein is overexpressed in the tumor cells, which can be detected with immunohistochemical stain. Another translocation associated marker is ERG, which is positive in cases with the *EWSR1–ERG* gene fusion.[11] However, both FLI1 and ERG are nonspecific and can be expressed in other lesions.

Ewing sarcoma shows patchy staining with keratin and can express other markers such as desmin, S100, CD57 and NFP.[12] In areas of rosette-formation, neural markers (NSE and CD57) are strongly positive. PAX7 expression has been recently described in Ewing sarcoma (90%), *ESWSR1-NAFTc2* fusion sarcomas and *BCOR–CCNB3* sarcomas.[13,14]

MOLECULAR FEATURES

Ewing sarcoma is characterized by recurrent translocation between a member of the RNA-

Table 1
Translocation-related immunohistochemical stains

Stains	Ewing Sarcoma	CIC-Rearranged Sarcoma	BCOR-Rearranged Sarcoma	Non–ETS-Fused Sarcoma	Other Tumors with Positive Staining
ETV4		Positive, nuclear[29]	Negative		WT, DSRCT, melanoma, small cell carcinoma[29]
NUT	Negative	Positive, nuclear[24]	Negative		NUT carcinoma[24]
DUX4		Positive, nuclear, in CIC-DUX4 sarcomas[31]			Subtype of pediatric B-cell precursor lymphoblastic leukemia[59]
FLI1	Positive, nuclear, in EWSR1-FLI1 sarcomas		Positive, nuclear		
ERG	Positive, nuclear, in EWSR1-ERG sarcomas	Positive, nuclear	Negative		Vascular tumor (ie, hemangiomas, angiosarcoma), extramedullary myeloid tumors[60]
BCOR		Negative	Positive, nuclear, including ITD		CCSK[39]
CCNB3		Negative	Positive, nuclear, in BCOR-CCNB3 sarcomas		

Blank cells indicate no available information on staining patterns for those markers.
Abbreviations: CCSK, clear cell sarcoma of the kidney; DSRCT, desmoplastic small round cell tumor; WT Wilms' tumor.

binding FET family (*EWSR1* or *FUS*), which are RNA binding proteins involved in transcription and slicing, with a member of ETS transcription family (*FLI1*, *ERG*, *ETV1*, *ETV4*, or *FEV*), which are involved in cell proliferation, differentiation, cell cycle control, angiogenesis, and apoptosis.

In the majority (85%) of Ewing sarcomas, the 5' portion of the *EWSR1* gene on chromosome 22 fuses to the 3' portion of the *FLI1* gene on chromosome 11, resulting in a t(11;22) (q24;q12) rearrangement.[1] The *EWSR1–FLI* fusion product is an active transcription factor that binds DNA via its *FLI*-derived ETS domain and regulates gene expression through the *EWSR1* portion of the fusion. Other less frequent fusion partners are *ERG*, *ETV1*, *ETV4*, and *FEV*. The *EWSR1–ERG* translocation, t(21;22) (q22;q12), is present in 5% to 10% of the cases, whereas the others are much less common (approximately 3%).[1,15]

Alternative gene rearrangements in Ewing sarcoma include *FUS* gene, resulting in *FUS–ERG* or *FUS–FEV* fusions, t(16;21) (p11;q24) or t(2;16) (q35;p11), respectively.[16] It is believed that *EWSR1* and *FUS* genes are functionally similar. Thus, *FUS* gene rearranged tumors show similar Ewing sarcoma morphology and positive CD99 membranous staining but lack the *EWSR1* rearrangement. Knowledge of these alternative gene arrangements is important to initiate further molecular testing to confirm Ewing sarcoma if *EWSR1* rearrangements are not found.

In addition to the variability of *EWSR1* fusion partners, the breakpoint locations within the genes can also differ. For example, 60% of *EWSR1–FLI1* translocations show fusion between *EWSR1* exon 7 and *FLI1* exon 6 (type 1), which were considered to have better outcome.[17] Recent treatment protocols eliminated prognostic differences based on these fusion types.[1,18] Knowledge of this exonic

---

Box 1
Pediatric tumors with round cell morphology

Small round cell tumors

  Neuroblastoma

  Non-Hodgkin lymphoma and leukemia

  Rhabdomyosarcoma

  Ewing sarcoma

  Ewing-like sarcoma

  Malignant rhabdoid tumor

  Desmoplastic small round cell tumor

Sarcomas with round cell component

  Ewing sarcoma

  Ewing-like sarcomas

  Mesenchymal chondrosarcoma

  Synovial sarcoma

  Small cell osteosarcoma

  Malignant peripheral nerve sheath tumor

Visceral tumors with round cell component (organ specific tumors and visceral presentation of sarcomas)

  Wilms tumor

  Hepatoblastoma, small cell variant

  Pleuropulmonary blastoma

  Ewing-like sarcoma (eg, *CIC*-rearranged sarcoma in kidney)

---

heterogeneity of *EWSR1* fusion transcripts, however, is essential when designing targeted molecular tests for detection of the gene products.

PROGNOSIS

Current Ewing sarcoma therapy includes multi-agent chemotherapy, surgical resection and local radiotherapy, which has significantly improved the outcome of this aggressive tumor. The 5-year overall survival rate in children with localized disease is 75% to 82%, and in metastatic or early relapsing cases is approximately 30%.[3,4] Between 20% and 25% of adult and pediatric patients have metastasis to lungs, bone, and/or bone marrow at diagnosis, rendering a much poorer prognosis.[4]

CIC-REARRANGED SARCOMAS

CIC-rearranged sarcoma is the most frequent (66%–68%) genetic subtype of *EWSR1* negative round cell sarcomas.[19,20] The *CIC* (capicua

transcriptional repressor) gene is located on chromosome 19q13.2. The most common fusion partner is *DUX4* or *DUX4L* gene, located on 4q35 or 10q26.3 respectively. Fusions with *FOXO4* and *NUTM1* genes have also been described in pediatric cases.[21–24]

CIC-rearranged sarcomas also occur in older patients with peak incidence between 20 and 40 years of age.[19,25,26] Twenty-two percent of patients are in the pediatric age group and there is a slight male predominance.[25] Most frequently, the tumor occurs in extraskeletal locations and predominantly in deep soft tissues of the trunk and limbs (86%). Occasionally, it has been reported in the head and neck region, retroperitoneum and pelvis.[3] Visceral involvement has also been described (12%). Primary bone involvement is rare (3%).[25,26]

CIC–NUTM1 sarcomas, which are aggressive tumors with a predilection for the central nervous system in pediatric patients, can infiltrate into the surrounding cranial bone and soft tissue[24,25] and

Table 2
Unique features of soft tissue tumors with round cell morphology

Soft Tissue Tumor	Features
Rhabdomyosarcoma, alveolar	Monomorphous round to oval mesenchymal cells, focal clear cell morphology, solid or nested pattern depending on presence of fibrous stroma Positive with desmin, myogenin, myoD1 t(2:13) *PAX3-FOXO1* and t(1;13) *PAX7-FOXO1* gene fusion; 20% translocation negative
Rhabdomyosarcoma, embryonal	Intratumoral heterogeneity, loose myxoid stroma, round and spindle mesenchymal cells with variable degree of morphologic skeletal muscle differentiation (strap, tadpole or spider cells) Positive with desmin, myogenin, myoD1 Highly variable karyotype, no recurrent translocation
Malignant rhabdoid tumor/ extrarenal rhabdoid tumor	Intratumoral heterogeneity, highly cellular discohesive sheets to myxoid areas, rhabdoid cells (might be inconspicuous), small cell variant Negative with INI-1, positive with desmin and keratin Homozygous inactivation of *SMARCB1* on chr 22q11.2
Desmoplastic small round cell tumor	Sharply outlined nests of small round cells set in desmoplastic stroma Polyphenotypic differentiation with expression of epithelial, myogenic and neural markers; positive with CD99 and WT1c t(11;22) *EWSR1-WT1* fusion resulting in overexpression of carboxyl terminal portion of WT1 protein
Mesenchymal chondrosarcoma	Biphasic tumor with round to oval, focally spindled cells admixed with hyaline cartilaginous islands, myopericytomatous vascular pattern Positive with SOX9, CD99 and NKX2-2 t(8;8) (q21;q13.3) *HEY1-NCOA2* fusion
Synovial sarcoma	Mono-or biphasic tumor with stromal and epithelial components, sheets and fascicles of plump ovoid cells and cuboidal/columnar epithelial cells, with/out hemangiopericytoma-like vascular pattern, myxoid stroma, poorly differentiated areas Positive with CD99, TLE1, keratin, t(X,18) translocation between *SS18* gene and *SSX* genes (*SSX1, SSX2, SSX4*)
Small cell osteosarcoma	Small cells with round to oval pleomorphic nuclei, fine to coarse chromatin, lace-like osteoid production Positive with SATB2, can be positive with CD99, No recurrent rearrangement
Malignant peripheral nerve sheath tumor	Diverse microscopic appearance, alternating hypo- and hypercellular areas, fascicular growth pattern, spindle cells, heterologous elements, branching hemangiopericytoma-like vessels Positive with TLE1, SOX10 and S100 (focal) Complex numerical and structural chromosomal alterations, mutations of *NF1, TP43, CDKN2A*, over expression of *EGFR*
Myoepithelial tumor of soft tissue	Variable morphology, epithelioid cells, abundant sclerotic stroma Positive with keratin, EMA, S100, negative with INI-1 *EWSR1* and *FUS* rearrangements with many partners

Fig. 2. Left temporal mass with *CIC-DUX4* positive tumor. (*A*) Gross photo of the resection specimen showing a solid gray tumor mass with marked hemorrhage and necrosis. (*B*) Tumor showing solid sheets of closely packed intermediate round to oval cells (original magnification ×100; stain: hematoxylin and eosin). (*C*) Mild nuclear pleomorphism, hyperchromatic nuclei, prominent nucleoli and small amounts of cytoplasm (original magnification ×200; stain: hematoxylin and eosin).

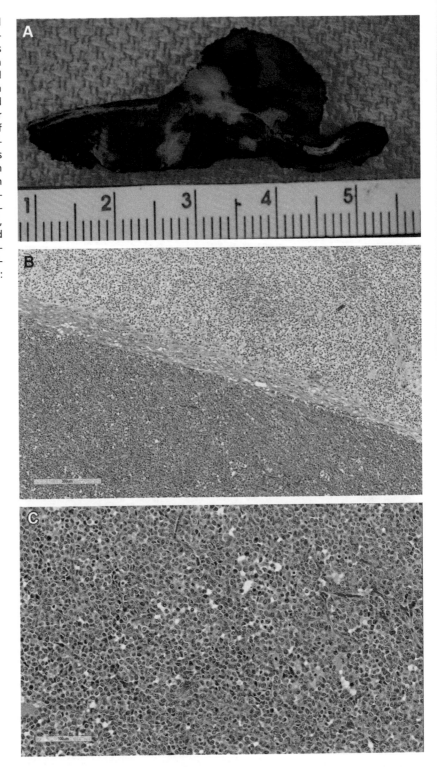

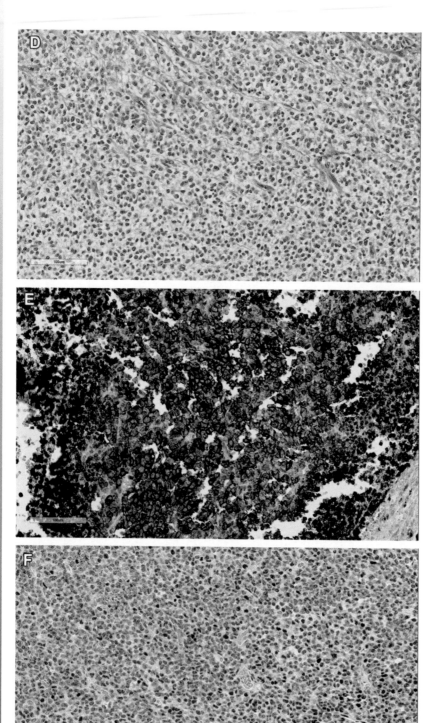

Fig. 2. (continued). (D) Tumor cells with similar nuclear features but with clear cytoplasm (original magnification ×200 stain: hematoxylin and eosin). (E) Immunohistochemical stain with CD99 showing positivity (original magnification ×200). (F) Immunohistochemical stain with WT1 showing focally positive nuclear staining (original magnification ×200).

Fig. 3. (*A*) BCOR-CCNB3 rearranged tumor. Solid sheets of round cells with delicate capillary network (original magnification ×200; stain: hematoxylin and eosin). (*B*) Post-treatment tumor shows less cellularity and more myxoid stroma (original magnification ×100; stain: hematoxylin and eosin). (*C*) Immunohistochemical stain with CD99 shows diffuse staining (original magnification ×200).

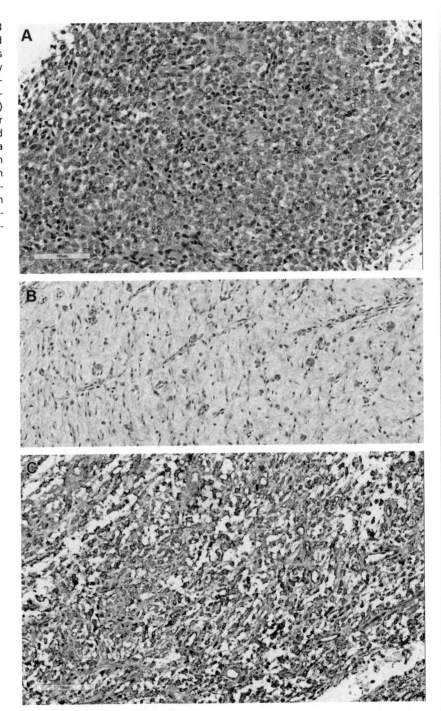

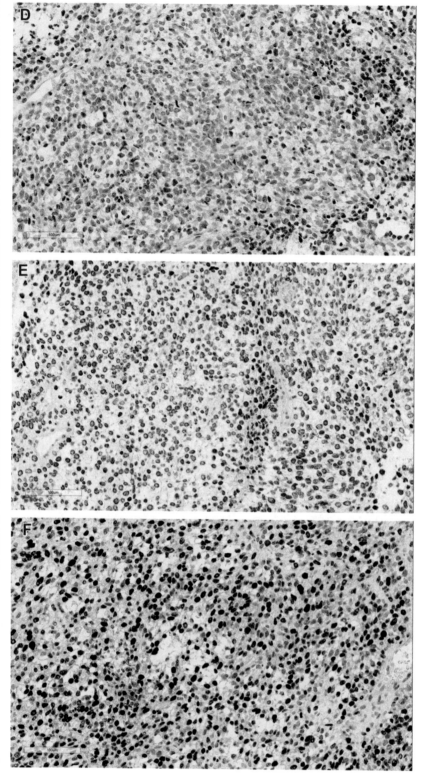

Fig. 3. (continued). (*D*) Immunohistochemical stain with BCOR showing diffuse staining with variable intensity (original magnification ×200). (*E*) Diffuse nuclear staining with SATB2 (original magnification ×200). (*F*) Nuclear staining with cyclin D1 (original magnification ×200).

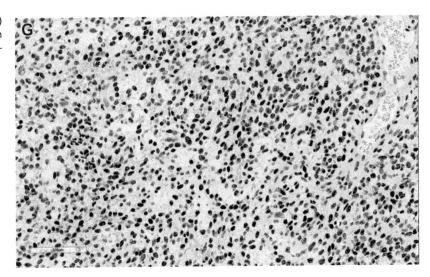

Fig. 3. *(continued).* *(G)* Nuclear staining with TLE1 (original magnification ×200).

should be considered as a possible diagnosis at this anatomic location.[24]

GROSS AND MICROSCOPIC FEATURES

Grossly, these tumors seem to be well-circumscribed, and comprise a white to gray fleshy mass with areas of hemorrhage and necrosis (Fig. 2A). The tumor size in published cases has varied from 3 to 14 cm.[3,8,27,28] *CIC*-rearranged tumors share similar morphologic features regardless the fusion partners.[22] The tumor is less monotonous than Ewing sarcoma and shows a mild degree of nuclear pleomorphism and intratumoral heterogeneity[29] (Fig. 2B). The tumor predominantly exhibits diffuse or vaguely lobular or nodular architecture.[25] The tumor cells are small to intermediate sized, round to ovoid with focal spindling. Epithelioid and rhabdoid cytomorphology has also been described.[25,26,30] The nuclei are finely hyperchromatic or vesicular with prominent nucleoli.[15,24] The cytoplasm is eosinophilic with focal clearing[3] (Fig. 2C, D). Mitotic figures are frequent. The stroma can be sclerotic, desmoplastic, or myxoid. Fibrocollagenous septae can focally delineate cellular tumor nodules, and prominent myxoid changes can result in reticular and pseudoalveolar architecture. Myxoid changes are seen in prechemotherapy and postchemotherapy specimens.[8] Geographic necrosis and hemorrhage can also be present.

IMMUNOHISTOCHEMISTRY

The CD99 staining pattern is mixed, membranous and cytoplasmic, and focal to patchy[16,19,26] (Fig. 2E). Only 23% of the cases show diffuse staining pattern.[25] Stains for FLI1, ERG, and ETV4 are positive in *CIC*-rearranged sarcomas.[27,29] DUX4 shows nuclear staining in CIC–DUX4 fused sarcomas.[31] NKX2-2, BCOR, and CCNB3 are negative.[29,30]

Nuclear and/or cytoplasmic WT1 staining is very useful, with high sensitivity (90%–95%) and specificity (80%–95%)[3,29] (Fig. 2F), although 1 series of pediatric cases suggests a lower rate of nuclear positivity (25%).[32] *CIC*-rearranged sarcomas show at least focal staining with calretinin,[3,27,29] some positivity with CD56,[8] and only a few cases have shown focal staining with AE1/AE3, desmin, and S100.[3,25,29] Sarcomas with *CIC-NUTM1* fusion show similar immunophenotype as mentioned. In addition, there is homogenous nuclear staining with NUT and some cases show focal expression of SOX2.

MOLECULAR FEATURES

The *CIC* gene is located on chromosome 19q13 and encodes a protein that belongs to a family of high mobility group box transcription repressors. The most common fusion partner is *DUX4* gene, which encodes the double homeobox 4 transcription factor on chromosome 4, or *DUX4L* gene (double homeobox 4-like gene) on chromosome 10, resulting in t(4;19) (q35;q13) or t(10;19) (q26;q13) translocations, respectively.[19,31] The *CIC* gene is largely preserved and fused with the C terminus of *DUX4*, which loses the majority of the *DUX4* sequence.[33] The C terminal end of *DUX4* enhances the transcriptional activity of *CIC* and the resultant protein dysregulates expression of the downstream targets.[19] For example, it upregulates *PEA3* family genes, including ETV1, 4, and 5.[1,16,26]

Other fusion partners are *FOXO4* on Xq13[22] leading to *CIC-FOXO4,* t(X;19) (q13;q13.3), and *NUTM1* (NUT midline carcinoma family member 1) on 15q14 fusing to form *CIC-NUTM1,* t(15;19) (q14;q13).[24] There are cases of *CIC*-rearranged tumors, in which the fusion partner is still unknown. *CIC* gene abnormalities have been also described in other type of tumors, including oligodendroglioma and angiosarcoma.[26]

PROGNOSIS

The *CIC*-rearranged sarcomas have a more aggressive clinical course and worse overall survival when compared with Ewing sarcoma. Lung metastases are common at diagnosis, and reports suggest a poor response to traditional Ewing sarcoma chemotherapy. The 5-year overall survival is 17% to 43%,[25] compared with 77% in Ewing sarcoma.[3,15,25] *CIC*-rearranged sarcomas also have a less favorable outcome than *BCOR*-rearranged sarcomas (as discussed elsewhere in this article). The *CIC-NUTM1* sarcoma, in particular, is highly aggressive.[24] It has a low mean survival of 18 months, whereas the mean survival in *CIC*-rearranged sarcoma is 139 months.[25]

Interestingly, tumors in superficial locations, such as the skin, subcutis, or submucosa, and 1 case involving an axillary lymph node, have shown better clinical outcomes.[8,28]

BCOR-REARRANGED SARCOMAS

BCOR-rearranged sarcomas are the second most frequent (4%–14%) subcategory of undifferentiated round cell sarcomas.[34,35] These tumors occur in long and flat bones (55.5%), such as the bones of pelvis, lower extremities, and paraspinal region, and less commonly in soft tissues (38.8%).[3,36] There is a strong male predominance and 81% of cases affect patients between 10 and 20 years of age.[36]

GROSS AND MICROSCOPIC FEATURES

Tumor size varies from 3 to 27 cm,[36] and tumors have a tan-grey fleshy appearance with focal areas of necrosis. Microscopically, *BCOR*-rearranged sarcomas show variable patterns. There are hypercellular solid sheets and nodules of round to oval cells (**Fig. 3A**). The spindle cell areas can be arranged into fascicles and small concentric whorls, and the cellular areas can show dyscohesion. The stroma is fibrocollagenous or myxoid[37] with a delicate capillary network.[3,16,34,37] Nuclei are pleomorphic and hyperchromatic with finely

dispersed chromatin and inconspicuous nucleoli.[16,38,39] The extent of necrosis and mitotic activity varies in published series. Myxoid and sclerotic changes are more prominent in post-treatment specimens[37] (**Fig. 3B**). Recurrent and metastatic lesions are noted to have increased cellularity and increased pleomorphism.[16,38,39]

IMMUNOHISTOCHEMISTRY

BCOR-rearranged sarcomas are usually strongly positive with CD99 (50%–60%), although patchy or absent staining has been reported[16,36,38] (**Fig. 3C**). The BCOR protein is strongly and diffusely expressed[3,36] (**Fig. 3D**). In *BCOR–CCNB3* fusion cases, CCNB3 is a useful immunohistochemical marker.[37,38] SATB2 (special AT-rich sequence-binding protein 2), which is a reliable marker of osteoblastic differentiation and was thought to be specific for osteosarcoma, has also been found to be helpful in these cases, with nuclear expression in 88.9% of *BCOR*-rearranged cases[37] (**Fig. 3E**).

Other helpful markers are cyclin D1 (90%) (**Fig. 3F**), TLE1 (transducin-like enhancer of split-1, a sensitive marker for synovial sarcoma) (80%) (**Fig. 3G**), bcl2 (100%, 90%), and CD117 (60%).[36,38] CD56 is positive, but AE1/AE3, S100, SMA, desmin, and myogenin are negative. There is no expression of ERG, WT1, or NKX2.2.[30]

MOLECULAR PATHOLOGY FEATURES

BCOR–CCNB3 gene rearrangement is the most frequent alteration (60%).[16] There is a paracentric inversion on the X chromosome between exon 15 of *BCOR* (BCL-6 corepressor) located on Xp11.14 and exon 5 of *CCNB3* located on Xp11.22.[25,35] *BCOR* encodes the BCL-6 corepressor gene, whereas *CCNB3* encodes testis specific cyclin B3 (a member of the cyclin family important in cell cycle regulation).[25] The resultant fusion protein results in overexpression of CCNB3.[16,36,37]

Additional recurrent genetic alterations are fusions with *MAML3* and *ZC3H7B* resulting in *BCOR–MAML3* and *ZC3H7B–BCOR* fusion transcripts.[40] *BCOR* internal tandem duplication, *BCOR–ITD*, results in tumors that are molecularly distinct from those with *BCOR* rearrangements. Kao and collegaues[41] studied infantile undifferentiated round cell sarcoma cases and they found that 9% of the cases had a *YWHAE–NUTM2B* fusion and 41% of the cases had *BCOR* ITD. Their results also demonstrated that *BCOR* ITD and *YWHAE–NUTM2B* fusion are mutually exclusive in undifferentiated round cell sarcoma in infants. This molecular phenomenon has also been reported in clear cell sarcoma of the kidney.[42] In the same cohort, 86% of primitive myxoid mesenchymal tumor of infancy cases also showed *BCOR* ITD.[41]

PROGNOSIS

BCOR-rearranged sarcomas are chemosensitive and have similar or even better prognosis than Ewing sarcoma.[38] The 5-year overall survival has been reported to be 72% to 75%,[36,37] similar to Ewing sarcoma (79%) and much better than *CIC*-rearranged sarcomas (43%).[36] Cases occurring in the extremities a have longer survival period than cases of axial skeleton and soft tissue disease.[38]

Non–*ETS*-FUSED ROUND CELL SARCOMAS

Non–*ETS*-fused sarcomas are extremely rare, and characterized by a fusion between *EWSR1* or *FUS* gene and a member of non-ETS family, such as *PATZ1* or *NFATc2*.[43,44] The reported age range is wide, between 12 and 67 years of age, with male predominance.[44–46] Anatomic locations and morphologic features depend on the underlying gene fusions. *EWSR1/FUS–NFATc2* sarcomas are commonly seen in the metaphysis or diaphysis of long bones,[43] whereas the *EWSR1–PATZ1* sarcomas tend to occur in the deep soft tissues of the chest wall and abdomen.[44,47]

GROSS FEATURES AND MICROSCOPY

EWSR1–NFATc2 sarcomas are solid fleshy masses, arising in the long bone, destroying the cortex and invading into the adjacent soft tissue. Tumor size ranges between 2 and 18 cm in published cases.[43] Histologically, the tumor shows microscopic heterogeneity. The tumor can comprise a fairly uniform population of small to medium sized round to epithelioid cells arranged in sheets, cords, thin trabeculae, and pseudoacinar structures. The cells have large pleomorphic hyperchromatic or vesicular nuclei, and prominent nucleoli. The cytoplasm is eosinophilic to clear.[43] The stroma can be abundant in myxohyaline with a "myoepithelial" appearance[48] or is collagenous with fibrous septa delineating cellular tumor nests. Alternatively, the tumor can comprise densely cellular solid sheets of hyperchromatic round cells often with nuclear pleomorphism and with small amount of intervening stroma.[49] Branching vascular networks have also been described.[16,45,49] Mitotic figures and necrosis are variable.[3]

EWSR1–PATZ1 sarcomas can also exhibit a variable histologic appearance. In additional to the features described, microcytic and macrocystic changes and focal infiltrates of plasma cells and lymphocytes within the tumor have been reported.[45]

IMMUNOHISTOCHEMISTRY

EWSR1/FUS–NFATc2 tumors, similarly to Ewing sarcoma, show focal or diffuse membranous staining with CD99. The tumor is positive with PAX7 and NKX2.2.[43] S100, synaptophysin, chromogranin, pan-cytokeratin, SMA, desmin, CD34, WT1, and ERG are negative. Positive staining with SATB2 has been reported in 2 cases.[43] *EWSR1–PATZ1* tumors show polyphenotypic staining. CD99, desmin myogenin, myoD1, S100, SOX10, CD34, and GFAP have all been reported positive. Epithelial markers, including EMA, AE1/3, and Cam5.2, are negative.[45]

MOLECULAR PATHOLOGY FEATURES

EWSR1–NFATc2 fusion t(20;22) (q13.2;q12.2) results in a truncated NFATc2 protein with loss of the first 2 exons, which encode the regulatory region. In the absence of negative phosphorylation signals, NFATc2 freely and constitutively translocates to the nucleus, targeting certain genes.[43] *EWSR1–PATZ1* fusion results from intrachromosomal inversion at 22q12. *PATZ1* encodes a zinc finger protein and plays role in chromatin remodeling and transcription regulation.[47,50] Other *EWSR1* fusions partners, including *SP3*[50] and *SMARCA5*,[51] have also been described.

PROGNOSIS

Owing to the rarity of this disease, there are limited data available on clinical behavior.[48]

DIFFERENTIAL DIAGNOSIS

Many pediatric tumors exhibit round cell morphology (see **Box 1**), and the differential diagnosis is broad. These include small round cell tumors, some of which are nonsarcomatous such as neuroblastoma, lymphomas, and leukemias. However, with a combination of clinical presentation, morphology and initial immunohistochemical panels, many nonsarcomatous neoplasms can be excluded. In small samples, such as needle core biopsies, tumors with a focal round cell component can be challenging to subclassify. However, with a similar approach to that described elsewhere in this article, nonsarcomatous tumors can usually be excluded before embarking on molecular testing.

Table 3
Summary of Ewing and Ewing-like sarcomas

	Ewing Sarcoma	CIC-Rearranged Sarcoma	BCOR-Rearranged Sarcoma	Non-ETS-Fused Sarcoma
Histology	Monomorphic Small, round light and dark cells round nuclei, fine chromatin, inconspicuous nucleoli, Small eosinophilic cytoplasm, occasional cytoplasmic vacuoles (periodic acid–Schiff positive), occasional rosettes Minimal intervening stroma; no myxoid stroma	Solid sheets or vaguely lobular Predominantly round cells, focal spindle or epithelioid cells Mild nuclear atypia/pleomorphism Hyperchromatic or vesicular nuclei with prominent nucleoli Eosinophilic or clear cytoplasm Sclerotic or myxoid stroma Necrosis common CIC-NUT sarcomas: myoepithelial features	Solid sheets of round cells, focal short fascicles of spindle cells Fibrocollagenous or myxoid stroma with delicate capillary network Hyperchromatic nuclei, finely dispersed chromatin, inconspicuous nucleoli Necrosis BCOR-ITD: variability in cellularity ranging from solid sheets of round cells to less cellular spindled areas,	*EWSR1/FUS-NFATc2*: round and/or spindle cells, variable growth patterns, uniform round to pleomorphic nuclei, hyperchromatic or vesicular chromatin with prominent nucleoli, clear or eosinophilic cytoplasm, Fibrocollagenous or myxoid stroma *EWSR1-PATZ1*: cystic changes, abundant intratumoral inflammatory Cells branching vascular network
IHC	CD99: strong, diffuse membranous staining NKX2-2, FLI1, ERG: positive in tumors with specific molecular rearrangements	CD99: focally positive ETV4, WT1: positive NKX2-2: negative	CD99: focal BCOR, CCNB3, TLE1, SATB2 and cyclinD1 positive	*EWSR1-NFATc2*: similar to Ewing sarcoma (positive with CD99, +/– NKX2-2, PAX7, focal pancytokeratin[2]) *EWSR1 - PATZ1*: polyphenotypic, positive with CD99, desmin, myogenin, MyoD1, S100, SOX10, CD34 positive
Location	Long bone, pelvis, ribs	Deep soft tissue of trunk and limbs; organs *CIC-NUT* sarcomas: brain	Long and flat bones (55.5%); soft tissues (38.8%)	*EWSR1/FUS - NFATc2*: bones *EWSR1 - PATZ1*: deep soft tissue of chest and abdomen

Molecular	EWSR1-FLI1 t(11;22) (q24;q12) EWSR1-ERG t(21;22) (q22;q12) FUS-ERG t(16;21) (p11;q24) FUS-FEV t(2;16) (q35;p11)	CIC-DUX4 t(4;19) (q35;q13.1) CIC-DUX4L t(10;19) (q26.3;q13.1) CIC-FOXO4 t(X;19) (q13;q13.3) CIC-NUTM1 t(15;19) (q14;q13.2)	BCOR-CCNB3 t(X;X) (p11;p11) BCOR-MAML3 BCOR-ITD ZC3H7B-BCOR	EWSR1-PATZ1 EWSR1-NFATc2 t(20;22) (q13.2;q12.2)
5-y overall survival	75%–82% (localized disease)	17%–43%	72%–75%	Insufficient data
Highlights on DD considerations	Other round cell sarcomas	CIC-NUTM1 vs NUT carcinomas (speckled nuclear staining with NUT in NUT carcinoma[52]) Myoepithelial carcinoma	BCOR-ITD sarcoma vs CCSK (similar histologic appearance) vs PMMTI SS	EWSR1-PATZ1 sarcoma vs DSRCT (dot like staining with desmin in DSRCT)

Abbreviations: CCSK, clear cell sarcoma of kidney; DD, differential diagnosis; IHC, immunohistochemistry; PMMTI, primitive myxoid mesenchymal tumor of infancy.

Table 4
Other useful immunohistochemical markers

Stains	Ewing Sarcoma	CIC-Rearranged Sarcoma	BCOR-Rearranged Sarcoma	Non-ETS-Fused Sarcoma	Other Tumors with Positive Staining
CD99	Positive (distinct membranous)	Focal to patchy, membranous and cytoplasmic[16,19,26]	Positive, variable extent and intensity	Positive in *EWSR1/FUS-NFATc2* sarcomas (similar to Ewing sarcoma) Positive in *EWSR1-PATZ1* sarcomas[44]	LBL/lymphoma, SS, RMS, DSRCT, mesenchymal chondrosarcoma
WT1	Negative	Positive, 70% nuclear[8]	Negative		
TLE1	Negative		Positive, nuclear[30]		SS; rarely, MPNST, SFT[61]
cyclinD1			Positive, nuclear[30]		
PAX7[13,14]	Positive, nuclear		Positive in *BCOR-CCNB3* sarcomas	Positive in *EWSR1/FUS-NFATc2* sarcomas	Alveolar RMS, SS, small cell osteosarcoma, DSRCT[14]
SATB2	Positive, nuclear (10%)		Positive, nuclear[36]	Positive in *EWSR1/FUS-NFATc2* sarcomas[42]	SS,[62,63] OS,[64] undifferentiated pleomorphic sarcoma (bone), fibrosarcoma (bone),[64] mesenchymal chondrosarcoma, DLBCL
NKX2-2[9]	Positive, nuclear	Positive (5%)	Negative	Positive in *EWSR1/FUS-NFATc2* sarcomas[42]	Olfactory neuroblastoma, mesenchymal chondrosarcoma, SS, poorly diff. unclassified round cell sarcoma
SOX10	Positive, nuclear			Positive in *EWSR1-PATZ1* sarcomas[44]	MPNST, clear cell sarcoma of soft tissue, myoepithelial tumors

Blank cells indicate no available information on staining patterns for those markers.
Abbreviations: DLBCL, diffuse large B-cell lymphoma; DSRCT, desmoplastic small round cell tumor; LBL, lymphoblastic lymphoma; MPNST, malignant peripheral nerve sheath tumor; OS, osteosarcoma; RMS, rhabdomyosarcoma; SFT, solitary fibrous tumor; SS, synovial sarcoma.

Visceral presentations have been described in Ewing sarcoma (eg, in the kidney), and with some of the new genetic subtypes (eg, CIC-rearranged sarcomas of the kidney).[32] Therefore, round cells sarcomas should also be considered in the differential diagnosis of visceral tumors with a round cell morphology. The characteristic morphologic immunohistochemical and molecular features of round cell sarcomas are summarized in **Table 2** and of the newcomers in **Table 3**.

MOLECULAR TECHNIQUES AND IMMUNOHISTOCHEMICAL STAINS

There are several ancillary investigations that aid in the diagnosis of round cell sarcomas. Novel immunohistochemical stains, detecting fusion gene proteins in tumor cells are helpful tools to triage cases for molecular testing, and enable us to target molecular testing to confirm the diagnosis.

Chromosomal karyotyping (traditional karyotyping and spectral karyotyping) is the classic method to provide global information about all chromosomes in a single assay. Both techniques have low resolution (3–5 Mb for conventional cytogenetics and 1–2 Mb for spectral karyotyping),[52,53] which limits their ability to detect small chromosomal translocations. Moreover, they require fresh sample, and are time consuming and costly. There is a failure rate owing to difficulty in culturing tumor cells.[54,55]

Fluorescence in situ hybridization (FISH) is a rapid test to detect translocations, amplifications and deletions for a given probe. In pediatric sarcomas, break-apart FISH is commonly used, which demonstrates any rearrangements of the locus probed, but does not identify the translocation partner. Therefore, it cannot discriminate between tumors with the same parent gene rearrangement (eg, tumors with EWSR1 rearrangement). The great advantage of FISH is that it can be applied on touch preparations, fresh tissue, frozen specimen and formalin-fixed paraffin-embedded tissues, and it has a relatively quick turn around time.[56]

Reverse transcription polymerase chain reaction is a highly sensitive and rapid technique to detect specific fusion transcripts. Each primer set detects a single fusion gene. Therefore, tumors with multiple fusion genes require multiple probe sets in the same reaction. It is not a screening test, and unusual or rare translocations can be missed. The assay requires small amount of fresh or snap frozen tissue.[54,55] Formalin-fixed paraffin-embedded tissues can also be used but success rate depends on the quality of extracted RNA.

Reverse transcription and amplification bias is also well-known. More recent technologies include NanoString RNA technology and next-generation sequencing (NGS), including whole genome and exon sequencing.

NanoString technology detects and counts up to several hundreds of fusion transcripts tagged with fluorescent barcodes (molecular barcode based system) in one hybridization reaction.[57] The technology requires a very small amount of RNA material and works well with formalin-fixed paraffin-embedded tissue. The technique does not require amplification or reverse transcription, is more sensitive than microarrays, and has similar sensitivity and accuracy to reverse transcription polymerase chain reaction.[58] Transcripts panels can be set up to help specific molecular analysis of pediatric sarcomas.[57]

NGS platforms perform parallel sequencing of millions of small fragments of DNA from multiple samples at fairly reduced cost. It can be used to sequence entire genome, specific areas of interest (eg, exome) or a subset of genes of interest (eg, targeted RNA sequencing). This latter approach is exemplified by the TruSight RNA pan cancer panel, which is an RNA sequencing technique using NGS, can assess all cancer related RNA transcripts in a single assay, and can identify rare or novel partner genes. However, compared with more simple multiplex techniques such as NanoString, the TruSight assay is more resource-intensive and has a longer turnaround time (10–14 days).

SUMMARY

BCOR-, CIC- and non–ETS-fused sarcomas are the most recent genetic subtypes of round cells sarcomas of soft tissue and bone. These tumors have overlapping histologic and immunohistochemical features and detection of their genetic alteration is essential in making an accurate diagnosis. Because certain recurrent translocations have been associated with worse prognosis, accurate subclassification has therapeutic and prognostic implications.

Immunochemical stains against chimeric oncoprotein (product of gene fusion) are helpful tools to narrow down the diagnoses and to decide on appropriate molecular testing to confirm the diagnosis. These immunohistochemical markers include BCOR, CCNB3, DUX4, ETV4, ERG, and FLI-1 (see **Table 1**). Other immunohistochemical stains commonly used in other sarcomas have also been proven to be helpful in pediatric round cell sarcomas, and include WT1, TLE1, cyclin-D1, PAX7, SATB2, and NKX2.2 (**Table 4**).

Molecular assays are essential to detect the presence of fusion genes. The type of assay ranges from simple, FISH-based test to NGS-based technologies. Whichever assay is chosen, knowledge of the possible rearrangements present will help guide interpretation of the results obtained, especially when nonmultiplexed assays return a negative result. In these instances, newer molecular techniques, such as NanoString technology and NGS, might be necessary to confirm the diagnosis.

CLINICS CARE POINTS

- Advances in the understanding of molecular abnormalities provide great promise for more accurate diagnosis for patients with undifferentiated round cell sarcomas.
- New genetic subtypes of undifferentiated round cell sarcomas are CIC-rearranged sarcomas, BCOR-rearranged sarcomas and non–ETS-fused round cell sarcomas.
- CIC-rearranged sarcomas behave more aggressively than Ewing sarcoma, whereas BCOR-rearranged sarcomas have a similar 5-year overall survival compared with Ewing sarcoma. Only limited data are available for non-ETS sarcomas.
- Spindle cells, nuclear pleomorphism, prominent nucleoli, and weak, focal, or negative staining with CD99 are not the features of classical Ewing sarcoma, and other sarcomas should be considered.
- In cases with Ewing sarcoma morphology, strong and diffuse membranous staining with CD99 and lack of EWSR1 rearrangement, alternative fusion transcripts (eg, FUS–ERG or FUS–FEV) should be considered.
- Ewing sarcomas are positive with CD99 and NKX2.2. ERG and FLI1 are also expressed in EWSR1–ERG and EWSR1–FLI1 fusion positive cases, respectively.
- Useful markers in CIC-rearranged sarcomas are CD99, WT1, ETV4, and DUX4, and in BCOR–CCNB3 rearranged sarcomas are CD99, BCOR, CCNB3, and TLE1.
- EWSR1–PATZ1 fusion positive tumor should be considered in spindle and round cell sarcomas with polyphenotypic immunohistochemical profile.
- Non ETS-rearranged tumor are positive with PAX7, NKX2.2, and CD99.
- Molecular studies to detect gene fusions include FISH, reverse transcription polymerase chain reaction, NanoString, and NGS technologies.

DISCLOSURE

The authors have nothing to disclose.

REFERENCES

1. Fletcher CDM, Bridge JA, Hogendoorn P, et al. WHO classification of tumours of soft tissue and bone. 4th edition. Lyon (France): IAPC Press; 2013.
2. Somers GR, Gupta AA, Doria AS, et al. Pediatric undifferentiated sarcoma of the soft tissues: a clinico-pathologic study. Pediatr Dev Pathol 2006;9(2):132–42.
3. Antonescu CR, Blay JY, Bovee JVMG, et al. WHO classification of tumours of soft tissue and bone. 5th edition. Lyon (France): IAPC Press; 2020. Available at: http://whobluebooks.iarc.fr/editorialboard/index.php.
4. Casali PG, Bielack S, Abecassis N, et al. Bone sarcomas: ESMO–PaedCan–EURACAN Clinical Practice Guidelines for diagnosis, treatment and follow-up. Ann Oncol 2018;29(Supplement 4):iv79–95.
5. Applebaum MA, Worch J, Matthay KK, et al. Clinical features and outcomes in patients with extra-skeletal Ewing sarcoma. Cancer 2011;117(13):3027–32.
6. Wardelmann E, Haas RL, Bovée JVMG, et al. Evaluation of response after neoadjuvant treatment in soft tissue sarcomas; the European Organization for Research and Treatment of Cancer–Soft Tissue and Bone Sarcoma Group (EORTC–STBSG) recommendations for pathological examination and reporting. Eur J Cancer 2016;53:84–95.
7. Gomez-Brouchet A, Mascard E, Siegfried A, et al. Assessment of resection margins in bone sarcoma treated by neoadjuvant chemotherapy: literature review and guidelines of the bone group (GROUPOS) of the French sarcoma group and bone tumor study group (GSF-GETO/RESOS). Orthop Traumatol Surg Res 2019;105(4):773–80.
8. Yoshida A, Goto K, Kodaira M, et al. CIC-rearranged sarcomas: a study of 20 cases and comparisons with Ewing sarcomas. Am J Surg Pathol 2016;40(3):313–23.
9. Hung Y, Fletcher C, Hornick J. Evaluation of NKX2-2 expression in round cell sarcomas and other tumors with EWSR1 rearrangement: imperfect specificity for Ewing sarcoma. Mod Pathol 2016;29:370–80.
10. Shibuya R, Matsuyama A, Nakamoto M, et al. The combination of CD99 and NKX2.2, a transcriptional target of EWSR1-FLI1, is highly specific for the diagnosis of Ewing sarcoma. Virchows Arch 2014;465(5):599–605.
11. Wang W, Patel N, Caragea M, et al. Expression of ERG, an ETS family transcription factor, identifies ERG-rearranged Ewing sarcoma. Mod Pathol 2012;25:1378–83.

12. Antonescu C. Round cell sarcomas beyond Ewing: emerging entities. Histopathology 2014;64:26–37.

13. Charville G, Wang W, Ingram D, et al. EWSR1 fusion proteins mediate PAX7 expression in Ewing sarcoma. Mod Pathol 2017;30:1312–20.

14. Toki S, Wakai S, Sekimizu M, et al. PAX7 immunohistochemical evaluation of Ewing sarcoma and other small round cell tumours. Histopathology 2018; 73(4):645–52.

15. Renzi S, Anderson ND, Light N, et al. Ewing-like sarcoma: an emerging family of round cell sarcomas. J Cell Physiol 2019;234:7999–8007.

16. Sbaraglia M, Righi A, Gambarotti M, et al. Ewing sarcoma and Ewing-like tumours. Virchows Arch 2020; 476:109–19.

17. de Alava E, Kawai A, Healey JH, et al. EWS-FLI1 fusion transcript structure is an independent determinant of prognosis in Ewing's sarcoma. J Clin Oncol 1998;16(4):1248–55.

18. van Doorninck JA, Ji L, Schaub B, et al. Current treatment protocols have eliminated the prognostic advantage of type 1 fusions in Ewing sarcoma: a report from the Children's Oncology Group. J Clin Oncol 2010;28(12):1989–94.

19. Italiano A, Sung YS, Zhang L, et al. High prevalence of CIC fusion with double-homeobox (DUX4) transcription factors in EWSR1-negative undifferentiated small blue round cell sarcomas. Genes Chromosomes Cancer 2012;51(3):207–18.

20. Graham C, Chilton-MacNeill S, Zielenska M, et al. The CIC-DUX4 fusion transcript is present in a subgroup of pediatric primitive round cell sarcomas. Hum Pathol 2012;43(2):180–9.

21. Solomon D, Brohl AK, Javed MM. Clinicopathologic Features of a Second Patient with Ewing-like Sarcoma Harboring CIC-FOXO4 Gene Fusion. Am J Surg Pathol 2014;38(12):1724–5.

22. Sugita S, Arai Y, Tonooka A, et al. A novel CIC-FOXO4 gene fusion in undifferentiated small round cell sarcoma: a genetically distinct variant of Ewing-like sarcoma. Am J Surg Pathol 2014; 38(11):1571–6.

23. Sugita S, Arai Y, Aoyama T, et al. NUTM2A-CIC fusion small round cell sarcoma: a genetically distinct variant of CIC-rearranged sarcoma. Hum Pathol 2017;65:225–30.

24. Le Loarer F, Pissaloux D, Watson S, et al. Clinicopathologic Features of CIC-NUTM1 Sarcomas, a New Molecular Variant of the Family of CIC-Fused Sarcomas. Am J Surg Pathol 2019;43(2):268–76.

25. Antonescu C, Owosho A, Zhang L, et al. Sarcomas with CIC-rearrangements are a distinct pathologic entity with aggressive outcome: a clinicopathologic and molecular study of 115 cases. Am J Surg Pathol 2017;41(7):941–9.

26. Gambarotti M, Benini S, Gamberi G, et al. CIC–DUX4 fusion-positive round-cell sarcomas of soft tissue and bone: a single-institution morphological and molecular analysis of seven cases. Histopathology 2016;69:624–34.

27. Smith S, Buehler D, Choi E, et al. CIC-DUX sarcomas demonstrate frequent MYC amplification and ETS-family transcription factor expression. Mod Pathol 2015;28:57–68.

28. Brčić I, Brodowicz T, Cerroni L, et al. Undifferentiated round cell sarcomas with CIC-DUX4 gene fusion: expanding the clinical spectrum. Pathology 2020;52(2):236–42.

29. Hung Y, Fletcher C, Hornick J. Evaluation of ETV4 and WT1 expression in CIC-rearranged sarcomas and histologic mimics. Mod Pathol 2016;29: 1324–34.

30. Yamada Y, Kuda M, Kohashi K, et al. Histological and immunohistochemical characteristics of undifferentiated small round cell sarcomas associated with CIC-DUX4 and BCOR-CCNB3 fusion genes. Virchows Arch 2017;470:373–80.

31. Siegele B, Roberts J, Black JO, et al. DUX4 Immunohistochemistry is a Highly Sensitive and Specific Marker for CIC-DUX4 Fusion-positive Round Cell Tumor. Am J Surg Pathol 2017;41(3):423–9.

32. Mangray S, Kelly DR, LeGuellec S, et al. Clinicopathologic Features of a Series of Primary Renal CIC-rearranged Sarcomas With Comprehensive Molecular Analysis. Am J Surg Pathol 2018;42(10): 1360–9.

33. Kawamura-Saito M, Yamazaki Y, Kawaguchi N, et al. Fusion between CIC and DUX4 up-regulates PEA3 family genes in Ewing-like sarcomas with t(4;19)(q35;q13) translocation. Hum Mol Genet 2006;15(13):2125–37.

34. Peters T, Kumar V, Polikepahad S, et al. BCOR–CCNB3 fusions are frequent in undifferentiated sarcomas of male children. Mod Pathol 2015;28: 575–86.

35. Pierron G, Tirode F, Lucchesi C, et al. A new subtype of bone sarcoma defined by BCOR-CCNB3 gene fusion. Nat Genet 2012;44:461–6.

36. Kao Y, Owosho AA, Sung Y, et al. BCOR-CCNB3 Fusion Positive Sarcomas. Am J Surg Pathol 2018; 42(5):604–15.

37. Ludwig K, Alaggio R, Zin A, et al. BCOR-CCNB3 Undifferentiated Sarcoma—Does Immunohistochemistry Help in the Identification? Pediatr Dev Pathol 2017;20(4):321–9.

38. Puls F, Niblett A, Marland G, et al. BCOR-CCNB3 (Ewing-like) sarcoma: a clinicopathologic analysis of 10 cases, in comparison with conventional Ewing sarcoma. Am J Surg Pathol 2014;38(10):1307–18.

39. Matsuyama A, Shiba E, Umekita Y, et al. Clinicopathologic diversity of undifferentiated sarcoma with BCOR-CCNB3 fusion. Am J Surg Pathol 2017; 41(12):1713–21.

40. Specht K, Zhang L, Sung Y, et al. Novel BCOR-MAML3 and ZC3H7B-BCOR gene fusions in undifferentiated small blue round cell sarcomas. Am J Surg Pathol 2016;40(4):433–42.

41. Kao Y, Sung Y, Zhang L, et al. Recurrent BCOR Internal Tandem Duplication and YWHAE-NUTM2B Fusions in Soft Tissue Undifferentiated Round Cell Sarcoma of Infancy. Am J Surg Pathol 2016;40(8):1009–20.

42. Karlsson J, Valind A, Gisselsson D. BCOR internal tandem duplication and YWHAE-NUTM2B/E fusion are mutually exclusive events in clear cell sarcoma of the kidney. Genes Chromosomes Cancer 2016;55(2):120–3.

43. Diaz-Perez JA, Nielsen GP, Antonescu C, et al. EWSR1/FUS-NFATc2 rearranged round cell sarcoma: clinicopathological series of 4 cases and literature review. Hum Pathol 2019;90:45–53.

44. Chougule A, Taylor MS, Nardi V, et al. Spindle and round cell sarcoma With EWSR1-PATZ1 gene fusion. Am J Surg Pathol 2019;43(2):220–8.

45. Koelsche C, Kriegsmann M, Kommoss FKF, et al. DNA methylation profiling distinguishes Ewing-like sarcoma with EWSR1–NFATc2 fusion from Ewing sarcoma. J Cancer Res Clin Oncol 2019;145:1273–81.

46. Bode-Lesniewska B, Fritz C, Exner GU, et al. EWSR1-NFATC2 and FUS-NFATC2 gene fusion-associated mesenchymal tumors: clinicopathologic correlation and literature review. Sarcoma 2019;2019:9386390.

47. Bridge JA, Sumegi J, Druta M, et al. Clinical, pathological, and genomic features of EWSR1-PATZ1 fusion sarcoma. Mod Pathol 2019;32:1593–604.

48. Cohen JN, Sabnis AJ, Krings G, et al. EWSR1-NFATC2 gene fusion in a soft tissue tumor with epithelioid round cell morphology and abundant stroma: a case report and review of the literature. Hum Pathol 2018;81:281–90.

49. Wang GY, Thomas DG, Davis JL, et al. EWSR1-NFATC2 Translocation-associated Sarcoma Clinicopathologic Findings in a Rare Aggressive Primary Bone or Soft Tissue Tumor. Am J Surg Pathol 2019;43(8):1112–22.

50. Wang L, Bhargava R, Zheng T, et al. Undifferentiated small round cell sarcomas with rare EWS gene fusions: identification of a novel EWS-SP3 fusion and of additional cases with the EWS-ETV1 and EWS-FEV fusions. J Mol Diagn 2007;9(4):498–509.

51. Sumegi J, Nishio J, Nelson M, et al. A novel t(4;22)(q31;q12) produces an EWSR1–SMARCA5 fusion in extraskeletal Ewing sarcoma/primitive neuroectodermal tumor. Mod Pathol 2011;24:333–42.

52. Shaffer LG, Bejjani BA. A cytogeneticist's perspective on genomic microarrays. Hum Reprod Update 2004;10(3):221–6.

53. Imataka G, Arisaka O. Chromosome analysis using spectral karyotyping (SKY). Cell Biochem Biophys 2012;62(1):13–7.

54. Bridge JA, Cushman-Vokoun AM. Molecular diagnostics of soft tissue tumors. Arch Pathol Lab Med 2011;135(5):588–601.

55. Igbokwe A, Lopez-Terrada DH. Molecular testing of solid tumors. Arch Pathol Lab Med 2011;135(1):67–82.

56. Lazar A, Lynne V, Abruzzo RE, et al. Molecular diagnosis of sarcomas: chromosomal translocations in sarcomas. Arch Pathol Lab Med 2006;130(8):1199–207.

57. Sheth J, Arnoldo A, Zhong Y, et al. Sarcoma subgrouping by detection of fusion transcripts using NanoString nCounter technology. Pediatr Dev Pathol 2019;22(3):205–13.

58. Geiss GK, Bumgarner RE, Birditt B, et al. Direct multiplexed measurement of gene expression with color-coded probe pairs. Nat Biotechnol 2008;26(3):317–25.

59. Lilljebjörn H, Henningsson R, Hyrenius-Wittsten A, et al. Identification of ETV6-RUNX1-like and DUX4-rearranged subtypes in paediatric B-cell precursor acute lymphoblastic leukaemia. Nat Commun 2016;7:11790.

60. Miettinen M, Wang Z, Paetau A, et al. ERG transcription factor as an immunohistochemical marker for vascular endothelial tumors and prostatic carcinoma. Am J Surg Pathol 2011;35(3):432–41.

61. Foo WC, Cruise MW, Wick MR, et al. Immunohistochemical staining for TLE1 distinguishes synovial sarcoma from histologic mimics. Am J Clin Pathol 2011;135(6):839–44.

62. Kao YC, Sung YS, Zhang L, et al. BCOR overexpression is a highly sensitive marker in round cell sarcomas with BCOR genetic abnormalities. Am J Surg Pathol 2016;40(12):1670–8.

63. Creytens D. SATB2 and TLE1 expression in BCOR-CCNB3 (Ewing-like) sarcoma, mimicking small cell osteosarcoma and poorly differentiated synovial sarcoma. Appl Immunohistochem Mol Morphol 2020;28(1):e10–2.

64. Davis JL, Horvai AE. Special AT-rich sequence-binding protein 2 (SATB2) expression is sensitive but may not be specific for osteosarcoma as compared with other high-grade primary bone sarcomas. Histopathology 2016;69(1):84–90.

Histopathologic and Molecular Features of Central Nervous System Embryonal Tumors for Integrated Diagnosis Reporting

Bonnie L. Cole, MD[a,b],
Christopher R. Pierson, MD, PhD[c,d,e],*

KEYWORDS

- Atypical teratoid rhabdoid tumor • CNS embryonal tumor
- Embryonal tumor with multilayered rosettes • Integrated diagnosis • Medulloblastoma
- Molecular testing • Subgroup

Key points

- Integrating histopathologic and molecular data in diagnostic reporting improves accuracy and, in turn, patient care.
- The integrated diagnosis provides needed flexibility to allow the incorporation of new knowledge into practice as the understanding of tumor biology increases.
- Pathologists must keep abreast of recent developments in order to report accurate integrated diagnoses for embryonal tumors.

ABSTRACT

Embryonal tumors of the pediatric central nervous system are challenging clinically and diagnostically. These tumors are aggressive, and patients often have poor outcomes even with intense therapy. Proper tumor classification is essential to patient care, and this process has undergone significant changes with the World Health Organization recommending histopathologic and molecular features be integrated in diagnostic reporting. This has especially impacted the workup of embryonal tumors because molecular testing has resulted in the identification of clinically relevant tumor subgroups and new entities. This review summarizes recent developments and provides a framework to workup embryonal tumors in diagnostic practice.

OVERVIEW

Embryonal tumors of the central nervous system (CNS) represent a heterogeneous group of

^a Department of Laboratories, Seattle Children's Hospital, OC.8.720, 4800 Sand Point Way Northeast, 1959 NE Pacific St., Box 357470, Seattle, WA 98105, USA; ^b Department of Anatomic Pathology, University of Washington School of Medicine, 1959 NE Pacific St., Box 357470, Seattle, WA 98195, USA; ^c Department of Pathology and Laboratory Medicine, Nationwide Children's Hospital, J0359, 700 Children's Drive, Columbus, OH 43205, USA; ^d Department of Pathology, The Ohio State University, 129 Hamilton Hall, 1645 Neil Avenue, Columbus, OH 43210, USA; ^e Department of Biomedical Education & Anatomy, The Ohio State University, 1645 Neil Avenue, Columbus, OH 43210, USA
* Corresponding author. Department of Pathology and Laboratory Medicine, Nationwide Children's Hospital, J0359, 700 Children's Drive, Columbus, OH 43205.
E-mail address: Christopher.pierson@nationwidechildrens.org

Surgical Pathology 13 (2020) 783–800
https://doi.org/10.1016/j.path.2020.08.005
1875-9181/20/© 2020 Elsevier Inc. All rights reserved.

neoplasms that are populated by poorly differentiated, highly proliferative cells that confer a small blue cell appearance to a tumor.[1] These tumors are histologically high grade and clinically aggressive. Brain tumors are the leading cause of cancer-related death in children, and embryonal tumors are the most common high-grade brain tumor in children; from birth to 4 years of age, they are the most common type of brain tumor.[2] These tumor types have several overlapping morphologic and immunophenotypic features, so they can be challenging to distinguish from each other and from nonembryonal brain tumors. Applying advances in molecular genetics to diagnostic practice has enhanced the ability to reliably distinguish embryonal tumors and is a reliable complement to morphologic diagnosis. Molecular testing has showed that these tumors are far more heterogeneous than previously imagined. The identification of unique driver mutations and epigenetic alterations has redefined tumor classification and demonstrated new relationships among existing tumor types. In the process, new entities were identified, and new categories, anchored to molecular-based subgroups, were established. The World Health Organization (WHO) recognized that incorporating molecular information with histopathology, grade, and immunohistochemical findings, using a layered approach known as the integrated diagnosis (example in **Table 1**), would improve diagnostic accuracy and patient care and be flexible enough to incorporate new information as it is discovered.[3] Here, the authors review advances in embryonal tumors that will facilitate the reporting of an integrated diagnosis by practicing pathologists.

MEDULLOBLASTOMA

CLINICOPATHOLOGIC FEATURES

Medulloblastoma accounts for about a quarter of all childhood brain tumors, making it the most common embryonal tumor. Medulloblastoma is far less common in adults. The WHO defines medulloblastoma as a grade IV, small round blue cell tumor of the cerebellum with 5 histologies recognized: classic, desmoplastic/nodular (DN), medulloblastoma with extensive nodularity (MBEN), and large cell, and anaplastic; the latter 2 patterns are combined into 1 histologic group, large cell/anaplastic (LCA).[1] Classic medulloblastoma shows densely cellular patternless sheets or large groups of poorly differentiated cells. The cells have inconspicuous cytoplasm and hyperchromatic nuclei without discernible nucleoli. Mitoses and karyorrhexis are typically abundant. Neuronal differentiation is typical in medulloblastomas, as reflected by Homer Wright rosettes (~40%) and immunohistochemically as synaptophysin, NeuN, or neurofilament expression (**Fig. 1A**). The DN type comprises ~20% of all medulloblastomas overall and ~50% of those in patients less than 3 years of age. Its architecture is mixed with densely cellular, poorly differentiated, mitotically active areas interrupted by variably sized nodules with comparatively more neuronal differentiation and lower proliferative rates (**Fig. 1B, C**). The internodular zones have abundant reticulin, whereas nodules lack reticulin, and this pattern is a diagnostic feature of DN (**Fig. 1D**). Nodules express relatively more neuronal markers than internodular zones (**Fig. 1E**). MBEN tends to occur in infants and can be thought of as a pronounced form of DN whereby nodules predominate and internodular zones are reduced (**Fig. 1F**). The nodules are large with irregular, lobulated configurations. The cell population within the nodules is typically arranged in linear streams and consists of neurocytic cells with small, round nuclei and scant cytoplasm.

The large cell type is seen in ~4% of medulloblastomas and is clinically aggressive. It shows large cells with vesicular nuclei and prominent nucleoli (**Fig. 1G**). The anaplastic type comprises ~15% of medulloblastomas and shows nuclear enlargement with pronounced pleomorphism. Several nuclei intimately wrap around a neighboring nucleus beyond the extent of nuclear molding often encountered in classic medulloblastomas (**Fig. 1H**). Multinucleated tumor cells may be seen. Anaplastic and large medulloblastomas are clinically aggressive, and both have high proliferation rates, atypical mitoses, and pronounced karyorrhexis/apoptosis, whereby

Table 1	
Sample embryonal tumor integrated diagnosis	
Integrated diagnosis:	Medulloblastoma, classic, WNT-activated WHO grade IV
Histologic classification:	Medulloblastoma, classic
WHO grade:	Grade IV
Molecular information:	Beta-catenin nuclear expression (immunohistochemistry [IHC]) Monosomy 6 positive (FISH) YAP1 expressed (IHC) GAB1 not expressed (IHC)

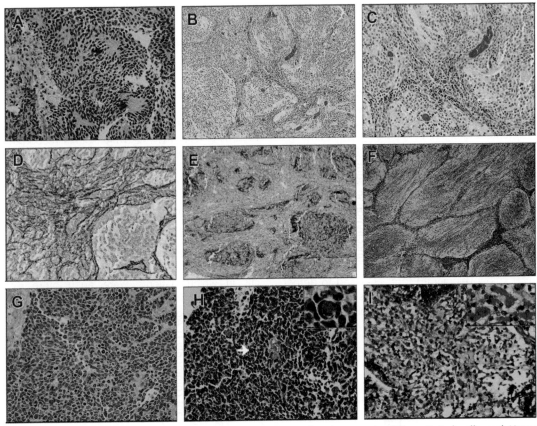

Fig. 1. Medulloblastoma histopathologic types. Classic type showing poorly differentiated cells and Homer Wright rosettes [hematoxylin-eosin, original magnification 200x] (*A*, *arrows*), (*B*) DN type with nodules and inter-nodular zones [B, hematoxylin-eosin, original magnification 200x; C, hematoxylin-eosin, original magnification 400x] (*B*, *C*), reticulin [hematoxylin-eosin, original magnification 200x] (*D*), and synaptophysin immunostaining [hematoxylin-eosin, original magnification 200x] (*E*) to demonstrate tumor architecture. MBEN histology [hematoxylin-eosin, original magnification 100x] (*F*) has back-to-back nodules with cells arranged in linear arrays, without intervening desmoplastic zones. Large cell type features large nuclei with open chromatin [hematoxylin-eosin, original magnification 400x] (*G*). Anaplastic type [hematoxylin-eosin, original magnification 400x] (*H*) shows marked pleomorphism, multinucleation, and wrapping (*arrow*). Medullomyoblastoma showing tumor cells with eosinophilic cytoplasm [hematoxylin-eosin, original magnification 400x] (*I*).

the dying cells amalgamate into little groups known as apoptotic lakes. For these reasons and because large cell and anaplastic histolopathologies may coexist in a given tumor, the WHO combines them into a single variant, LCA. LCA histopathology may occur within other histologic types, but it must predominate in a given tumor for it to be a true LCA medulloblastoma.

Finally, myogenic or melanotic differentiation may be encountered and is known as medullomyoblastoma or melanocytic medulloblastoma. The WHO considers them morphologic variants and not distinct entities.[1] Myogenic differentiation takes the form of rhabdomyoblasts with variable eosinophilic cytoplasm containing striations that express skeletal muscle proteins, such as desmin (**Fig. 1I**). Melanotic differentiation mimics melanocytes or retinal pigment epithelium morphologically with pigmentation and melanocytic marker (HMB-45) expression.

Histopathology, although helpful, does not capture the full extent of medulloblastoma heterogeneity and is susceptible to interobserver variability, so more informative and reliable classification methods were needed.[4] Several studies showed that molecular testing reproducibly identifies subgroups within medulloblastoma that reflect tumor heterogeneity better than histopathology. Each subgroup is distinct biologically and in terms of patient demographics and outcomes. The WHO recognizes medulloblastoma molecular subgroups: WNT-activated; SHH-activated, *TP53*-wildtype; SHH-activated, *TP53*-mutant; non-WNT/non-SHH (group 3); and group 4; all have different mutation, gene expression, DNA methylation, and cytogenetic profiles (**Table 2**).[1] Histopathology poorly

Table 2
Genetically defined medulloblastoma at a glance

WHO Recognized Subtypes	WNT-Activated	SHH-Activated, TP53-Mutant	SHH-Activated, TP53-Wildtype	Non-WNT/Non-SHH Group 3	Non-WNT/Non-SHH Group 4
Age	Mostly children and some adults; uncommon in infants	Primarily infants and adults; fewer children		Mostly children, sometimes infants, uncommon in adults	Mostly children, sometimes infants and adults
Gender	Male = Female		Male > Female	Male > Female	Male > Female
Prognosis	Very good	Very poor	Intermediate overall; Infants good	Poor	Intermediate
Risk category	Low if <16 y old. May not be as favorable over 16 y of age	Very high: either metastatic or nonmetastatic	Standard: no $MYCN$ amplification and nonmetastatic. High: has either or both $MYCN$ amplification and metastasis	Standard: No MYC amplification and nonmetastatic. Very high: metastatic	Low: Nonmetastatic and chromosome 11 loss. Standard: Nonmetastatic, no chromosome 11 loss. High: Metastatic
Histology	Classic >> LCA	Classic (~40%), DN (~35%), MBEN (~10%), LCA (~15%) SHH-activated, TP53-wildtype commonly DN SHH-activated, TP53-mutant commonly LCA		Classic, LCA	Classic, LCA
Immunohistochemistry for subtyping	Nuclei beta-catenin and YAP1 positive	GAB1, filamin A, and YAP1 positive		YAP1 negative; nuclei beta-catenin negative and GAB1 negative IHC can distinguish non-WNT/non-SHH tumors from WNT- and SHH-activated tumors but it cannot distinguish group 3 and 4 tumors from each other	

	WNT	SHH	Group 3	Group 4

Genetic testing	Profiling
	WNT pattern by DNA methylation or gene expression profiling
	SNV
	  CTNNB1 exon 3 gof or *APC* lof
	Cytogenetics
	  Monosomy 6
		Profiling
		SHH *pattern* by DNA methylation or gene expression profiling
		SNV/deletions
		  PTCH1 (del, lof): all ages
		  SUFU (del, lof): infants
		  SMO (gof): adults
		  TP53 deletions/lof mutations
		Amplifications
		  GLI1, GLI2, or *MYCN*
		Cytogenetics
		  9q or 10q loss
			Profiling
			Group 3 *pattern by* DNA methylation or gene expression profiling
			Cytogenetics
			  i17q
			Amplifications
			  MYC, OTX2
			SNV
			  In 5%+ of cases:
			    SMARCA4, KBTBD4, CTDNEP1, and *KMT2D* cases
				Profiling
				Group 4 pattern by DNA *methylation* or gene expression profiling
				Cytogenetics
				  i17q, loss 11q
				Amplification
				  MYCN
				Duplication
				  SNCAIP
				SNV
				  In <10% of cases:
				    KDM6A, ZMYM3, KTM2C, and *KBTBD4*

Differential diagnosis	CNS embryonal tumor Atypical teratoid rhabdoid tumor Embryonal tumor with multilayered rosettes Ependymoma, anaplastic High-grade astrocytoma			
Practice points	Medulloblastoma, NOS is used by WHO if a tissue artifact or sample inadequacy precludes classification of the medulloblastoma further and other entities (eg, ATRT, ETMR, gliomas) are excluded. A small proportion of non-WNT/non-SHH medulloblastomas that have overlapping molecular profiling data and are intermediate in the sense that they could be assigned to either group 3 or to group 4 data, which suggests that they may have a better prognosis than group 3 and group 4 tumors overall.			

Abbreviations: Del, deletion; gof, gain of function; lof, loss of function; NOS, not otherwise specified.

aligns with subgroup. WNT-activated medulloblastomas are almost always classic with rare LCA tumors. DN and MBEN are essentially always SHH-activated; however, all histopathologies are possible in the SHH-activated group. The SHH-activated, TP53-wildtype subgroup is commonly DN, whereas the SHH-activated, TP53-mutant group is often LCA. Group 3 and group 4 medulloblastomas may be classic or LCA.[4–9]

The recognized subgroups were initially identified by transcriptional profiling, which remains an effective means of subgroup determination clinically, although DNA methylation profiling has probably emerged as the best test for subgroup determination, owing to the fact that each subgroup can be robustly identified using small amounts of DNA from archival tissues.[10–13] In these assays, the gene expression or methylation profile of the tumor undergoing testing is compared with profiles of known medulloblastomas from each subgroup to determine the best match. Unfortunately, these assays are not widely available, so other testing strategies are used, and these too will be discussed.[14,15]

Subgroup classification is likely to evolve. It follows that studying larger numbers of tumors using more sensitive assays with better data interpretation algorithms would be capable of resolving greater complexity within the recognized subgroups. Therefore, as progress advances, it is expected that distinct subsets within the currently recognized subgroups will emerge and classification systems will change accordingly. This change is already occurring, and the emerging subsets within the subgroups are termed "subtypes" and designated by Greek letters until more data become available.[4] The WHO does not recognize subtypes, so they will not be detailed here, but this will likely be of future importance.[12,16]

MOLECULAR SUBGROUPS

WNT-Activated Medulloblastoma

WNT-activated tumors comprise ~10% of medulloblastomas, affect male and female patients equally, and often arise in patients over 4 years old with a peak incidence ~10 years. They make up ~15% of adult medulloblastomas and are rare in infants. WNT-activated tumors arise along the dorsal brainstem, just off the fourth ventricular midline, where they may involve the cerebellar peduncles or cerebellopontine angle.[17] WNT-activated medulloblastomas have survival rates of 95% in children; however, in patients older than 16 years old, the prognosis may not be as favorable. The underlying reason for the excellent prognosis in this subgroup is unknown, but they metastasize infrequently (~10%), rarely recur, and rarely show LCA histopathology; however, even if they are LCA, the prognosis remains favorable.[18]

Gene expression or DNA methylation profiling can identify WNT-activated medulloblastomas. If these assays are unavailable, a tumor may be classified as WNT-activated if two of the following are supportive: beta-catenin nuclear immunolabeling, CTNNB1 mutation analysis, or monosomy chromosome 6 detection.[15] Somatic CTNNB1 exon 3 mutations are found in ~90% of WNT-activated medulloblastomas, whereas ~10% have somatic APC mutations.[19,20] Germline APC mutations (familial adenomatous polyposis) are also possible. These mutations converge on beta-catenin to upregulate WNT-signaling. CTNNB1 encodes beta-catenin, and mutations stabilize the protein, so it accumulates in the nucleus. APC regulates beta-catenin degradation, and loss-of-function mutations result in beta-catenin persistence and its subsequent nuclear accumulation. Beta-catenin nuclear accumulation is the hallmark of WNT-signaling, and it is detectable immunohistochemically. Beta-catenin nuclear labeling is typically diffuse in WNT-activated medulloblastoma, but occasionally it is limited to a few percent of tumor cells.[14] Monosomy of chromosome 6 occurs in ~80% of WNT-activated tumors and is more common in tumors with CTNNB1 mutations. Monosomy 6 can be detected using fluorescence in situ hybridization (FISH) or DNA copy number arrays, and it provides evidence to support classification as WNT-activated; however, it is occasionally encountered in other subgroups, making it a suboptimal stand-alone test.[15] Other than monosomy of chromosome 6, WNT-activated tumors generally have balanced genomes without large amplifications or deletions.

SHH-Activated Medulloblastoma

SHH-activated tumors have a balanced gender ratio and show a bimodal age distribution, most commonly affecting infants (0–3 years) and adults (>16 years). These tumors are thought to originate from granular cell precursors and tend to arise in the cerebellar hemispheres.[17] SHH-activated medulloblastoma comprise ~30% of all medulloblastomas and are classified using TP53 status because mutations confer very poor outcomes in this subgroup.[1]

Gene expression and DNA methylation profiling are considered the best means to identify SHH-activated medulloblastomas. SHH-activated tumors harbor characteristic somatic or germline mutations or copy number changes in genes that encode SHH-pathway proteins, which result in enhanced SHH-signaling. Somatic loss-of-function mutations or deletions in *PTCH1* (~40%) or *SUFU* (~10%), activating *SMO* mutations (~9%) and amplification of *GLI1* or *GLI2* (~9%) and *MYCN* (~7%), are recurring alterations.[12,19] Germline mutations in *PTCH1* (Gorlin syndrome) or *SUFU* predispose to SHH-activated medulloblastoma. The genomes of SHH-activated tumors are balanced, aside for losses of chromosomes 9q or 10q, which lead to loss of heterozygosity for *PTCH1* (9q22) and *SUFU* (10q24). *TERT* promoter mutations are more prevalent (~39% of SHH-activated tumors) in this subgroup than the others, especially in adults.

GAB1 and filamin A expression is increased in SHH-activated tumors, but not in other medulloblastomas. If expression or methylation profiling or gene testing cannot be performed, GAB1 or filamin A immunohistochemistry may be supportive of SHH-activation, but it should probably not be regarded as definitive.[14,15] *TP53* mutations may be somatic or germline (Li-Fraumeni syndrome). Testing should especially be performed in patients 4 to 17 years old with SHH-activated tumors, because *TP53* mutations are enriched in this age range. Immunohistochemical staining for p53 may show strong, diffuse labeling in *TP53*-mutant tumors, but it should be considered a surrogate to gene testing and not definitive.

Non-WNT, Non-SHH Medulloblastoma: Group 3 and Group 4

Medulloblastoma transcriptome and methylome profiling consistently identified 2 subgroups that, unlike WNT- and SHH-activated tumors, lacked obvious drivers but were reproducibly identified.[12,19] These tumors are collectively referred to as non-WNT/non-SHH or as group 3 and group 4 individually. In contrast to WNT- and SHH-activated medulloblastomas, these subgroups characteristically have unbalanced genomes, and recurrent somatic single nucleotide variations (SNV) are less frequent.

Group 3 comprises ~30% of all medulloblastomas and has a poor prognosis overall because they are commonly metastatic at presentation (~40%). Male patients predominate, and young children or infants tend to be affected. Group 3 tumors involve the vermis and grow into the fourth ventricle. They characteristically show MYC expression: ~17% have *MYC* amplification, whereas some have *PVT1-MYC* fusions. Aneuploidy is common with 25% to 50% harboring isochromosome 17q. Gains of chromosome 7

and 1q and loss of 8, 10q, and 16q are common. In group 3 medulloblastomas, the presence of metastatic disease, isochromosome 17q, or *MYC* amplification is associated with increased risk. In fact, patients with metastatic disease and *MYC* amplification are considered very high risk.[21]

Group 4 comprise ~40% of medulloblastomas, are more frequent in male patients, and occur during childhood and adolescence. Like group 3 tumors, group 4 tumors tend to involve the vermis. Metastasis occurs in up to 40% of cases at diagnosis, but patient outcome is intermediate when compared with group 3. The most common driver mutation is overexpression of the chromatin modifier, PRDM6, associated with *SNCAIP* tandem duplication. Loss-of-function mutations or deletions in certain histone modifier genes occur in less than 10% of cases.[19] *MYCN*, *OTX2*, and *CDK6* amplifications may occur. Typical chromosomal alterations include isochromosome 17q, gains of chromosome 7 and 18q, and losses of 8p, 8q, and 11p. Group 4 tumors in most female patients show loss of one X chromosome.[7,22] Isochromosome 17q occurs in ~66% of group 4 tumors and is not predictive of outcome as it is in group 3. Group 4 tumors with chromosome 11 loss and/or 17 gain have a good outcome even in the presence of metastatic disease.[23]

Gene expression or methylation profiling is needed to subgroup a medulloblastoma, particularly for group 3 or 4 because SNV are infrequent and drivers are unclear. If these assays are unavailable, an immunohistochemical staining panel, including beta-catenin, GAB1 or filamin A, and YAP1, may be used (**Fig. 2**).[14] This panel can separate WNT (beta-catenin immunoreactive nuclei) and SHH (increased GAB1 or filamin A expression) tumors from non-WNT/non-SHH medulloblastomas, but it cannot distinguish group 3 and 4 tumors from each other. In the panel non-WNT/non-SHH, medulloblastomas lack beta-catenin nuclear labeling, and GAB1, filamin A, and YAP1 expression, whereas YAP1 is expressed in both WNT- and SHH-activated medulloblastoma subgroups. The panel is convenient and economical, but it is not considered definitive.

EMBRYONAL TUMOR WITH MULTILAYERED ROSETTES

CLINICOPATHOLOGIC FEATURES

The typical embryonal tumor with multilayered rosettes (ETMR) patient is less than 4 years old, and most are under 2 years of age (**Table 3**). The gender ratio is equal. ETMRs arise in the cerebrum

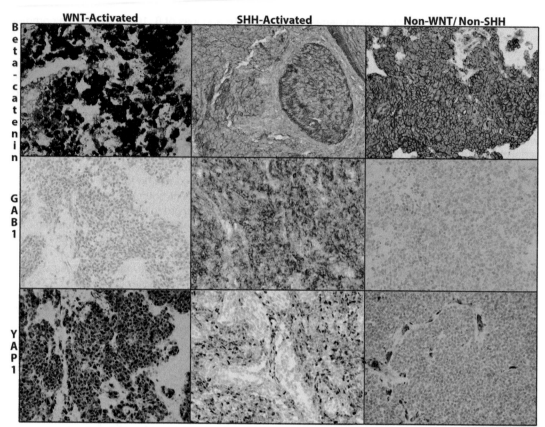

Fig. 2. Medulloblastoma genetic subgroups demonstrating representative immunostaining using subgrouping antibody panel (hematoxylin-eosin, original magnification 400x).

Table 3
Embryonal tumor with multilayered rosettes at a glance

Age	Most are <2 y old, almost all are <4 y
Gender	Male = Female
Location	Supratentorial > Infratentorial; spinal cord and ocular locations are possible
Prognosis	Poor
Histology	Richly cellular WHO grade IV neoplasm with embryonal cell population, neuropil-like areas, multilayered or true rosettes, anaplasia, abundant mitoses, and karyorrhexis
Genetics	Chromosome 19q13.42 *C19MC* alterations (amplifications or fusions) are defining of ETMR
Immunohistochemistry	Diffuse, strong LIN28A expression, used as a surrogate marker
Differential diagnosis	CNS embryonal tumor Medulloblastoma, for cerebellar tumors Atypical teratoid rhabdoid tumor Ependymoma, anaplastic Immature teratoma with neuroepithelial elements
Practice points	ETMR, NOS refers to an ETMR in which *C19MC* has not been tested ETMR, not elsewhere classified, refers to a tumor with histologic and immunohistochemical features of ETMR where molecular testing was negative for *C19MC*-alteration

(70% of cases), cerebellum, or brainstem (combined 30% of cases).[24] These tumors are clinically aggressive, and the prognosis is poor. The incidence of ETMR is unknown due in part to diagnostic variability related to differences in past terminology used for various histopathologic patterns. Now all of these patterns are known to harbor a molecular alteration in *C19MC*, which unifies them as ETMRs.[1,25–28]

ETMR is populated by poorly differentiated cells with high-grade cytologic features, including brisk mitoses and abundant karyorrhexis, although this is not universal, and some examples are bland cytologically (**Fig. 3**A).[26,28] Tumor cells can grow

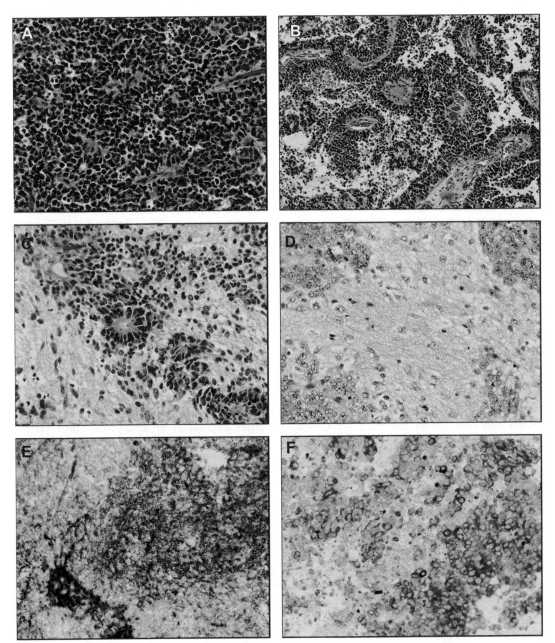

Fig. 3. ETMR histopathology showing poorly differentiated cell population [hematoxylin-eosin, original magnification 200x] (*A*), papillary architecture [hematoxylin-eosin, original magnification 200x] (*B*), multilayered rosettes [hematoxylin-eosin, original magnification 400x] (*C*), and neuropil-like tissue [hematoxylin-eosin, original magnification 400x] (*D*). Representative synaptophysin [hematoxylin-eosin, original magnification 400x] (*E*) and LIN28A [hematoxylin-eosin, original magnification 400x] (*F*) immunohistochemistry.

in sheets, papillae, or trabeculae (**Fig.** 3B). There are characteristic rosettes with multiple layers of cells and distinct luminal borders; however, rosettes may be rare or focally present (**Fig.** 3C). The histopathologic patterns include embryonal tumor with abundant neuropil and true rosettes (ETANTR), ependymoblastoma, and medulloepithelioma; multiple histologic patterns may be encountered in the same tumor. The ETANTR pattern has true rosettes and prominent neuropil.[24,29] Ependymoblastoma has an embryonal cell component, which characteristically abuts or merges with the periphery of multilayered rosettes, forming a so-called ependymoblastic rosette. Neuropil-like tissue may be sparse in ependymoblastoma. Unlike true ependymomas, ependymoblastoma shows little to no Epithelial membrane antigen (EMA) expression, and if observed, it will be limited to the lumen edge and typically lack the dotlike pattern of ependymoma. Medulloepithelioma has embryonal cells growing in trabecular, tubular, or papillary structures. Medulloepithelioma may have evidence of neuronal, ependymal, astrocytic, and oligodendroglial differentiation, and multilayered rosettes are variable.

The neuropil-like tissue and, if present, neurocytic cells are strongly immunoreactive for synaptophysin and variably immunolabel with NeuN and neurofilament (**Fig.** 3D, E). Glial fibrillary acidic protein (GFAP) expression is minimal or absent. ETMR expresses pluripotency proteins, and one of them, LIN28A, is used as a surrogate diagnostic marker. Cytoplasmic LIN28A immunolabeling is characteristically diffuse and intense in *C19MC*-altered tumors (**Fig.** 3F). LIN28A not entirely specific for ETMR because other embryonal tumors may express it albeit focally or weakly. Nonetheless, LIN28A can help gauge the need for *C19MC* testing, which is diagnostic.

MOLECULAR FEATURES

The characteristic alteration in ETMR consists of fusions and amplifications of the *C19MC* microRNA cluster on chromosome 19q13.4.[30,31] This chromosomal region is thought to be relatively unstable and prone to fusion of *TTYH1* with *C19MC*.[32] A subset of ETMRs lacks rosettes and neuropil and consists exclusively of embryonal cells, making molecular testing important for accurate diagnosis.

ATYPICAL TERATOID RHABDOID TUMOR

CLINICOPATHOLOGIC FEATURES

Atypical teratoid rhabdoid tumors (ATRTs) tend to arise in the first 5 years of life, making them the most common brain tumor of infants. ATRT is uncommon after age 10 years. ATRT preferentially affects male patients, and they arise with equal frequency in the cerebrum and cerebellum, but are less common in the brainstem and spinal cord. Posterior fossa ATRTs are more common in the first 2 years of life. ATRT patients may present with multifocal disease, and tumor may spread via cerebrospinal fluid pathways. Intense treatment approaches are required, and the prognosis is generally poor. Approximately 30% of cases arise in the setting of rhabdoid tumor predisposition syndrome (RTPS) 1, which is due to inactivating germline *SMARCB1* mutation. Rarely, cases are associated with RTPS 2, owing to inactivating germline *SMARCA4* mutation. Predisposition syndrome patients are at risk for multifocal disease at presentation in either the brain or elsewhere (commonly renal) or in combination.

ATRT is a WHO grade IV embryonal tumor defined by biallelic inactivation of *SMARCB1* and corresponding loss of expression for the encoding protein, INI-1. Rarely, *SMARCA4* biallelic inactivation with loss of its corresponding encoded protein, BRG1, is observed.[33,34] ATRT has a wide variety of histopathologic appearances. Typically there is a population of poorly differentiated, embryonal cells that often includes rhabdoid cells (**Fig.** 4A, B). The characteristic rhabdoid cell has an eccentrically situated vesicular nucleus with a prominent nucleolus and eosinophilic cytoplasm. Rhabdoid cells are often easier to appreciate in smear preparations or at low magnification, whereby an eosinophilic background is noted. Sometimes rhabdoid cells are inconspicuous or absent among a much larger population of embryonal cells. ATRT is capable of significant heterogeneity, and cells may differentiate along glial (including ependymal), mesenchymal, or epithelial lines, so tumor architecture is variable and can be mixed with sheets, nests, trabeculae, cords, fascicles, and glandlike or papillary structures. Immunohistochemistry shows loss of INI-1 expression in virtually every tumor nucleus, which is diagnostic, whereas expression is retained in nonneoplastic elements (vessels and inflammatory cells) (**Fig.** 4C). Most ATRTs show membranous or cytoplasmic EMA immunoreactivity (**Fig.** 4D). Immunohistochemistry for neuronal (synaptophysin, neurofilament) and glial (GFAP) markers is often at least focally positive (**Fig.** 4E). ATRT may show immunoreactivity for cytokeratins, smooth muscle actin, and vimentin, but not for desmin.

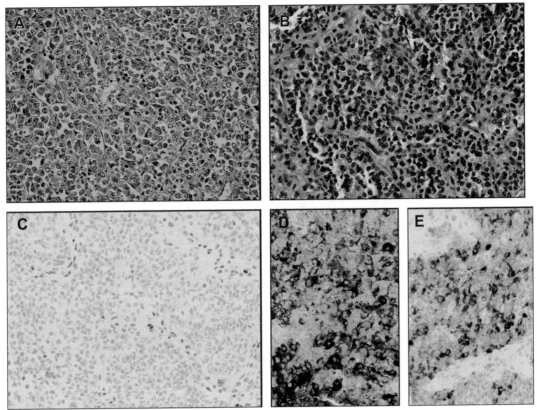

Fig. 4. ATRT histopathology demonstrating rhabdoid [hematoxylin-eosin, original magnification 400x] (*A*) and poorly differentiated cells [hematoxylin-eosin, original magnification 400x] (*B*). Immunohistochemistry shows loss of INI-1 expression in tumor but not endothelial cell nuclei [hematoxylin-eosin, original magnification 400x] (*C*), membranous and cytoplasmic EMA [hematoxylin-eosin, original magnification 400x] (*D*), and synaptophysin expression [hematoxylin-eosin, original magnification 400x] (*E*).

MOLECULAR FEATURES

SMARCB1 (rarely *SMARCA4*) biallelic loss-of-function alterations are due to mutations and/or deletions. Deletions may be large and encompass the *SMARCB1* locus at 22q. An integrated diagnosis of ATRT requires *SMARCB1* (*SMARCA4*) gene testing or INI-1 (BRG1) immunohistochemistry. INI-1 and BRG1 are subunits of the SWI/SNF chromatin remodeling complex, and when either is missing, epigenetic dysregulation results.[35] How this drives ATRT pathogenesis is unknown; however, it is potent because studies show that ATRTs have quiet genomes with *SMARCB1* as the only recurrent alteration in some tumors.[36] Transcriptomic and methylation profiling studies have revealed ATRT subgroups that differ in patient demographics, tumor location, and *SMARCB1* genotype (**Table 4**).[37–39] Currently, ATRT molecular subgrouping is not recognized by the WHO, but it may in the future.[40,41] Three subgroups are acknowledged: (1) ATRT-SHH, with increased SHH signaling; (2) ATRT-TYR, which shows overexpression of certain melanosomal markers including tyrosinase; (3) ATRT-MYC, with increased MYC expression.[37,42] Studies show that ATRT-SHH and ATRT-MYC tumors may have a worse prognosis than ATRT-TYR tumors, and tyrosinase expression may be a useful ATRT-TYR marker.[37,41] Expression of ASCL1, a NOTCH1 signaling regulator, may be a prognostic marker because it correlated with better prognosis in 1 study.[39]

CENTRAL NERVOUS SYSTEM EMBRYONAL TUMORS

CLINICOPATHOLOGIC AND MOLECULAR FEATURES

Central nervous system embryonal tumors account for ~2% of pediatric CNS neoplasms (**Table 5**). The mean age of presentation is ~6 years, and overall, they are more common in male patients. Most arise in the cerebral hemispheres, but the cerebellum, brainstem, and spinal cord can be involved. The overall 5-year survival rate is 20% to 30%. Broadly speaking, all

Table 4
Atypical teratoid rhabdoid tumors at a glance

Subgroups (Not Recognized by WHO) Preferred Methodology: DNA Methylation Profiling	ATRT-TYR	ATRT-SHH	ATRT-MYC
Age (median)	12 mo	20 mo	27 mo
Location	Infratentorial > Supratentorial	Supratentorial > Infratentorial	Supratentorial > Infratentorial; spinal
Prognosis	Relatively better: TYR > SHH and MYC; relatively worse		
Genetics: SMARCB1 alterations	Point mutations and focal deletions	Compound heterozygous point mutations, some focal deletions	Large deletions
Histology	Densely cellular, WHO grade IV tumor with variable population of rhabdoid cells and a poorly differentiated, embryonal cell component		
Immunohisto-chemistry	INI-1 loss Possible diagnostic marker: tyrosinase	INI-1 loss Possible prognostic marker: ASCL1	INI-1 loss
Differential diagnosis	Embryonal tumor with multilayered rosettes CNS embryonal tumors Medulloblastoma, for cerebellar tumors Choroid plexus carcinoma Ependymoma, anaplastic Composite rhabdoid tumors, such as meningioma or glioma with rhabdoid cells		
Practice points	Up to 4% of ATRT cases will have intact SMARCB1 alleles and retained INI-1 expression; many of these will show biallelic loss-of-function mutations in SMARCA4 and loss of BRG1 expression CNS embryonal tumor with rhabdoid features refers to an embryonal tumor with rhabdoid cells and other morphologic features of ATRT (eg, polyphenotypic differentiation) in which SMARCB1/INI-1 and SMARCA4/BRG1 are intact or not tested		

Table 5
Central nervous system embryonal tumors at a glance

Emerging Subgroups (Not WHO Recognized)	CNS NB-FOXR2	CNS EFT-CIC	CNS HGNT-BCOR ITD	CNS HGNET-MN1
Age	Infants to young adults	More common in infants	More common in infants	More common in adolescence and adults
Gender ratio	Male < Female	Male > Female	Might be more common in males	Male << Female
Location	Supratentorial	Supratentorial	Supratentorial or infratentorial	Supratentorial > Infratentorial
Prognosis	Fair	Fair	Poor	Favorable
Histology	CNS neuroblastoma CNS ganglioneuroblastoma	Alveolar, fascicular	Spindle to ovoid cells Pseudopallisading necrosis	Diverse: solid and pseudopapillary Stromal hyalinization
Genetics	Rearrangements that increase FOXR2 expression	ETS transcription factors upregulated due to CIC rearrangement Subset with CIC-NUTM1 fusion	Internal tandem duplication in BCOR exon 15	MN1 rearrangements
Immunohisto-chemistry	Synaptophysin and OLIG2 positive	Lack neuronal and glial differentiation NUTM1 expression in CIC-NUTM1 fused tumors	GFAP-positive perivascular pseudorosettes Synaptophysin negative OLIG2 positive BCOR nuclear expression, uncertain specificity	Limited expression of glial and neuronal markers
Differential diagnosis	Embryonal tumor with multilayered rosettes Medulloblastoma, for cerebellar tumors Atypical teratoid rhabdoid tumor Ependymoma, especially anaplastic High-grade astrocytoma Astroblastoma vs CNS HGNT-BCOR ITD and CNS HGNET-MN1			

members of this group are WHO grade IV, densely cellular neoplasms populated by actively proliferating, poorly differentiated small blue cells that commonly show some degree of neuronal differentiation and possibly glial or occasional epithelial, myogenic, or melanocytic differentiation (**Fig. 5**A–C). Mitotic activity is readily evident, and necrosis is common. In the past, these tumors were classified as primitive neuroectodermal tumors (PNET) because they arose in children, morphologically resembled embryonic cells, and lacked defining features of other embryonal tumors. The term PNET has recently been abandoned by the WHO and replaced with CNS neuroblastoma, CNS ganglioneuroblastoma, medulloepithelioma, and CNS embryonal tumor, NOS (**Fig. 5**A, D).[1] These tumors are diagnostically challenging because of a lack of distinguishing morphologic and immunohistochemical features and overlapping features shared with other high-grade CNS tumors. Molecular groups, which have recently been described, include CNS neuroblastoma with *FOXR2*

activation, CNS high-grade neuroepithelial tumor with *BCOR* internal tandem duplication, CNS high-grade neuroepithelial tumor with *MN1* alteration, and CNS Ewing sarcoma family tumor with *CIC* alteration.[43–46] These newly identified molecular alterations are not recognized by the WHO as subgroup defining; however, this area of classification is rapidly evolving, and it is likely that these entities will be incorporated in future editions of the WHO classification system.

HISTOLOGIC MIMICS OF CENTRAL NERVOUS SYSTEM EMBRYONAL TUMORS

Although most brain tumors with embryonal histology can be classified into the categories previously described, it is important to be aware of histologic mimics (**Fig. 6**). Because this diverse group of tumors is not the focus of this article, they will only be mentioned here briefly. Anaplastic ependymomas and high-grade gliomas are the most common tumors mistaken for CNS

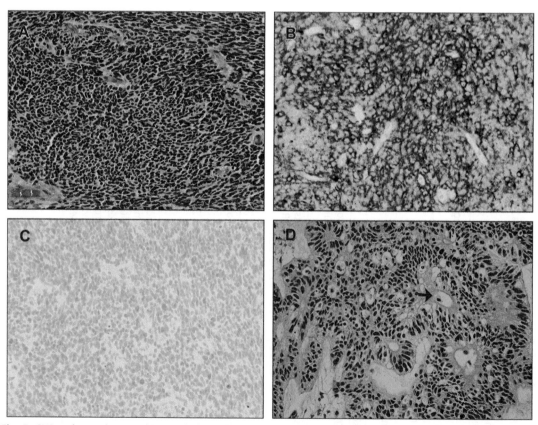

Fig. 5. CNS embryonal tumor histopathology showing sheets of poorly differentiated cells [hematoxylin-eosin, original magnification 200x] (*A*) that express synaptophysin [hematoxylin-eosin, original magnification 400x] (*B*), but not OLIG2 [hematoxylin-eosin, original magnification 400x] (*C*). Medulloepithelioma showing rosettes (*arrow*) and trabecular architecture [hematoxylin-eosin, original magnification 400x] (*D*).

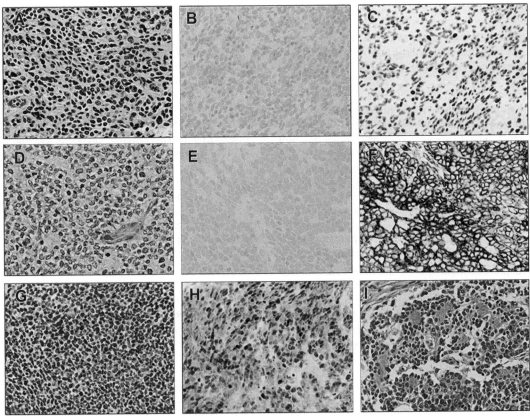

Fig. 6. Histologic mimics of CNS embryonal tumors. High-grade glioma with *H3F3A* mutation [hematoxylin-eosin, original magnification 400x] (*A*); GFAP is essentially negative [original magnification 400x] (*B*), but tumor cell nuclei are positive for H3 K27M by immunohistochemistry. [original magnification 400x] (*C*) This RELA-fusion positive anaplastic ependymoma lacks perivascular pseudorosettes [hematoxylin-eosin, original magnification 400x] (*D*), and lost GFAP immunoreactivity [original magnification 400x] (*E*); diffuse L1CAM staining was retained [original magnification 400x] (*F*). A primary alveolar rhabdomyosarcoma of the CNS with *PAX3-FOXO1* fusion [hematoxylin-eosin, original magnification 400x] (*G*) displays diffuse myogenin staining [original magnification 400x] (*H*). Peripheral neuroblastoma [hematoxylin-eosin, original magnification 400x] (*I*) may either directly extend or metastasize to the CNS.

embryonal tumors.[45,47] Although high-grade gliomas have glial processes and typically express GFAP, these tumors can lose GFAP expression and even display focal synaptophysin staining. Many high-grade gliomas that mimic CNS embryonal tumors have characteristic histone alterations, such as *H3F3A* G34 or K27M mutations; therefore, immunohistochemistry and/or molecular profiling may help with the diagnosis. Anaplastic ependymomas similarly may lose their characteristic histologic and immunohistochemical features. They may not display classic perivascular pseudorosettes and may lack their typical GFAP and dotlike EMA immunolabeling.[48] In evaluation of supratentorial tumors, molecular identification of *RELA* or *YAP* fusions can help ensure that the correct diagnosis of ependymoma is rendered.

Pineal tumors can appear histologically similar to other CNS embryonal tumors; however, the WHO considers them to be in a separate tumor category.[1] Nevertheless, these tumors should be kept in mind when faced with any tumor that radiologically involves the pineal region. Pineoblastoma and other pineal tumors may have immunohistochemical features indistinguishable from other CNS embryonal neoplasms. Clinical and radiologic correlation is a key part of diagnostic practice. Other common pediatric small round blue cell tumors may rarely occur as primary neoplasms of the CNS or as metastases. These tumors include rhabdomyosarcoma, Ewing sarcoma, lymphoma, peripheral neuroblastoma, and others. Starting with a broad differential can help pathologists avoid many of the pitfalls involved in making these challenging diagnoses.

SUMMARY

Molecular testing is certain to increase in importance in embryonal brain tumor diagnostics and patient prognostication; however, histopathology still provides important information so it is unlikely to be supplanted. Molecular testing is powerful, but it cannot classify every tumor. Molecular data also need to be interpreted within a biologic context. For example, *MN1* alterations are not specific for 1 tumor type and may be encountered in certain embryonal tumors or in astroblastoma, and different *BCOR* alterations have been described in different classes of brain tumors.[43–45,49,50] Histopathology, therefore, provides the biological context needed to understand the relevance of an identified molecular alteration, which positions pathologists as the ideal professionals to integrate molecular and histopathological findings in a clinically meaningful way. Because of the growing importance of reporting an integrated diagnosis, the role of pathologists as a member of a multidisciplinary care team will likely only grow going forward.

DISCLOSURE

The authors have no commercial or financial relationship with a direct interest in the subject matter or materials discussed in the article. The authors have no funding sources to report.

REFERENCES

1. Louis DN, Ohgaki H, Wiestler OD, et al. WHO classification of tumours of the central nervous system. Revised 4th edition. Lyon (France): IARC; 2016.
2. Ostrom QT, Gittleman H, Truitt G, et al. CBTRUS statistical report: primary brain and other central nervous system tumors diagnosed in the United States in 2011-2015. Neuro Oncol 2018; 20(suppl_4):iv1–86.
3. Louis DN, Perry A, Reifenberger G, et al. The 2016 World Health Organization classification of tumors of the central nervous system: a summary. Acta Neuropathol 2016;131(6):803–20.
4. Taylor MD, Northcott PA, Korshunov A, et al. Molecular subgroups of medulloblastoma: the current consensus. Acta Neuropathol 2012;123(4):465–72.
5. Cho YJ, Tsherniak A, Tamayo P, et al. Integrative genomic analysis of medulloblastoma identifies a molecular subgroup that drives poor clinical outcome. J Clin Oncol 2011;29(11):1424–30.
6. Kool M, Koster J, Bunt J, et al. Integrated genomics identifies five medulloblastoma subtypes with distinct genetic profiles, pathway signatures and clinicopathological features. PLoS One 2008;3(8): e3088.
7. Northcott PA, Korshunov A, Witt H, et al. Medulloblastoma comprises four distinct molecular variants. J Clin Oncol 2011;29(11):1408–14.
8. Remke M, Hielscher T, Northcott PA, et al. Adult medulloblastoma comprises three major molecular variants. J Clin Oncol 2011;29(19):2717–23.
9. Thompson MC, Fuller C, Hogg TL, et al. Genomics identifies medulloblastoma subgroups that are enriched for specific genetic alterations. J Clin Oncol 2006;24(12):1924–31.
10. Capper D, Jones DTW, Sill M, et al. DNA methylation-based classification of central nervous system tumours. Nature 2018;555(7697):469–74.
11. Capper D, Stichel D, Sahm F, et al. Practical implementation of DNA methylation and copy-number-based CNS tumor diagnostics: the Heidelberg experience. Acta Neuropathol 2018;136(2): 181–210.
12. Hovestadt V, Ayrault O, Swartling FJ, et al. Medulloblastomics revisited: biological and clinical insights from thousands of patients. Nat Rev Cancer 2020; 20(1):42–56.
13. Schwalbe EC, Williamson D, Lindsey JC, et al. DNA methylation profiling of medulloblastoma allows robust subclassification and improved outcome prediction using formalin-fixed biopsies. Acta Neuropathol 2013;125(3):359–71.
14. Ellison DW, Dalton J, Kocak M, et al. Medulloblastoma: clinicopathological correlates of SHH, WNT, and non-SHH/WNT molecular subgroups. Acta Neuropathol 2011;121(3):381–96.
15. Gottardo NG, Hansford JR, McGlade JP, et al. Medulloblastoma Down Under 2013: a report from the third annual meeting of the International Medulloblastoma Working Group. Acta Neuropathol 2014; 127(2):189–201.
16. Cavalli FMG, Remke M, Rampasek L, et al. Intertumoral heterogeneity within medulloblastoma subgroups. Cancer Cell 2017;31(6):737–54.e6.
17. Gibson P, Tong Y, Robinson G, et al. Subtypes of medulloblastoma have distinct developmental origins. Nature 2010;468(7327):1095–9.
18. Ellison DW, Kocak M, Dalton J, et al. Definition of disease-risk stratification groups in childhood medulloblastoma using combined clinical, pathologic, and molecular variables. J Clin Oncol 2011;29(11):1400–7.
19. Northcott PA, Robinson GW, Kratz CP, et al. Medulloblastoma. Nat Rev Dis Primers 2019;5(1):11.
20. Surun A, Varlet P, Brugieres L, et al. Medulloblastomas associated with an APC germline pathogenic variant share the good prognosis of CTNNB1-mutated medulloblastomas. Neuro Oncol 2020; 22(1):128–38.
21. Ramaswamy V, Remke M, Bouffet E, et al. Risk stratification of childhood medulloblastoma in the

molecular era: the current consensus. Acta Neuropathol 2016;131(6):821–31.

22. Kool M, Korshunov A, Remke M, et al. Molecular subgroups of medulloblastoma: an international meta-analysis of transcriptome, genetic aberrations, and clinical data of WNT, SHH, group 3, and group 4 medulloblastomas. Acta Neuropathol 2012;123(4): 473–84.

23. Shih DJ, Northcott PA, Remke M, et al. Cytogenetic prognostication within medulloblastoma subgroups. J Clin Oncol 2014;32(9):886–96.

24. Eberhart CG, Brat DJ, Cohen KJ, et al. Pediatric neuroblastic brain tumors containing abundant neuropil and true rosettes. Pediatr Dev Pathol 2000;3(4): 346–52.

25. Korshunov A, Remke M, Gessi M, et al. Focal genomic amplification at 19q13.42 comprises a powerful diagnostic marker for embryonal tumors with ependymoblastic rosettes. Acta Neuropathol 2010;120(2):253–60.

26. Korshunov A, Sturm D, Ryzhova M, et al. Embryonal tumor with abundant neuropil and true rosettes (ETANTR), ependymoblastoma, and medulloepithelioma share molecular similarity and comprise a single clinicopathological entity. Acta Neuropathol 2014;128(2):279–89.

27. Sin-Chan P, Mumal I, Suwal T, et al. A C19MC-LIN28A-MYCN oncogenic circuit driven by hijacked super-enhancers is a distinct therapeutic vulnerability in ETMRs: a lethal brain tumor. Cancer Cell 2019;36(1):51–67.e7.

28. Spence T, Sin-Chan P, Picard D, et al. CNS-PNETs with C19MC amplification and/or LIN28 expression comprise a distinct histogenetic diagnostic and therapeutic entity. Acta Neuropathol 2014;128(2): 291–303.

29. Gessi M, Giangaspero F, Lauriola L, et al. Embryonal tumors with abundant neuropil and true rosettes: a distinctive CNS primitive neuroectodermal tumor. Am J Surg Pathol 2009;33(2):211–7.

30. Nobusawa S, Yokoo H, Hirato J, et al. Analysis of chromosome 19q13.42 amplification in embryonal brain tumors with ependymoblastic multilayered rosettes. Brain Pathol 2012;22(5):689–97.

31. Wang Y, Chu SG, Xiong J, et al. Embryonal tumor with abundant neuropil and true rosettes (ETANTR) with a focal amplification at chromosome 19q13.42 locus: further evidence of two new instances in China. Neuropathology 2011; 31(6):639–47.

32. Kleinman CL, Gerges N, Papillon-Cavanagh S, et al. Fusion of TTYH1 with the C19MC microRNA cluster drives expression of a brain-specific DNMT3B isoform in the embryonal brain tumor ETMR. Nat Genet 2014;46(1):39–44.

33. Hasselblatt M, Gesk S, Oyen F, et al. Nonsense mutation and inactivation of SMARCA4 (BRG1) in an

atypical teratoid/rhabdoid tumor showing retained SMARCB1 (INI1) expression. Am J Surg Pathol 2011;35(6):933–5.

34. Hasselblatt M, Nagel I, Oyen F, et al. SMARCA4-mutated atypical teratoid/rhabdoid tumors are associated with inherited germline alterations and poor prognosis. Acta Neuropathol 2014;128(3):453–6.

35. Roberts CW, Orkin SH. The SWI/SNF complex–chromatin and cancer. Nat Rev Cancer 2004;4(2): 133–42.

36. Lee RS, Stewart C, Carter SL, et al. A remarkably simple genome underlies highly malignant pediatric rhabdoid cancers. J Clin Invest 2012;122(8): 2983–8.

37. Johann PD, Erkek S, Zapatka M, et al. Atypical teratoid/rhabdoid tumors are comprised of three epigenetic subgroups with distinct enhancer landscapes. Cancer Cell 2016;29(3):379–93.

38. Torchia J, Golbourn B, Feng S, et al. Integrated (epi)-genomic analyses identify subgroup-specific therapeutic targets in CNS rhabdoid tumors. Cancer Cell 2016;30(6):891–908.

39. Torchia J, Picard D, Lafay-Cousin L, et al. Molecular subgroups of atypical teratoid rhabdoid tumours in children: an integrated genomic and clinicopathological analysis. Lancet Oncol 2015;16(5):569–82.

40. Fruhwald MC, Biegel JA, Bourdeaut F, et al. Atypical teratoid/rhabdoid tumors-current concepts, advances in biology, and potential future therapies. Neuro Oncol 2016;18(6):764–78.

41. Fruhwald MC, Hasselblatt M, Nemes K, et al. Age and DNA methylation subgroup as potential independent risk factors for treatment stratification in children with atypical teratoid/rhabdoid tumors. Neuro Oncol 2020;22(7):1006–17.

42. Ho B, Johann PD, Grabovska Y, et al. Molecular subgrouping of atypical teratoid/rhabdoid tumors-a reinvestigation and current consensus. Neuro Oncol 2020;22(5):613–24.

43. Ferris SP, Velazquez Vega J, Aboian M, et al. High-grade neuroepithelial tumor with BCOR exon 15 internal tandem duplication-a comprehensive clinical, radiographic, pathologic, and genomic analysis. Brain Pathol 2020;30(1):46–62.

44. Lucas CG, Solomon DA, Perry A. A review of recently described genetic alterations in central nervous system tumors. Hum Pathol 2020;96:56–66.

45. Sturm D, Orr BA, Toprak UH, et al. New brain tumor entities emerge from molecular classification of CNS-PNETs. Cell 2016;164(5):1060–72.

46. Yoshida Y, Nobusawa S, Nakata S, et al. CNS high-grade neuroepithelial tumor with BCOR internal tandem duplication: a comparison with its counterparts in the kidney and soft tissue. Brain Pathol 2018; 28(5):710–20.

47. Hwang EI, Kool M, Burger PC, et al. Extensive molecular and clinical heterogeneity in patients with

histologically diagnosed CNS-PNET treated as a single entity: a report from the Children's Oncology Group Randomized ACNS0332 trial. J Clin Oncol 2018;36(34):3388–95. JCO2017764720.

48. Hasselblatt M, Paulus W. Sensitivity and specificity of epithelial membrane antigen staining patterns in ependymomas. Acta Neuropathol 2003;106(4): 385–8.

49. Tauziede-Espariat A, Pages M, Roux A, et al. Pediatric methylation class HGNET-MN1: unresolved issues with terminology and grading. Acta Neuropathol Commun 2019;7(1):176.

50. Torre M, Meredith DM, Dubuc A, et al. Recurrent EP300-BCOR fusions in pediatric gliomas with distinct clinicopathologic features. J Neuropathol Exp Neurol 2019;78(4):305–14.

Updates in Pediatric Glioma Pathology

Melanie H. Hakar, DO[a], Matthew D. Wood, MD, PhD[b],*

KEYWORDS

• Glioma • Pediatric • Astrocytoma • Glioblastoma • Molecular profiling

Key points

- Pediatric gliomas are histologically diverse and have a wide range of clinical behaviors.

- Diagnosis and characterization of pediatric gliomas can be aided by molecular testing to identify characteristic molecular features, stratify risk groups, and reveal potentially targetable molecular alterations.

- Tumor histologic classification and clinical information can guide molecular testing to maximize yield.

- Consensus recommendations for molecular testing in some pediatric glioma subtypes have been published and are likely to be incorporated into the next World Health Organization Classification of Central Nervous System Tumors.

ABSTRACT

Gliomas are a diverse group of primary central nervous system tumors with astrocytic, oligodendroglial, and/or ependymal features and are an important cause of morbidity/mortality in pediatric patients. Glioma classification relies on integrating tumor histology with key molecular alterations. This approach can help establish a diagnosis, guide treatment, and determine prognosis. New categories of pediatric glioma have been recognized in recent years, due to increasing application of molecular profiling in brain tumors. The aim of this review is to alert pediatric pathologists to emerging diagnostic concepts in pediatric glioma neuropathology, emphasizing the incorporation of molecular features into diagnostic practice.

OVERVIEW

Primary central nervous system (CNS) tumors are the most common solid tumor in children in the United States and the leading cause of cancer-related death in this age group.[1] CNS tumors are classified by histologic and molecular criteria set forth by the World Health Organization (WHO) and published in a reference book of international standards on histologic and genetic typing of tumors, currently in a revised fourth edition, published in 2016.[2] Historically, CNS tumor classification was based on the tumor histomorphology and immunophenotype. The histologic classification of a tumor defined the WHO grade, ranging from nonmalignant grade I tumors that potentially are curable by resection (such as pilocytic astrocytoma [PA] and ganglioglioma) to clinically aggressive grade IV tumors (such as glioblastoma [GBM] and medulloblastoma). In 2016, the WHO incorporated molecular criteria into some of the CNS tumor diagnostic categories, thereby requiring molecular information to support an "integrated diagnosis" in certain tumors.[3,4] For pediatric CNS tumors, this approach has had an impact on the classification of diffuse intrinsic pontine gliomas (DIPGs), medulloblastomas, atypical teratoid rhabdoid tumor, embryonal tumor

[a] Department of Pathology, Oregon Health & Science University, 3181 Southwest Sam Jackson Park Road, L-113, Portland, OR 97239, USA; [b] Department of Pathology, Oregon Health & Science University and Knight Cancer Institute, 3181 Southwest Sam Jackson Park Road, L-113, Portland, OR 97239, USA
* Corresponding author.
E-mail address: woodmat@OHSU.edu

Surgical Pathology 13 (2020) 801–816
https://doi.org/10.1016/j.path.2020.08.006
1875-9181/20/© 2020 Elsevier Inc. All rights reserved.

surgpath.theclinics.com

Abbreviations	
CNS	Central nervous system
DIPG	Diffuse intrinsic pontine glioma
DNA	Deoxyribonucleic acid
ERK	Extracellular signal-related kinase
FISH	Fluorescence in situ hybridization
GBM	Glioblastoma
GFAP	Glial fibrillary acidic protein
IDH	Isocitrate dehydrogenase
MAPK	Mitogen-activated protein kinase
NF	Neurofibromatosis
PA	Pilocytic astrocytoma
PF-EPN-A	Posterior fossa ependymoma type A
PF-EPN-B	Posterior fossa ependymoma type B
PMA	Pilomyxoid astrocytoma
PXA	Pleomorphic xanthoastrocytoma
WHO	World Health Organization

with multilayered rosettes, and supratentorial ependymoma.[3] Integrated classification of diffuse hemispheric gliomas is based on isocitrate dehydrogenase (IDH) mutations and presence or absence of copy number loss of chromosome arms 1p and 19q (1p/19q-codeletion), alterations that are common in adult tumors but comparatively rare in pediatrics.[5]

Large-scale molecular profiling efforts on cohorts of pediatric gliomas—both low-grade and high-grade and across histologic classification—have brought insight into the genetic drivers of these tumors, revealing a complex relationship between histomorphology, molecular alterations, and clinical behavior. Molecular profiling, therefore, is an increasingly important piece of the brain tumor diagnostic and therapeutic puzzle.[6–8] On the other hand, not all tumors fit neatly into a specific diagnostic category; there still are histologic and molecular gray areas that raise diagnostic challenges.[9,10] The goal of this review is to discuss some recent advancements in the molecular characterization and subgrouping of pediatric gliomas, a broadly defined group of distinct entities that together form the most common type of pediatric CNS tumor. Emphasis is placed on recognition of the more common pediatric gliomas and their associated molecular features and on radiologic findings, histologic features, and immunophenotypic markers that can help guide diagnostically

relevant molecular testing. Some newly identified tumor subcategories that are not yet incorporated into the WHO classification system are discussed, and the review concludes with a discussion of DNA methylation–based brain tumor profiling, a powerful tool for classifying CNS tumors that already has proved valuable for identifying distinct tumor subgroups in medulloblastomas and in poorly differentiated CNS embryonal tumors.[11,12] Many of the glioma subgroupings discussed in this review are based on insights from DNA methylation–based profiling.

GENERAL DIAGNOSTIC PRINCIPLES

Gliomas are primary CNS neoplasms thought to arise from glial progenitors or neuroectodermal stem cells. In the mature CNS, the glia comprise astrocytes, oligodendroglial cells, ependymal cells, choroid plexus cells, and microglia. Historically, gliomas were categorized by their morphologic, immunophenotypic, or ultrastructural resemblance to a differentiated glial cell type. This system, however, raised challenges. Some gliomas have ambiguous morphology that lowered diagnostic reproducibility between pathologists, and tumors with mixed features or primitive/undifferentiated morphology did not fit into a single category. In addition, a few rare gliomas do not align neatly with any differentiated glial cell type, such as chordoid glioma and angiocentric glioma—both of which have characteristic molecular alterations—and astroblastoma, a rare tumor that probably represents a morphologic pattern rather than a specific diagnostic entity.[13–16] One goal in incorporating molecular features into CNS tumor classification is to define more objective criteria for CNS tumor diagnosis so that distinct tumor entities are defined precisely, creating more homogeneous subgroups to align with treatment options and prognosis.[3]

A tumor's location, patient age, presenting symptoms, and the tumor's relationship to the uninvolved brain all can be helpful in establishing a differential diagnosis. As a framework for this review, the pediatric gliomas are categorized by growth pattern (circumscribed or diffuse), tumor location (hemispheric or midline), and histologic grade (low vs high). Circumscribed gliomas have a compact growth pattern and a relatively sharp border to uninvolved brain tissue and potentially are curable by resection alone. Diffuse gliomas grow as individual neoplastic cells percolating through the background CNS parenchyma, infiltrating gray and white matter and forming characteristic secondary structures around neurons, capillaries, and in the subpial compartment. Gliomas of WHO grade I or grade II collectively are considered low-grade, whereas high-grade gliomas are WHO grade III or grade IV. The specific histologic criteria for tumor grading depends on the tumor subtype; for example, an ependymoma with mitotic activity, necrosis, and vascular proliferation is designated WHO grade III, whereas those same microscopic features in a diffuse astrocytic glioma make the tumor WHO grade IV (ie, GBM). Certain molecular features can override a tumor's histologic grade, with diffuse midline glioma a commonly encountered example in pediatric pathology (discussed later). Key diagnostic features for specific pediatric gliomas are discussed herein. Readers seeking a broader overview of glioma diagnosis are referred to recent reviews that have detailed the histologic classification and useful immunohistochemical markers for practical diagnostic practice.[17–19]

Applying a strict definition, pure gliomas do not include neuronal or mixed glial-neuronal tumors or poorly differentiated CNS embryonal tumors, such as medulloblastoma and atypical teratoid/rhabdoid tumor. Glioneuronal tumors and embryonal tumors, however, can overlap histologically with the gliomas, and, conversely, gliomas can show neuronal, neurocytic, or embryonal features, further complicating the differential diagnosis. Due to the overlapping clinical presentation and histologic similarities between these categories,

common glioneuronal tumors, such as ganglioglioma, dysembryoplastic neuroepithelial tumor, and rosette-forming glioneuronal tumor, often are studied concurrently with pediatric low-grade gliomas in the literature.[20–23] In a seminal study of histologically defined CNS embryonal tumors (or, CNS primitive neuroectodermal tumors, in the old nomenclature), approximately 35% of cases were proved to be gliomas through molecular analysis, demonstrating the significant diagnostic challenge posed by these cases and the utility of having robust molecular markers for tumor classification.[24] Fortunately, these tumors are comparatively rare, and the most common tumors encountered by pediatric pathologists are histologically low-grade, circumscribed gliomas with recurrent genetic alterations that can be identified through routine molecular testing. Glioneuronal tumors and CNS embryonal tumors were reviewed in detail in a recent edition of the *Surgical Pathology Clinics*, and an accompanying review of pediatric gliomas from the same edition provides another perspective on this tumor category.[25–27]

A cancer diagnosis in a pediatric patient raises consideration of a tumor predisposition syndrome. The frequency of a predisposing germline variant in childhood cancer patients overall is estimated at 7% to 8%.[28] Absence of a family history does not necessarily exclude a germline predisposition in a pediatric patient, due to de novo mutation. The frequency of predisposing germline alterations in pediatric CNS tumor patients varies by the type of tumor. A comprehensive discussion of pediatric germline alterations across all pediatric CNS tumors is beyond the scope of this review, but this topic recently was covered in detail by Muskens and colleagues.[29] Pediatric high-grade diffuse gliomas can be associated with Li-Fraumeni syndrome, mismatch repair deficiency syndromes, neurofibromatosis type 1 (NF1), melanoma-astrocytoma syndrome, and other conditions, whereas low-grade gliomas can be associated with conditions including NF1, Noonan syndrome, and tuberous sclerosis complex. Nonglial CNS tumors also have germline/syndromic underpinnings, for example, medulloblastomas associated with Gorlin syndrome and atypical teratoid/rhabdoid tumor associated with rhabdoid tumor predisposition syndrome.

PILOCYTIC ASTROCYTOMA, PLEOMORPHIC XANTHOASTROCYTOMA, AND TECTAL GLIOMA

PA is the most common childhood CNS tumor.[1] It carries an excellent prognosis, with greater than

90% 10-year survival.[30] PA shows a predilection for the posterior fossa (**Fig. 1**A) but can occur throughout the CNS. For example, PA accounts for a majority of pediatric spinal low-grade gliomas.[31] Histologically, PAs generally have discrete borders with only limited infiltrative growth and variable microscopic or macroscopic cyst formation (**Fig. 1**B). Classic PA displays biphasic architecture, with loosely structured, microcystic zones often harboring eosinophilic granular bodies alternating with compact fibrillary areas with frequent Rosenthal fibers (**Fig. 1**C).[2] Intraoperative smear preparations show distinctive hairlike (piloid) fibrillary processes extending from a monomorphic population of atypical astrocytic cells, and Rosenthal fibers can be identified in some intraoperative smear preparations (**Fig. 1**D). PAs display a broad range of morphologic characteristics, including some features associated with higher-grade gliomas in other histologic contexts. For example, tufts of glomeruloid microvascular proliferation, pleomorphic or multinucleated cells, scattered mitotic figures, and/or necrosis may be present and do not confer a higher-grade designation. Pilomyxoid astrocytoma (PMA) is a variant of PA that typically occurs in the hypothalamic region in infants. Histologically, the tumor shows a mucinous background and prominent perivascular orientation of tumor cells and absent or only very rare Rosenthal fibers and eosinophilic granular bodies (**Fig. 1**E).[32] PMA originally was designated WHO grade II based on reports of increased likelihood of local recurrence and cerebrospinal fluid dissemination.[33] Their clinical behavior is unpredictable, however, possibly due to their unfavorable location that precludes complete surgical resection. PMA is not assigned a definite grade in the current version of the

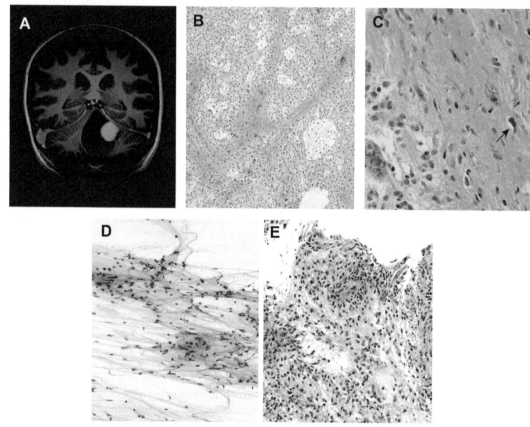

Fig. 1. PA and PMA. Coronal T1-weighted postcontrast imaging shows a posterior fossa cystic lesion with an enhancing mural nodule (*A*). Microscopic examination shows a biphasic astrocytic neoplasm with numerous microcystic spaces [Hematoxylin-eosin] (*B*) and densely fibrillar zones with numerous Rosenthal fibers [Hematoxylin-eosin] (*arrow* [*C*]). The classic intraoperative smear preparation for PA is a histologically bland astrocytic proliferation with elongated bipolar processes. Rosenthal fibers further support the diagnosis once piloid gliosis has been considered and excluded [Hematoxylin-eosin] (*D*). PMA shows a myxoid background and prominent perivascular arrangement of tumor cells [Hematoxylin-eosin] (*E*); Rosenthal fibers and eosinophilic granular bodies are characteristically absent.

WHO classification system; further study on the behavior of this tumor is required.[32]

Alterations in the mitogen-activated protein kinase (MAPK)/extracellular signal-related kinase (ERK) pathway have been identified in up to 90% of PAs.[34] The most common alteration is an approximately 2-Mb chromosome 7q34 tandem duplication resulting in a *KIAA1549-BRAF* fusion. This results in replacement of the BRAF N-terminal autoregulatory domain with the N-terminus of the KIAA1549 protein, leading to constitutive activity of the in-frame BRAF C-terminal catalytic domain.[35] *KIAA1549-BRAF* fusion is found in a majority of PAs outside the setting of NF1, most commonly in posterior fossa and optic pathway tumors.[35,36] Many other *BRAF* fusion partners have been described, including *FAM131B*, *MACF1*, and *FXR1*, all retaining the BRAF C-terminal kinase domain and thus sharing a mechanism with KIAA1549-BRAF.[20] Fluorescence in situ hybridization (FISH) can suggest a *BRAF* rearrangement but has the limitation of not identifying the specific rearrangement partner. Some laboratories use additional FISH probes to detect the KIAA1549-BRAF rearrangement, when present. *BRAF* point mutations are the next most frequent molecular alteration in PA, most commonly a single base-pair substitution affecting amino acid position 600 (p.V600E), leading to constitutive MAPK pathway activation, with other variants rarely reported.[34,37] PAs with *BRAF* V600E mutation are more common in supratentorial locations than in the posterior fossa, but *KIAA1549-BRAF* is the more common alteration in both compartments.[20] Alternative MAPK pathway alterations have been described in PA, including fusions involving *RAF1*, *NTRK2*, and *FGFR1* and activating point mutations in *FGFR1* and *PTPN11*.[38] Less frequently, PAs may harbor *PTPN11*, *KRAS*, *TP53*, or *PTEN* mutations.[39,40] PA is the most common glioma in patients with NF1.[41] Mutations resulting in loss of the *NF1* gene product neurofibromin lead to constitutive activation of the MAPK/ERK pathway, and PAs in NF1 patients generally lack *BRAF* alterations seen in sporadic cases.[42]

Recent studies have attempted to shed light on the biologic underpinnings of PAs based on anatomic location through DNA methylation–based profiling.[43] The data indicate that there is a distinct difference in the subgrouping of infratentorial versus supratentorial PAs. As patient-specific targeted therapies continue to improve, a directed method of identifying molecular alterations will be imperative to direct treatment, and consensus recommendations for molecular profiling of pediatric gliomas—including PA—

have been proposed.[8,21] Although the WHO 2016 revised fourth edition currently does not impart an integrated diagnosis for PA, future revisions may see an updated diagnostic schema integrating molecular data into PA classification.

Pleomorphic xanthoastrocytoma (PXA), WHO grade II, is another circumscribed astrocytic glioma that is more common in children and adolescents compared with adults. A vast majority are supratentorial, and they often are superficial and involve the temporal lobe and may be cystic. Anaplastic PXA (WHO grade III) is defined by 5 or more mitotic figures per 10 high-power fields, usually accompanied by necrosis and a sometimes with paradoxically less pleomorphism than PXA.[2,44] *BRAF* point mutations are found in approximately 50% to 75% of PXAs, with nearly all being p.V600E.[2] The differential diagnosis of anaplastic PXA versus epithelioid GBM, an entity that was added to the WHO classification system in 2016, can be difficult because of the histologic overlap, shared molecular features, and similar demographics between these 2 entities.[45] The precise relationship between anaplastic PXA and epithelioid GBM is uncertain at this time.

Tectal gliomas are a distinct type of pediatric glioma defined by the tumor location and low-grade histology. When biopsied, the tumors align histologically with PA in most cases or less commonly with diffuse astrocytoma.[46] *BRAF* fusion and p.V600E mutations can be identified in approximately 25% and 7.5% of cases, respectively, and may co-occur with activating point mutations in the *KRAS* oncogene.[46,47] Molecular subgrouping by DNA methylation–based profiling supports that tectal gliomas are a distinct entity from conventional PA or diffuse astrocytoma. The tumor is associated with favorable overall survival, although significant long-term morbidity can occur, and cerebrospinal fluid dissemination is rare.[46]

HISTONE H3 AND ISOCITRATE DEHYDROGENASE–MUTANT CENTRAL NERVOUS SYSTEM TUMORS

Recurrent mutations in histone-encoding genes define 2 recently identified CNS tumor types with particular relevance in pediatric patients. Sequencing studies on biopsy or autopsy material from children with DIPG revealed recurrent mutations in histone H3 encoding genes at lysine position 27.[48,49] The most common alteration is a missense mutation that changes the lysine (K) at position 27 to methionine (M), abbreviated as K27M-mutant. Lysine position 27 is conserved in several histone H3 isoforms. To date, K27M mutations are reported in *H3F3A*, *HIST1H3B/C*, and very rarely in *HIST2H3C*.[5,50] Other H3F3A missense mutations also occur and may be more common in spinal cord diffuse gliomas.[51] A methionine residue at position 27 cannot be trimethylated, and the mutant H3 protein has a dominant negative effect on methyltransferase enzymes, leading to widespread dysregulation of H3 K27 trimethylation and deregulation of gene expression.[52,53] Clinicopathologic studies of H3 K27M–mutant diffuse gliomas later revealed their occurrence across a broad age range, occurring in midline locations, such as the brainstem, spinal cord, cerebellum, pineal region, and thalamus.[54,55] The presence of H3 K27M mutation is associated with a worse prognosis in pediatric diffuse glioma patients, although this may not hold true in adults.[55,56] The 2016 WHO revised fourth edition introduced the integrated diagnosis of "Diffuse midline glioma, H3 K27M–mutant, WHO grade IV," thus recognizing this as a distinct entity from other types of diffuse glioma. Initially, H3 K27M mutations were thought to be exclusive to diffuse midline gliomas, but this alteration now is recognized in tumors with other histologic patterns, such as PA and ganglioglioma, sometimes co-occurring with *BRAF* p.V600E.[57–59] The prognosis of these rare, circumscribed K27M-mutant glioma variants is suggested to be better than for diffuse midline glioma but worse than H3–wild-type counterparts with similar histology. Current recommendations are to reserve the diffuse midline glioma diagnosis for midline tumors with a convincing diffusely infiltrative growth pattern and proven H3 K27M mutation.[60] Diffuse midline glioma accounts for approximately 80% of radiographically defined DIPGs (**Fig.** 2A). Histologically, tumors show a diffusely infiltrative growth pattern (**Fig.** 2B), with varying levels of mitotic activity, vascular proliferation, and necrosis. By histologic criteria, diffuse midline gliomas can meet criteria for diffuse astrocytoma, anaplastic astrocytoma, GBM, or any morphologic variant thereof. The presence of the H3 K27M mutant protein effectively overrides the histologic grade and defines the tumor as WHO grade IV. Mutation-specific antibodies for H3 K27M mutant protein are commercially available and can secure the diagnosis (**Fig.** 2C). The K27M mutant epitopes are conserved in *H3F3A*, *HIST1H3B*, and *HIST1H3C*, so H3 K27M immunoreactivity does not determine which histone H3 gene is mutated; DNA sequencing may be required if this information is needed.

Mutations in *H3F3A* (encoding histone H3.3) affecting guanine position 34 leading to guanine-to-arginine or guanine-to-valine substitution (p.G3 R/V; generally, p.G34-mutant) occur in cerebral hemispheric high-grade neuroepithelial tumors of adolescents and young adults (**Fig.** 2D). Two morphologic patterns are described. Some cases show morphologic features of GBM and immunoreactivity for glial fibrillary acidic protein (GFAP) and limited to no immunoreactivity for Olig2, another commonly used glial marker (**Fig.** 2E, F). Other cases show primitive neuronal or embryonal morphology, including high nuclear-to-cytoplasmic ratios, brisk mitotic activity, and nuclear molding, with limited to absent immunoreactivity for GFAP and occasionally with reactivity for antibodies against neuronal markers (**Fig.** 2G). In 1 study of 81 H3.3 G3–mutant tumors, the median age at diagnosis was 19 years; all tumors were located in the cerebral hemispheres, and approximately one-quarter of cases showed primitive neuronal morphology with strong immunoreactivity for neuronal markers and relatively few astrocytic features.[61] Therefore, histone H3.3 p.G34–mutant neuroepithelial tumor enters the differential diagnosis for a poorly differentiated CNS embryonal tumor. In a seminal study of 323 histologically defined CNS embryonal tumors, 5% were found to be *H3F3A* p.G34–mutant.[24] Approximately 75% of histone H3 p.G34R/V–mutant tumors show *MGMT* promoter methylation, much higher than the rate of approximately 15% to 25% in pediatric GBM overall.[9,10] Recently, the morphologic spectrum of *H3F3A* p.G34–mutant neuroepithelial tumors was expanded in a report of 2 hemispheric tumors in male adolescents who had both glial and dysplastic ganglion cell components.[62] At this time, neuroepithelial tumors with H3.3 p.G34R/V mutation are not a separate entity in the WHO classification, but, due to their distinctive features, it is likely that this will be defined as a separate entity by the WHO in the near future.

Diffuse gliomas with IDH gene mutations account for approximately 6% to 7% of diffuse gliomas in children, occurring mostly in adolescence and likely representing an early presentation of what conventionally is considered an adult tumor.[50] The histologic spectrum ranges from WHO grade II to grade IV diffuse astrocytic gliomas and WHO grade II or grade III oligodendrogliomas, with tumors usually located in the cerebral hemispheres (**Fig.** 3A). Immunohistochemistry for the most common form of IDH mutant protein, IDH1-R132H, is a helpful diagnostic aid, and convincing immunoreactivity confirms an IDH-mutant diffuse glioma (**Fig.** 3B, C). If the immunostain is negative, sequencing of *IDH1* and *IDH2* is required to exclude alternative *IDH1* mutations or mutations in the homologous *IDH2*

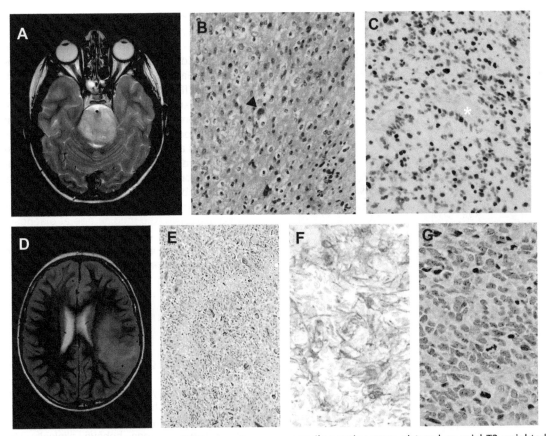

Fig. 2. Histone H3-mutant gliomas. DIPG presents as an expansile pontine mass, pictured on axial T2-weighted imaging (*A*). Histology shows a moderately cellular astrocytic neoplasm infiltrating parenchyma and surrounding the native pontine neurons [Hematoxylin-eosin] (*arrowhead* [*B*]). Immunohistochemistry for histone H3 K27M–mutant protein is positive in tumor cell nuclei, whereas the background non-neoplastic endothelial cell nuclei are nonreactive [Histone H3 p.K27M immunostain] ([*C*] *asterisk* marks a small vessel and endothelial cells). Histone H3.3 mutations at guanine position 34 occur in a subset of cerebral hemispheric tumors ([*D*] T2-weighted imaging). This case showed histologic features of GBM, with marked cellularity, cytologic atypia, and palisading necrosis [Hematoxylin-eosin] (*E*). Immunoreactivity for GFAP highlights tumor cell bodies and associated fibrillary processes [Glial fibrillary acidic protein immunostain] (*F*); Olig2 was negative (not pictured). Histone H3.3 p.G34–mutant tumors can show a dedifferentiated embryonal phenotype, with high nuclear-to-cytoplasmic ratios, brisk mitotic activity, and frequent apoptotic cells [Hematoxylin-eosin] (*G*). Immunohistochemistry for GFAP and Olig2 was negative in this case (not pictured).

gene. Confirmation of an IDH gene mutation in a pediatric patient could suggest an underlying cancer predisposition syndrome, such as Li-Fraumeni.[63] Oligodendrogliomas account for approximately 10% to 15% of adult diffuse gliomas, and evidence of both IDH gene mutation and chromosome arm 1p and 19q copy number loss is required for the integrated diagnosis.[2] Although some pediatric low-grade diffuse gliomas have oligodendroglioma-like morphology, genetically confirmed oligodendrogliomas with IDH mutation and 1p/19q-codeletion are exceptionally rare in patients under 18.[64,65] When the histologic features of a pediatric brain tumor align with oligodendroglioma, diffuse gliomas with

oligodendroglial morphology and MAPK pathway alterations—especially tumors with *FGFR1* alterations—should be considered (discussed later), and IDH mutation and 1p/19q-codeletion can be excluded by molecular studies.

CLINICS CARE POINTS: HISTONE H3 AND ISOCITRATE DEHYDROGENASE–MUTANT GLIOMAS

- Diffuse midline glioma, WHO grade IV, is a recently identified glioma entity defined by infiltrative growth, midline anatomic location, and recurrent mutations at lysine position 27 in histone H3 encoding genes.

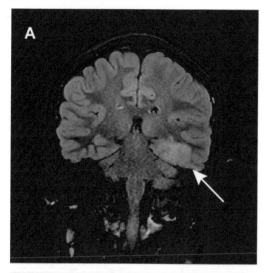

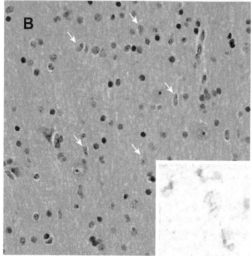

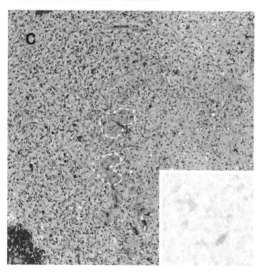

- Assessment of histone H3 lysine 27 mutation by immunohistochemistry or sequencing should be considered in pediatric gliomas with a midline location, including the brainstem, thalamus, cerebellum, and spinal cord.
- Midline diffuse astrocytic gliomas with K27M mutation are WHO grade IV, even if they lack the conventional histologic criteria of vascular proliferation and necrosis.
- Mutations at guanine position 34 in the *H3F3A* gene are identified in some hemispheric high-grade gliomas in children and adolescents and may be seen in tumors with embryonal morphology and limited immunoreactivity for glial markers.
- Diffuse gliomas with IDH gene mutation are rare in children but may be encountered in adolescent patients.

ISOCITRATE DEHYDROGENASE AND H3 WILD-TYPE PEDIATRIC HIGH-GRADE GLIOMAS

Pediatric high-grade gliomas lacking histone H3 or IDH gene mutations, hereafter collectively grouped as H3/IDH–wild-type, show a surprising range of clinical behavior that not always is predictable from tumor histology. Some histologically high-grade pediatric gliomas behave clinically like WHO grade I or grade II tumors, and molecular profiling studies support that such cases have molecular similarity to lower-grade neoplasms in some cases.[5,9,10] There is a pressing need for advancement of reliable, accessible testing methods to identify this more favorable subset of histologically high-grade tumors. Current CNS tumor profiling studies suggest that most of the remaining H3/IDH–wild-type pediatric high-grade gliomas fall into 1 of several molecular categories,

◄─────────────────────

Fig. 3. IDH-mutant gliomas. T2-weighted FLAIR imaging showed a signal abnormality in the left temporal lobe of a 15-year-old boy with seizures (*A* [*arrow*]). Histology showed a diffuse glioma of low cellularity with mild nuclear atypia (Hematoxylin-eosin, and isocitrate dehydrogenase 1 p.R132H immunostain [inset]) (*B* [*arrows*]). Immunoreactivity for IDH1 p.R132H mutant protein was positive (*B* [*inset*]), and the mutation was confirmed by Sanger sequencing. GBM histology with microvascular proliferation (*dashed lines*) is demonstrated in another case from a recurrent cerebellar tumor in a patient who had an initial resection at age 17 (Hematoxylin-eosin, and isocitrate dehydrogenase 1 p.R132H immunostain [inset]) (*C*). IDH1 p.R132H immunohistochemistry is positive (*C* [*inset*]).

with evidence for distinct prognoses in different tumor subgroups.[5,10] The exact number of molecular subgroups, and their defining alterations, are being investigated. Subgroups of pediatric H3/IDH–wild-type GBM enriched for tumors with *PDGFRA* amplification, *EGFR* amplification, and *MYC* or *MYCN* amplifications have been suggested based on the most recent data, but there is no single unifying alteration within each subgroup.[5,66] Gliomas with oncogene amplification account for some histone H3–wild-type DIPGs (Fig. 4), and this can also occur in hemispheric high-grade gliomas.

Gene fusions increasingly are recognized as drivers in childhood solid tumors, and pediatric gliomas are no exception.[67] Recurrent fusion alterations involving the *ALK*, *ROS1*, *MET*, and *NTRK* genes all are reported in pediatric high-grade

and low-grade CNS tumors, across a spectrum from pure gliomas to mixed glioneuronal tumors. Recent data from large multi-institutional cohorts showed that there is a particularly high rate of pathogenic fusions in hemispheric infantile high-grade gliomas, with approximately 60% to 80% of these cases showing fusions involving *ALK*, *ROS1*, *NTRK*, or *MET*.[68,69] Fusion detection has the potential to be of clinical significance. CNS tumor response to targeted therapy with NTRK inhibitors has been reported, and preclinical studies suggest that *MET*, *ALK*, and *ROS1* alterations potentially are targetable.[70–72]

PEDIATRIC LOW-GRADE DIFFUSE GLIOMAS

Low-grade diffuse gliomas are uncommon in children when compared with the circumscribed

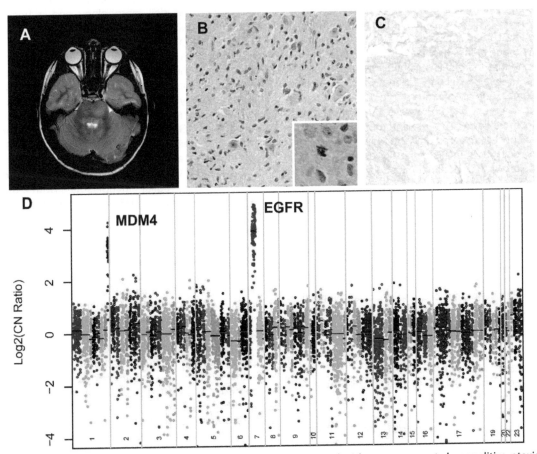

Fig. 4. DIPG without histone H3 mutation. A 5-year-old girl presented with eye movement abnormalities, ataxia, headaches, and vomiting. Imaging showed a nonenhancing T2 signal abnormality in the left pons and cerebellum ([A] T2-weighted imaging). Biopsy revealed an infiltrative astrocytic neoplasm with mitotic activity [Hematoxylin-eosin] ([B] *inset*) but no vascular proliferation or necrosis, supporting a histologic diagnosis of anaplastic astrocytoma, WHO grade III. Histone H3 K27M immunohistochemistry was negative for nuclear reactivity [Histone H3 p.K27M immunostain] (C). Next-generation sequencing revealed wild-type *IDH1*, *IDH2*, and *H3F3A* genes, with focal amplifications of *EGFR* on chromosome 7 and *MDM2* on distal 1q (D). ([D] *Courtesy of* Dr. Christopher Corless, Knight Diagnostic Laboratories, Portland, OR.)

astrocytic gliomas and mixed glial-neuronal tumors. Sequencing studies of pediatric low-grade diffuse gliomas have shown that a majority of these tumors lack pathogenic IDH and histone H3 mutations, and instead show alterations that activate the MAPK and/or phosphatidylinositol 3-kinase pathways.[20,73,74] A consensus group of neuropathologists recently recommended that these so-called pediatric-type diffuse gliomas can be subclassified by their underlying molecular alteration, providing useful diagnostic and prognostic information and suggesting potential therapeutic targets, such as *BRAF* p.V600E.[75] Correlation between the histologic pattern and underlying molecular alteration is unclear at this time, although, in some cohorts, tumors with oligodendroglial features are enriched for MAPK pathway activation due to *FGFR1* alterations (**Fig. 5**A–D) whereas MAPK activation due to *BRAF, MYB,* or *MYLB1* alterations correlate with astrocytic features (**Fig. 5**E, F).[73] A recent recommendation on criteria for an integrated diagnosis of pediatric low-grade diffuse gliomas has been issued, recognizing that there still is significant histologic overlap between diffuse gliomas, circumscribed gliomas, and glioneuronal tumors and that molecular features may not always reliably distinguish these entities.[75] This recommendation reinforces the concept that pediatric-type low-grade gliomas are distinct from histologically similar tumors in adults and have distinct molecular drivers. Future studies will address how these tumors should be classified and graded.

CLINICS CARE POINTS: PEDIATRIC H3/ ISOCITRATE DEHYDROGENASE–WILD-TYPE DIFFUSE GLIOMAS

- Pathogenic fusions and oncogene amplifications are common drivers of pediatric high-grade gliomas.
- Preclinical evidence and case reports suggest that gliomas with fusion alterations may respond to targeted therapies.
- Low-grade diffuse gliomas in children are enriched for MAPK pathway activating alterations including, but not limited to, *BRAF, FGFR1, MYB,* and *MYBL1,* and an integrated diagnosis to incorporate these molecular findings has been proposed.

EPENDYMOMAS

Ependymomas occur at any age and are located throughout the neural axis, and large-scale profiling studies suggest they consist of at least 9 distinct clinical-pathologic subtypes.[76] Ependymomas account for approximately 10% of pediatric CNS tumors and occur more commonly in the posterior fossa or supratentorial compartment than in the spinal cord. Supratentorial ependymomas with rearrangements involving the *RELA* gene now are recognized as a distinct entity and receive an integrated diagnosis per the 2016 WHO criteria. This rearrangement activates the nuclear factor-κB pathway, and immunohistochemistry for L1CAM and/or p65 are sensitive and specific surrogate markers for pathway activation.[77,78] The *RELA* rearrangement can be confirmed by FISH or sequencing analysis, which shows good correlation with immunohistochemistry and DNA methylation–based profiling.[79] Nearly all ependymomas with *RELA* rearrangement are anaplastic by histologic criteria, and tumors can have clear cell morphology and a background of delicate branching capillaries that mimic oligodendroglial or neurocytic tumors (**Fig. 6**A). Due to their supratentorial location, GBM enters the differential diagnosis for supratentorial anaplastic ependymomas. Unlike most GBMs, ependymal tumors are relatively circumscribed and not diffusely infiltrative. Immunostaining for GFAP can highlight perivascular pseudorosettes, and epithelial membrane antigen immunostaining can show paranuclear dot-like staining (**Fig. 6**B, C). Unlike most astrocytic and oligodendroglial neoplasms (with the exception of histone H3.3 p.G34–mutant tumors), Olig2 is negative or shows only limited staining in ependymoma (**Fig. 6**D). Rearrangements involving *YAP1* occur in approximately 10% of supratentorial ependymomas overall and are highly enriched in infants and children.[76] Other rare fusions also have been reported in supratentorial ependymomas, so absence of a *RELA* or *YAP1* fusion does not exclude an ependymoma diagnosis.[79]

Molecular classification of posterior fossa ependymomas identified a subset of tumors restricted mostly to infants and young children, referred to as posterior fossa ependymoma type A (PF-EPN-A).[76] Histologically, these tumors resemble traditional ependymomas and show loss of immunoreactivity for trimethylated histone H3 K27 (H3 K27me3 [**Fig. 6**E, F]).[80] Notably, diffuse gliomas with H3 K27M mutation also show reduced H3 K27me3, but mutations in histone H3-encoding genes are rare in ependymomas.[81] Rather, PF-EPN-A ependymomas have increased expression of a previously uncharacterized protein encoded by *EZHIP* (or *CXORF67*).[81] Mechanistic studies suggest that

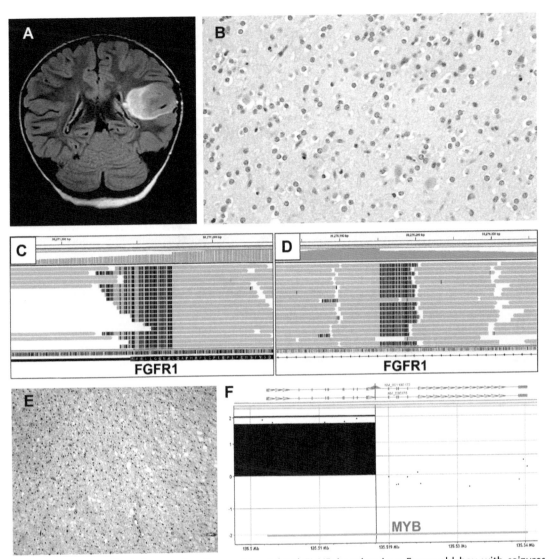

Fig. 5. Diffuse hemispheric low-grade glioma. T2-weighted FLAIR imaging in a 5-year-old boy with seizures showed a left parietal and insular cortex mass (*A*). Histologically the tumor showed infiltrating glial cells with rounded nuclei, crisp nuclear borders, delicate chromatin, and perinuclear cytoplasmic clearing [Hematoxylin-eosin] (*B*). Dysmorphic, or floating, neurons and nodular architecture were not identified, arguing against dysembryoplastic neuroepithelial tumor. Molecular profiling revealed tandem duplication of *FGFR1* as the only pathogenic alteration (*C, D*), with 3′ duplication boundary within exon 19 and 5′ boundary within intron 10-11. In a separate case, histology from a left temporal tumor in a 9-year-old boy with headaches showed moderately cellular infiltrative isomorphic cells with a myxoid background [Hematoxylin-eosin] (*E*). Genome-wide copy number profiling by single nucleotide polymorphism microarray showed focal copy number gain at chromosome 6q23.3, spanning approximately 828 kilobases and encompassing the first 9 exons of *MYB* (*F*). (*Courtesy of* [*C, D*] Dr. David Solomon, University of California San Francisco, San Francisco, CA; and [*F*] Dr. Yassmine Akkari, Legacy Laboratory Services, Portland, OR.)

this protein mimics the effect of the histone H3 K27M–mutant protein, inhibiting polycomb repressive complex 2 and leading to a global reduction in histone H3 K27 trimethylation with focal retention of H3 K27 trimethylation at specific gene-regulatory elements.[82] Despite the evidence for distinct molecular underpinning for

PF-EPN-A compared with the subgroup of posterior fossa ependymomas with retained H3 K27me3 (referred to as posterior fossa ependymoma type B [PF-EPN-B]), the clinical relevance of this subgrouping is unclear.[83,84] It is now suggested that molecular subgrouping—particularly with identification of *RELA* and *YAP1* subgroups

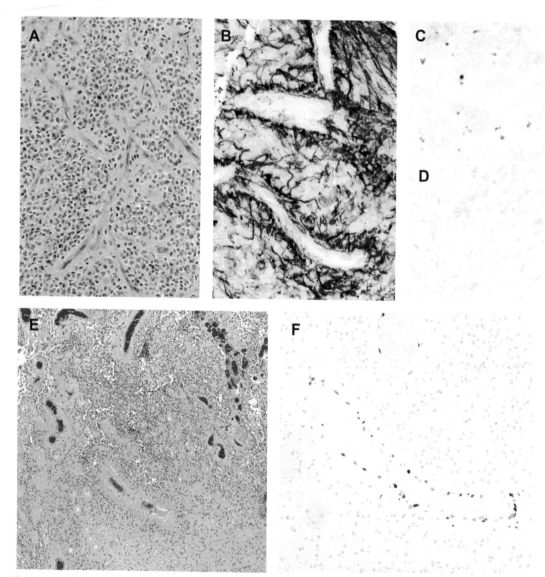

Fig. 6. Ependymomas. Histology from a supratentorial solid and cystic occipital lobe mass in a 6 year old with nausea showed a compact glial neoplasm with perivascular nucleus-free zones and cells with clear cytoplasm [Hematoxylin-eosin] (*A*). The tumor showed increased mitotic activity, necrosis, and microvascular proliferation. Immunostaining for GFAP was positive and highlighted perivascular fibrillary processes [Glial fibrillary acidic protein immunostain] (*B*). Epithelial membrane antigen staining showed a perinuclear dotlike staining pattern, a helpful but nonspecific finding supporting ependymal differentiation [Epithelial membrane antigen immunostain] (*C*). Most ependymomas show little to no immunoreactivity for Olig2 [Olig2 immunostain] (*D*). Molecular testing of this tumor by FISH was positive for *RELA* rearrangement. A separate case of a recurrent posterior fossa ependymoma in an 8-year-old boy shows well-formed perivascular pseudorosettes [Hematoxylin-eosin] (*E*). The patient's tumor was first diagnosed at 1 year of age. Immunohistochemistry for trimethylated histone H3 lysine 27 (H3K27me3) shows global loss of trimethylation in tumor nuclei, with retained immunoreactivity in the background non-neoplastic endothelial cells serving as an internal positive control [Trimethylated histone H3 lysine 27 immunostain] (*F*). Global loss of immunoreactivity for H3K27me3 supports a PF-EPN-A in this patient.

of supratentorial ependymomas and differentiation H3 K27me3-deficient PF-EPN-A from PF-EPN-B—be incorporated into clinical trials to help address this and other questions.[85]

DNA METHYLATION–BASED PROFILING

As emphasized in this review, there are distinct molecular subgroups within gliomas that do not correlate well with histology and clinical/radiologic features. Molecular information in the form of histone H3 K27 mutation status, *RELA* rearrangement, and IDH gene mutation status is incorporated into glioma diagnosis, but there are many more key alterations arising from molecular studies on CNS tumors. DNA methylation–based profiling is a technology that groups similar tumors together based on similar patterns of cytosine methylation, which is thought to reflect the tumor cell of origin and effects of the driving molecular alterations.[86] DNA methylation–based profiling is established as a research tool, and recent studies support its use on a clinical basis in both adult and pediatric CNS tumor diagnosis.[11,87] The platform has high utility for tumor subtyping, classification of histologically ambiguous or challenging cases, and identification of new tumor entities. Like any molecular testing approach, there are some limitations to this platform, such as a requirement for adequately cellular tumor and the potential need for other ancillary testing to confirm a defining tumor alteration like H3 K27 mutation. Still, DNA methylation–based profiling has significant potential to aid in pediatric CNS tumor classification and management.[11]

SUMMARY

Pediatric glioma classification is complex and challenging and increasingly relies on molecular information about a tumor to determine an integrated diagnosis that combines the tumor histologic appearance with key molecular alterations. Molecular profiling strongly supports that pediatric gliomas are distinct from adult gliomas and may be amenable to targeted therapeutic approaches in some cases. There are strong arguments for incorporating molecular subgrouping of tumors into clinical trials to help guide therapy and improve patient outcomes. Pediatric gliomas, therefore, are at the forefront of personalized medicine, and pathologists play a critical role by recognizing emerging tumor subgroups and guiding tumor molecular profiling.

DISCLOSURE

No disclosures.

REFERENCES

1. Ostrom QT, Cioffi G, Gittleman H, et al. CBTRUS Statistical Report: Primary Brain and Other Central Nervous System Tumors Diagnosed in the United States in 2012-2016. Neuro Oncol 2019;21(Supplement_5): v1–100.

2. Louis DN, Ohgaki H, Wiestler OD, et al. World Health Organization Classification of Tumours of the Central Nervous System. Lyon, France: International Agency for Research on Cancer; 2016.

3. Louis DN, Perry A, Reifenberger G, et al. The 2016 World Health Organization Classification of Tumors of the Central Nervous System: a summary. Acta Neuropathol 2016;131(6):803–20.

4. Louis DN, Perry A, Burger P, et al. International Society Of Neuropathology–Haarlem consensus guidelines for nervous system tumor classification and grading. Brain Pathol 2014;24(5):429–35.

5. Mackay A, Burford A, Carvalho D, et al. Integrated Molecular Meta-Analysis of 1,000 Pediatric High-Grade and Diffuse Intrinsic Pontine Glioma. Cancer Cell 2017;32(4):520–37.e5.

6. Horbinski C, Ligon KL, Brastianos P, et al. The medical necessity of advanced molecular testing in the diagnosis and treatment of brain tumor patients. Neuro Oncol 2019;21(12):1498–508.

7. Kline CN, Joseph NM, Grenert JP, et al. Targeted next-generation sequencing of pediatric neuro-oncology patients improves diagnosis, identifies pathogenic germline mutations, and directs targeted therapy. Neuro Oncol 2017;19(5):699–709.

8. Miklja Z, Pasternak A, Stallard S, et al. Molecular profiling and targeted therapy in pediatric gliomas: review and consensus recommendations. Neuro Oncol 2019;21(8):968–80.

9. Mackay A, Burford A, Molinari V, et al. Molecular, Pathological, Radiological, and Immune Profiling of Non-brainstem Pediatric High-Grade Glioma from the HERBY Phase II Randomized Trial. Cancer Cell 2018;33(5):829–42.e5.

10. Korshunov A, Ryzhova M, Hovestadt V, et al. Integrated analysis of pediatric glioblastoma reveals a subset of biologically favorable tumors with associated molecular prognostic markers. Acta Neuropathol 2015;129(5):669–78.

11. Pickles JC, Fairchild AR, Stone TJ, et al. DNA methylation-based profiling for paediatric CNS tumour diagnosis and treatment: a population-based study. Lancet Child Adolesc Health 2020; 4(2):121–30.

12. Korshunov A, Sahm F, Zheludkova O, et al. DNA methylation profiling is a method of choice for molecular verification of pediatric WNT-activated medulloblastomas. Neuro Oncol 2019;21(2):214–21.

13. Goode B, Mondal G, Hyun M, et al. A recurrent kinase domain mutation in PRKCA defines chordoid glioma of the third ventricle. Nat Commun 2018; 9(1):810.

14. Rosenberg S, Simeonova I, Bielle F, et al. A recurrent point mutation in PRKCA is a hallmark of chordoid gliomas. Nat Commun 2018;9(1):2371.

15. Bandopadhayay P, Ramkissoon LA, Jain P, et al. MYB-QKI rearrangements in angiocentric glioma

drive tumorigenicity through a tripartite mechanism. Nat Genet 2016;48(3):273–82.

16. Wood MD, Tihan T, Perry A, et al. Multimodal molecular analysis of astroblastoma enables reclassification of most cases into more specific molecular entities. Brain Pathol 2018;28(2):192–202.

17. Perry A, Wesseling P. Histologic classification of gliomas. Handb Clin Neurol 2016;134:71–95.

18. Velazquez Vega JE, Brat DJ. Incorporating Advances in Molecular Pathology Into Brain Tumor Diagnostics. Adv Anat Pathol 2018;25(3):143–71.

19. Wood MD, Halfpenny AM, Moore SR. Applications of molecular neuro-oncology - a review of diffuse glioma integrated diagnosis and emerging molecular entities. Diagn Pathol 2019;14(1):29.

20. Zhang J, Wu G, Miller CP, et al. Whole-genome sequencing identifies genetic alterations in pediatric low-grade gliomas. Nat Genet 2013;45(6):602–12.

21. Jones DTW, Kieran MW, Bouffet E, et al. Pediatric low-grade gliomas: next biologically driven steps. Neuro Oncol 2018;20(2):160–73.

22. Lassaletta A, Zapotocky M, Bouffet E, et al. An integrative molecular and genomic analysis of pediatric hemispheric low-grade gliomas: an update. Childs Nerv Syst 2016;32(10):1789–97.

23. Packer RJ, Pfister S, Bouffet E, et al. Pediatric low-grade gliomas: implications of the biologic era. Neuro Oncol 2017;19(6):750–61.

24. Sturm D, Orr BA, Toprak UH, et al. New Brain Tumor Entities Emerge from Molecular Classification of CNS-PNETs. Cell 2016;164(5):1060–72.

25. Blessing MM, Alexandrescu S. Embryonal Tumors of the Central Nervous System: An Update. Surg Pathol Clin 2020;13(2):235–47.

26. Chen J, Dahiya SM. Update on Circumscribed Gliomas and Glioneuronal Tumors. Surg Pathol Clin 2020;13(2):249–66.

27. Ahrendsen J, Alexandrescu S. An Update on Pediatric Gliomas. Surg Pathol Clin 2020;13(2):217–33.

28. Grobner SN, Worst BC, Weischenfeldt J, et al. The landscape of genomic alterations across childhood cancers. Nature 2018;555(7696):321–7.

29. Muskens IS, Zhang C, de Smith AJ, et al. Germline genetic landscape of pediatric central nervous system tumors. Neuro Oncol 2019;21(11):1376–88.

30. Collins VP, Jones DT, Giannini C. Pilocytic astrocytoma: pathology, molecular mechanisms and markers. Acta Neuropathol 2015;129(6):775–88.

31. Carey SS, Sadighi Z, Wu S, et al. Evaluating pediatric spinal low-grade gliomas: a 30-year retrospective analysis. J Neurooncol 2019;145(3):519–29.

32. Kulac I, Tihan T. Pilomyxoid astrocytomas: a short review. Brain Tumor Pathol 2019;36(2):52–5.

33. Louis DN, Ohgaki H, Wiestler OD, and Cavenee WK. World Health Organization Classification of Tumours of the Central Nervous System. Lyon, France: International Agency for Research on Cancer; 2007.

34. Jones DT, Gronych J, Lichter P, et al. MAPK pathway activation in pilocytic astrocytoma. Cell Mol Life Sci 2012;69(11):1799–811.

35. Jones DT, Kocialkowski S, Liu L, et al. Tandem duplication producing a novel oncogenic BRAF fusion gene defines the majority of pilocytic astrocytomas. Cancer Res 2008;68(21):8673–7.

36. Tatevossian RG, Lawson AR, Forshew T, et al. MAPK pathway activation and the origins of pediatric low-grade astrocytomas. J Cell Physiol 2010;222(3):509–14.

37. Khater F, Langlois S, Cassart P, et al. Recurrent somatic BRAF insertion (p.V504_R506dup): a tumor marker and a potential therapeutic target in pilocytic astrocytoma. Oncogene 2019;38(16):2994–3002.

38. Jones DT, Kocialkowski S, Liu L, et al. Oncogenic RAF1 rearrangement and a novel BRAF mutation as alternatives to KIAA1549:BRAF fusion in activating the MAPK pathway in pilocytic astrocytoma. Oncogene 2009;28(20):2119–23.

39. Jones DT, Hutter B, Jager N, et al. Recurrent somatic alterations of FGFR1 and NTRK2 in pilocytic astrocytoma. Nat Genet 2013;45(8):927–32.

40. Horbinski C, Hamilton RL, Nikiforov Y, et al. Association of molecular alterations, including BRAF, with biology and outcome in pilocytic astrocytomas. Acta Neuropathol 2010;119(5):641–9.

41. Rodriguez FJ, Perry A, Gutmann DH, et al. Gliomas in neurofibromatosis type 1: a clinicopathologic study of 100 patients. J Neuropathol Exp Neurol 2008;67(3):240–9.

42. Nix JS, Blakeley J, Rodriguez FJ. An update on the central nervous system manifestations of neurofibromatosis type 1. Acta Neuropathol 2019;139(4):625–41.

43. Sexton-Oates A, Dodgshun A, Hovestadt V, et al. Methylation profiling of paediatric pilocytic astrocytoma reveals variants specifically associated with tumour location and predictive of recurrence. Mol Oncol 2018;12(8):1219–32.

44. Ida CM, Rodriguez FJ, Burger PC, et al. Pleomorphic Xanthoastrocytoma: Natural History and Long-Term Follow-Up. Brain Pathol 2015;25(5):575–86.

45. Alexandrescu S, Korshunov A, Lai SH, et al. Epithelioid Glioblastomas and Anaplastic Epithelioid Pleomorphic Xanthoastrocytomas–Same Entity or First Cousins? Brain Pathol 2016;26(2):215–23.

46. Liu APY, Harreld JH, Jacola LM, et al. Tectal glioma as a distinct diagnostic entity: a comprehensive clinical, imaging, histological and molecular analysis. Acta Neuropathol Commun 2018;6(1):101.

47. Chiang J, Li X, Liu APY, et al. Tectal glioma harbors high rates of KRAS G12R and concomitant KRAS and BRAF alterations. Acta Neuropathol 2019;139(3):601–2.

48. Schwartzentruber J, Korshunov A, Liu XY, et al. Driver mutations in histone H3.3 and chromatin

remodelling genes in paediatric glioblastoma. Nature 2012;482(7384):226–31.

49. Wu G, Broniscer A, McEachron TA, et al. Somatic histone H3 alterations in pediatric diffuse intrinsic pontine gliomas and non-brainstem glioblastomas. Nat Genet 2012;44(3):251–3.

50. Castel D, Philippe C, Calmon R, et al. Histone H3F3A and HIST1H3B K27M mutations define two subgroups of diffuse intrinsic pontine gliomas with different prognosis and phenotypes. Acta Neuropathol 2015;130(6):815–27.

51. Sloan EA, Cooney T, Oberheim Bush NA, et al. Recurrent non-canonical histone H3 mutations in spinal cord diffuse gliomas. Acta Neuropathol 2019;138(5):877–81.

52. Lewis PW, Muller MM, Koletsky MS, et al. Inhibition of PRC2 activity by a gain-of-function H3 mutation found in pediatric glioblastoma. Science 2013; 340(6134):857–61.

53. Bender S, Tang Y, Lindroth AM, et al. Reduced H3K27me3 and DNA hypomethylation are major drivers of gene expression in K27M mutant pediatric high-grade gliomas. Cancer Cell 2013;24(5): 660–72.

54. Solomon DA, Wood MD, Tihan T, et al. Diffuse Midline Gliomas with Histone H3-K27M Mutation: A Series of 47 Cases Assessing the Spectrum of Morphologic Variation and Associated Genetic Alterations. Brain Pathol 2016;26(5):569–80.

55. Schreck KC, Ranjan S, Skorupan N, et al. Incidence and clinicopathologic features of H3 K27M mutations in adults with radiographically-determined midline gliomas. J Neurooncol 2019;143(1):87–93.

56. Karremann M, Gielen GH, Hoffmann M, et al. Diffuse high-grade gliomas with H3 K27M mutations carry a dismal prognosis independent of tumor location. Neuro Oncol 2018;20(1):123–31.

57. Pratt D, Natarajan SK, Banda A, et al. Circumscribed/non-diffuse histology confers a better prognosis in H3K27M-mutant gliomas. Acta Neuropathol 2018;135(2):299–301.

58. Kleinschmidt-DeMasters   BK,   Donson   A, Foreman NK, et al. H3 K27M Mutation in Gangliogliomas can be Associated with Poor Prognosis. Brain Pathol 2017;27(6):846–50.

59. Hochart A, Escande F, Rocourt N, et al. Long survival in a child with a mutated K27M-H3.3 pilocytic astrocytoma. Ann Clin Transl Neurol 2015;2(4): 439–43.

60. Louis DN, Giannini C, Capper D, et al. cIMPACT-NOW update 2: diagnostic clarifications for diffuse midline glioma, H3 K27M-mutant and diffuse astrocytoma/anaplastic astrocytoma, IDH-mutant. Acta Neuropathol 2018;135(4):639–42.

61. Korshunov A, Capper D, Reuss D, et al. Histologically distinct neuroepithelial tumors with histone 3 G34 mutation are molecularly similar and comprise a single nosologic entity. Acta Neuropathol 2016; 131(1):137–46.

62. Andreiuolo F, Lisner T, Zlocha J, et al. H3F3A-G34R mutant high grade neuroepithelial neoplasms with glial and dysplastic ganglion cell components. Acta Neuropathol Commun 2019;7(1):78.

63. Sumerauer D, Krskova L, Vicha A, et al. Rare IDH1 variants are common in pediatric hemispheric diffuse astrocytomas and frequently associated with Li-Fraumeni syndrome. Acta Neuropathol 2020;139(4):795–7.

64. Lee J, Putnam AR, Chesier SH, et al. Oligodendrogliomas, IDH-mutant and 1p/19q-codeleted, arising during teenage years often lack TERT promoter mutation that is typical of their adult counterparts. Acta Neuropathol Commun 2018;6(1):95.

65. Rodriguez FJ, Tihan T, Lin D, et al. Clinicopathologic features of pediatric oligodendrogliomas: a series of 50 patients. Am J Surg Pathol 2014;38(8):1058–70.

66. Korshunov A, Schrimpf D, Ryzhova M, et al. H3-/IDH-wild type pediatric glioblastoma is comprised of molecularly and prognostically distinct subtypes with associated oncogenic drivers. Acta Neuropathol 2017;134(3):507–16.

67. Jones DTW, Banito A, Grunewald TGP, et al. Molecular characteristics and therapeutic vulnerabilities across paediatric solid tumours. Nat Rev Cancer 2019;19(8):420–38.

68. Guerreiro Stucklin AS, Ryall S, Fukuoka K, et al. Alterations in ALK/ROS1/NTRK/MET drive a group of infantile hemispheric gliomas. Nat Commun 2019; 10(1):4343.

69. Clarke M, Mackay A, Ismer B, et al. Infant High-Grade Gliomas Comprise Multiple Subgroups Characterized by Novel Targetable Gene Fusions and Favorable Outcomes. Cancer Discov 2020;10(7):942–63.

70. Davare MA, Henderson JJ, Agarwal A, et al. Rare but Recurrent ROS1 Fusions Resulting From Chromosome 6q22 Microdeletions are Targetable Oncogenes in Glioma. Clin Cancer Res 2018;24(24): 6471–82.

71. Ziegler DS, Wong M, Mayoh C, et al. Brief Report: Potent clinical and radiological response to larotrectinib in TRK fusion-driven high-grade glioma. Br J Cancer 2018;119(6):693–6.

72. International Cancer Genome Consortium PedBrain Tumor P. Recurrent MET fusion genes represent a drug target in pediatric glioblastoma. Nat Med 2016;22(11):1314–20.

73. Qaddoumi I, Orisme W, Wen J, et al. Genetic alterations in uncommon low-grade neuroepithelial tumors: BRAF, FGFR1, and MYB mutations occur at high frequency and align with morphology. Acta Neuropathol 2016;131(6):833–45.

74. Sturm D, Pfister SM, Jones DTW. Pediatric Gliomas: Current Concepts on Diagnosis, Biology, and Clinical Management. J Clin Oncol 2017;35(21):2370–7.

75. Ellison DW, Hawkins C, Jones DTW, et al. cIMPACT-NOW update 4: diffuse gliomas characterized by MYB, MYBL1, or FGFR1 alterations or BRAF(V600E) mutation. Acta Neuropathol 2019; 137(4):683–7.

76. Pajtler KW, Witt H, Sill M, et al. Molecular Classification of Ependymal Tumors across All CNS Compartments, Histopathological Grades, and Age Groups. Cancer Cell 2015;27(5):728–43.

77. Gessi M, Capper D, Sahm F, et al. Evidence of H3 K27M mutations in posterior fossa ependymomas. Acta Neuropathol 2016;132(4):635–7.

78. Parker M, Mohankumar KM, Punchihewa C, et al. C11orf95-RELA fusions drive oncogenic NF-kappaB signalling in ependymoma. Nature 2014; 506(7489):451–5.

79. Pages M, Pajtler KW, Puget S, et al. Diagnostics of pediatric supratentorial RELA ependymomas: integration of information from histopathology, genetics, DNA methylation and imaging. Brain Pathol 2019; 29(3):325–35.

80. Panwalkar P, Clark J, Ramaswamy V, et al. Immunohistochemical analysis of H3K27me3 demonstrates global reduction in group-A childhood posterior fossa ependymoma and is a powerful predictor of outcome. Acta Neuropathol 2017;134(5):705–14.

81. Pajtler KW, Wen J, Sill M, et al. Molecular heterogeneity and CXorf67 alterations in posterior fossa group A (PFA) ependymomas. Acta Neuropathol 2018;136(2):211–26.

82. Jain SU, Do TJ, Lund PJ, et al. PFA ependymoma-associated protein EZHIP inhibits PRC2 activity through a H3 K27M-like mechanism. Nat Commun 2019;10(1):2146.

83. Junger ST, Mynarek M, Wohlers I, et al. Improved risk-stratification for posterior fossa ependymoma of childhood considering clinical, histological and genetic features - a retrospective analysis of the HIT ependymoma trial cohort. Acta Neuropathol Commun 2019;7(1):181.

84. Upadhyaya SA, Robinson GW, Onar-Thomas A, et al. Molecular grouping and outcomes of young children with newly diagnosed ependymoma treated on the multi-institutional SJYC07 trial. Neuro Oncol 2019;21(10):1319–30.

85. Pajtler KW, Mack SC, Ramaswamy V, et al. The current consensus on the clinical management of intracranial ependymoma and its distinct molecular variants. Acta Neuropathol 2017;133(1):5–12.

86. Capper D, Jones DTW, Sill M, et al. DNA methylation-based classification of central nervous system tumours. Nature 2018;555(7697):469–74.

87. Jaunmuktane Z, Capper D, Jones DTW, et al. Methylation array profiling of adult brain tumours: diagnostic outcomes in a large, single centre. Acta Neuropathol Commun 2019;7(1):24.

UNITED STATES POSTAL SERVICE®
Statement of Ownership, Management, and Circulation
(All Periodicals Publications Except Requester Publications)

1. Publication Title	2. Publication Number		3. Filing Date
SURGICAL PATHOLOGY CLINICS	025 – 478		9/18/2019

4. Issue Frequency	5. Number of Issues Published Annually	6. Annual Subscription Price
MAR, JUN, SEP, DEC	4	$213.00

7. Complete Mailing Address of Known Office of Publication (Not printer) (Street, city, county, state, and ZIP+4®)

ELSEVIER INC.
230 Park Avenue, Suite 800
New York, NY 10169

Contact Person
STEPHEN R. BUSHING

Telephone (Include area code)
215-239-3688

8. Complete Mailing Address of Headquarters or General Business Office of Publisher (Not printer)

ELSEVIER INC.
230 Park Avenue, Suite 800
New York, NY 10169

9. Full Names and Complete Mailing Addresses of Publisher, Editor, and Managing Editor (Do not leave blank)

Publisher (Name and complete mailing address)

DOLORES MELONI, ELSEVIER INC.
1600 JOHN F KENNEDY BLVD. SUITE 1800
PHILADELPHIA, PA 19103-2899

Editor (Name and complete mailing address)

KATERINA HEIDHAUSEN ELSEVIER INC.
1600 JOHN F KENNEDY BLVD. SUITE 1800
PHILADELPHIA, PA 19103-2899

Managing Editor (Name and complete mailing address)

PATRICK MANLEY, ELSEVIER INC.
1600 JOHN F KENNEDY BLVD. SUITE 1800
PHILADELPHIA, PA 19103-2899

10. Owner (Do not leave blank. If the publication is owned by a corporation, give the name and address of the corporation immediately followed by the names and addresses of all stockholders owning or holding 1 percent or more of the total amount of stock. If not owned by a corporation, give the names and addresses of the individual owners. If owned by a partnership or other unincorporated firm, give its name and address as well as those of each individual owner. If the publication is published by a nonprofit organization, give its name and address.)

Full Name	Complete Mailing Address
WHOLLY OWNED SUBSIDIARY OF REED/ELSEVIER, US HOLDINGS	1600 JOHN F KENNEDY BLVD. SUITE 1800 PHILADELPHIA, PA 19103-2899

11. Known Bondholders, Mortgagees, and Other Security Holders Owning or Holding 1 Percent or More of Total Amount of Bonds, Mortgages, or Other Securities. If none, check box ▶ ☐ None

Full Name	Complete Mailing Address
N/A	

12. Tax Status (For completion by nonprofit organizations authorized to mail at nonprofit rates) (Check one)
The purpose, function, and nonprofit status of this organization and the exempt status for federal income tax purposes:
☒ Has Not Changed During Preceding 12 Months
☐ Has Changed During Preceding 12 Months (Publisher must submit explanation of change with this statement)

PS Form 3526, July 2014 [Page 1 of 4 (see instructions page 4)] PSN: 7530-01-000-9931   PRIVACY NOTICE: See our privacy policy on www.usps.com.

---

13. Publication Title	14. Issue Date for Circulation Data Below
SURGICAL PATHOLOGY CLINICS	JUNE 2020

15. Extent and Nature of Circulation			Average No. Copies Each Issue During Preceding 12 Months	No. Copies of Single Issue Published Nearest to Filing Date
a. Total Number of Copies (Net press run)			319	306
b. Paid Circulation (By Mail and Outside the Mail)	(1)	Mailed Outside-County Paid Subscriptions Stated on PS Form 3541 (Include paid distribution above nominal rate, advertiser's proof copies, and exchange copies)	226	226
	(2)	Mailed In-County Paid Subscriptions Stated on PS Form 3541 (Include paid distribution above nominal rate, advertiser's proof copies, and exchange copies)	0	0
	(3)	Paid Distribution Outside the Mails Including Sales Through Dealers and Carriers, Street Vendors, Counter Sales, and Other Paid Distribution Outside USPS®	68	67
	(4)	Paid Distribution by Other Classes of Mail Through the USPS (e.g., First-Class Mail®)	0	0
c. Total Paid Distribution (Sum of 15b (1), (2), (3), and (4))		▶	296	293
d. Free or Nominal Rate Distribution (By Mail and Outside the Mail)	(1)	Free or Nominal Rate Outside-County Copies included on PS Form 3541	23	13
	(2)	Free or Nominal Rate In-County Copies included on PS Form 3541	0	0
	(3)	Free or Nominal Rate Copies Mailed at Other Classes Through the USPS (e.g., First-Class Mail)	0	0
	(4)	Free or Nominal Rate Distribution Outside the Mail (Carriers or other means)	0	0
e. Total Free or Nominal Rate Distribution (Sum of 15d (1), (2), (3) and (4))		▶	23	13
f. Total Distribution (Sum of 15c and 15e)		▶	319	306
g. Copies not Distributed (See Instructions to Publishers #4 (page #3))		▶	0	0
h. Total (Sum of 15f and g)		▶	319	306
i. Percent Paid (15c divided by 15f times 100)		▶	92.78%	95.75%

* If you are claiming electronic copies, go to line 16 on page 3. If you are not claiming electronic copies, skip to line 17 on page 3.

16. Electronic Copy Circulation	Average No. Copies Each Issue During Preceding 12 Months	No. Copies of Single Issue Published Nearest to Filing Date
a. Paid Electronic Copies ▶		
b. Total Paid Print Copies (Line 15c) + Paid Electronic Copies (Line 16a) ▶		
c. Total Print Distribution (Line 15f) + Paid Electronic Copies (Line 16a) ▶		
d. Percent Paid (Both Print & Electronic Copies) (16b divided by 16c × 100) ▶		

☒ I certify that 50% of all my distributed copies (electronic and print) are paid above a nominal price.

17. Publication of Statement of Ownership
☒ If the publication is a general publication, publication of this statement is required. Will be printed   ☐ Publication not required.
in the DECEMBER 2019 issue of this publication.

18. Signature and Title of Editor, Publisher, Business Manager, or Owner

Malathi Samayan

Malathi Samayan - Distribution Controller

Date
9/18/2019

I certify that all information furnished on this form is true and complete. I understand that anyone who furnishes false or misleading information on this form or who omits material or information requested on the form may be subject to criminal sanctions (including fines and imprisonment) and/or civil sanctions (including civil penalties).

PS Form 3526, July 2014 (Page 3 of 4)   PRIVACY NOTICE: See our privacy policy on www.usps.com

Printed and bound by CPI Group (UK) Ltd, Croydon, CR0 4YY

03/10/2024

01040372-0004